CHIROPRACTIC
The Science of Spinal Adjustment

———

A SERIES OF LESSONS CORRELATING AND
SYSTEMATIZING THE KNOWLEDGE NECESSARY
TO PRACTICE CHIROPRACTIC

Nature's Greatest Ally

IN RESTORING DISEASED CONDITIONS OF THE
BODY TO PERFECT HEALTH, WITHOUT THE AID
OF DRUGS OR SURGERY

———

BOOK 1
Physiology and Digestion
Lessons 1, 2, 3 and 4

———

ORIGINALLY PUBLISHED BY
AMERICAN UNIVERSITY
CHICAGO, ILLINOIS, U.S.A.

Disclaimer

We are proud to republish this series of books on chiropractic medicine. Originally published as a home-study course in 1913 by American University in Chicago, the 16 volumes give us an historical look at the theory and practice of chiropractic medicine in the early part of the 20th century.

This series is republished for historical interest only. The modern practice of chiropractic has advanced significantly in the century since these books were published. If you want to actually learn modern chiropractic techniques, please consult one of the many fine schools in this country.

The materials in these books are not intended to diagnose or treat disease. If you believe you are ill consult a licensed practitioner for care immediately. The publishers assume no liability for the use, misuse or nonuse of the materials in these books.

Thank you
OrganicMD Media

Table of Contents

Chiropractic The Science of Spinal Adjustment

EXTENSION COURSE
IN CHIROPRACTIC
AMERICAN UNIVERSITY
CHICAGO, Ill., U.S.A.

LESSON 1

"Our delight in any particular study, art, or science, rises and improves in proportion to the application which we bestow upon it. Thus, what was a first an exercise, becomes at length, an entertainment."

--Addison.

And thus, do we bid you welcome. You have taken the step that can only lead to a harvest of golden benefits for you to reap. Master these lessons, and your standing among the profession will be recognize at once. Get to work, and leave the issue to us. Your success can safely be left in our hands, for your hopes and ambitions for yourself are no higher than our aims and true resolves to help you. We want you to succeed as much as you can; and if you follow us faithfully you will.

At the outset, let us impress upon you the fact that we have a definite system or method of teaching, and a purpose in our work. As you proceed, more of that system will appear. It is only important now that you have confidence in our words, and

7

work faithfully. Don't allow outside influences to interfere, or we shall not be responsible for the results you accomplish. Follow us closely, and your confidence will grow.

Your moral obligations with us necessarily imply that you do not pass your lessons to others. With these lessons, we are teaching YOU alone. Would it not be unfair to us, if you loan them to others? It is evident, also, that the mere reading of a part of this course could not profit in itself as much as the systematic study of it all. Again, you, or we—perhaps both of us—might be wrongly judged by a person who knows only a little of our methods; whereas, a more extended study or investigation, such as you have made, would change opinions greatly. Hence, to loan your lessons to the "curious" means a possible wrong to the borrower, to yourself, and to us.

TO GET THE MOST FROM YOUR STUDY

It may be unnecessary to tell you how to study, and yet we feel it advisable to offer the following suggestions. You may have your own method of study, depending on your available time, opportunities and custom; but "a word to the wise is sufficient."

Have regular hours for study if possible, and keep them faithfully. This will help to methodize and systematize your work, and it will improve your powers of concentration. It is advisable to go into a room by yourself, where you will be undisturbed.

Master each lesson before attempting to write the examination. If you do this, you will have no difficulty with the test questions. Don't be in a hurry to get into Lesson 2 until you have learned all that is contained in Lesson

Read reflectively. Absorb the spirit of the work as well as the facts stated. Do not skim over the text matter, nor try to get ahead faster than is dependent on your thorough comprehension. You will only cheat yourself. Memorize the most important.

Never mind if you devote a week to each of the first lessons—later in the course, the work will be easier. The better foundation you lay in the beginning, the easier the work will be as you progress. To gain the greatest success you must build from the ground upward.

There is nothing more discouraging than to find it necessary to turn back and review that which should have been mastered thoroughly at first. There is enough in every lesson to challenge your deep interest from first to last.

"The greatest study of mankind is Man." It is a study full of intense interest, yet it can be easily learned. All true science is simple in its elements. You will find that each subject will charm your mind in proportion to the care you use in understanding it as you go along.

When writing your test examinations, always make your answers as short as possible and right to the point. This will develop your ability to express your ideas, to crystallize your thoughts. Say just enough, then stop.

"Don't give up the ship." Stick to the end, for every race is WON at the finish. Be resolute. Be patient and preserving. You want to make a BIG success, therefore you must make the necessary BIG effort. Determine to complete this course, and you will come out triumphant. Nothing can stand in your way.

You will find us loyal to your interests at all times, and we shall expect the same loyalty from you. With our help, you can WIN what you WILL.

> Yours to command,
> YOUR INSTRUCTORS
> American University

PHYSIOLOGY

This is the first subject to be studied, because it is the science that treats of the phenomena of normal living matter. It tells you of the functions of the body in health; later, we will learn the action of the body in disease.

BLOOD

Is the internal medium that circulates throughout the body. It carries digested food or nourishment and oxygen to every part; it collects and takes away to the organs of elimination refuse and waste products; it keeps the body moist; it is also a heat regulator, equalizing and regulating the normal temperature of the body, which is about 98.6 deg. Fahrenheit; and pure blood is considered a positive protection against disease infection, as no disease germ or bacteria can live in it. These are its functions.

The chemical reaction of blood is slightly alkaline, due to the presence of sodium carbonate and sodium phosphate, which give it a salty taste. This alkalinity is lessened by vigorous exercise which draws the acid from the muscles that is created by increased activity; also by and during the process of digestion; by lactation; and by various diseases which cause acid blood. Persons who have pimples and skin eruptions, redness, etc., usually have acid blood.

Blood is of two kinds; **arterial**, bright red in color, the purest in the body, flowing from the lungs and heart through the arteries, and **venous**, the "loaded," dark red or bluish, opaque blood flowing in the lunch and heart in the veins. Arterial blood contains more oxygen, while venous blood carries more carbon dioxide, and coagulates more readily. The odor of blood is peculiarly characteristic; and the specific gravity is 1,055 to 1,065, or a little heavier than water. Its temperature is normally about 100 deg. Fahrenheit

The composition of blood is approximately one-half liquid or plasma, and one-half solids; 90% of the liquid is water; .2% is sugar; and the balance is dissolved salts (flourides, chlorides, sulphates, phosphates, carbonates, etc.), and dissolved solids (fibrinogen, serum globulin, serum albumin). Blood plasma is white, sometimes yellowish in color.

The 50% solids in the blood are made up of red cells (Erythrocytes), white cells (Leukocytes), and platelets or simple blood disks.

Red cells are round, bi-concave disks, 1/3200 inch in diameter and number about 5,000,000 to the cubic millimeter. They are formed in the bone marrow, and are destroyed there also, as well as in the liver and spleen. Their color is due to hemoglobin, a colloidal proteid containing iron and Sulphur. These have a strong affinity for oxygen; consequently red cells carry oxygen from the lungs to the tissues.

White cells are larger, about 1/2500 inch in diameter, and are capable of ameboid motion, i.e., constantly changing in shape and position. This enables them to escape through the blood vessel walls and protect the body against the invasion of germs. They are the policeman and protectors or guards of the body. Though numbering only about 5,000 to 10,000 per cubic millimeter, their mobility enables them to exert a great protective power. They migrate to an affected part and surround the infectious substance, thereby preventing further intoxication. Besides attacking and destroying bacteria of nearly every kind

Lesson 1: Introduction

(called phagocytosis), they aid materially in the coagulation of the blood, carry fat and proteids to the tissues and assist preparing proteid food for absorption. Of the principal kinds white cells, about 20% are known as small lymphocytes (lymph cells), 7% large lymphocytes, 69% polymorphonuclears (mull nucleated cells), and 2% eosinophils (cells stainable with eosin dye).

Coagulation. The power of the blood to clot or coagulate is very beneficial and necessary, especially in cases of hemorrhage (bleeding). When first shed, it is perfectly fluid, but in a few moments becomes thick and sticky, then jelly-like and firmer. The blood serum—a faint yellowish liquid—appears on the surface of the clot, and increases until the clot floats.

A scientific description of coagulation may be given as follows. Normally the blood contains three substances, thrombogen, calcium, salts, and fibronogen. When blood is shed, the white cells break down, and a substance called thrombokinase is formed. This uniformed with thromgoben and calcium salts to form thrombin, which is the fibrin ferment. Thrombin unites with the fibrogen to form fibrin, which makes a network that entangles the blood cells and causes to clot. The student should learn this description.

After death, the blood clots first in the large vessels, and after several hours, in the smaller ones.

From 13 to 17 pounds or about 1/10 to 1/13 the body weight is composed of blood. It is distributed, ¼ to the heart, lungs, and large vessels, ¼ to the liver, ¼ to the muscles, and ¼ to the rest of the body. Two-thirds of the whole quantity may be lost, even suddenly by hemorrhage without causing death. Rectal injections of salt water will help make up lost blood.

When passing through the kidneys, the blood gives up uric acid, various salts, and water, all of which goes to make the urine. It then becomes venous blood, because it also loses oxygen and takes up carbon dioxide and other poisons.

In passing through the lungs, the blood loses the carbon dioxide nitrogen, and volatile organic substances taken up in circulation, and takes up oxygen which purifies it again for re-circulation. It also loses some of its heat.

While life lasts, the muscles of the heart contract and expand continuously. Its action is controlled by the sympathetic (involuntary) nervous system, the largest nerve of which running directly to the heart, is the vagus or pneumogastric. The heart has been called "a muscular pump," and it is the force of its strokes, due to the contraction of its muscular fibres, that causes the blood to flow throughout the body. The same amount of blood that is forced into the arteries at each heartbeat is emptied from the veins into the heart chambers. In circulation, blood travels about thirty-five feet per second.

The circulation is purely an automatic, mechanical process. It is caused by the contraction of the heart of cardiac muscles, reinforced by the tonicity of the arteries and the negative pressure in the veins. We will learn later how the heart beats my be increased or diminished by simple pressure on the vagus nerve, or a thrust given on the backbone, which causes a stimulation or depression of the controlling nerves of the heart.

Lesson 1: Introduction

The cardiac cycle is as follows: the heart auricles contract, increasing the blood pressure therein which forces open the auricolo-ventricular or mid-heart valves and sends the blood into the ventricles. Next the ventricles contract, increasing the pressure, which closes the auriculo-ventricular valves and opens the aortic and pulmonic or semi-lunar vlaves, and the blood rushes into the arteries. The heart contracted is called Systole. Its dilatation is called Diastole. Systole of the ventricles is the active state of the heart, because they are the largest cavities. As soon as this ceases, the muscles relax, the auricles enlarge and the ventricles are said to dilate, causing diastole. Between these actions is a rest period.

Blood pressure is the tension of the blood vessel walls, derived by the blood current, and usually equals 120 to 160 millimeters of mercury. Arterial blood pressure is raised by increased muscular activity. Arterial blood pressure is raised by increased muscular activity and the force of the heartbeat, also at times of digestion, exercise, emotion, and rapid respiration. The venous current is maintained by the force of the heart transmitted to the arteries and capillaries, the contraction of the surrounding muscles, and the action of little valves in the veins which prevent the blood from flowing back.

The pulse represents the cardiac impulse transmitted to the peripheral artery. The pulse wave, due to the amount of blood in the vessels, is about 9 ½ feet. At each heartbeat, additional tension is caused on the already filled vessels. There is no pulsation in the veins, except in some diseased conditions.

In healthy, normal adult life, the pulse beats about 72 times per minute. In females, it is from four to eight beats faster than in males. In youth, it is about 80 to 90; in infancy and at birth, 15 to 130 per minute.

A steady, slow pulse is generally strong; and a rapid pulse is usually weak and feeble. The fingers are ordinarily placed on the radial artery at the wrist, to feel the pulse, but it can be as easily felt at several other places in the body, perhaps the most convenient one being a point close to and immediately in front of the tragus of the ear.

The Sphygmograph is an instrument for graphical recording the pulse wave. It consists of a piece of wood or other material held by a spring over the radial artery. A system of levers transmits the movements of the artery to a delicate pointer which records the movement on a smoked surface. The record thus made is a Sphygmogram.

RESPIRATION

Life in the body is maintained by means of combustions, paradoxical as it may sound. The various processes that go on within our bodily house, constantly manufacture certain waste products and poisonous gases. We shall learn how to eliminative organs rid the system of the vast bulk of refuse, but the blood may be "screened" and purified continually, because it is being constantly contaminated. Nature uses combustion to burn up the waste products and it is by the organs of respiration and the act of breath that the oxygen necessary for Nature's purposes, is secured.

In the process of combustion, a poisonous gas, carbon dioxide is formed. It is absorbed by the blood, and by a chemical process is replaced by oxygen breathed into the lungs. The blood

Lesson 1: Introduction

then carries the oxygen to all parts of the body, where combustion utilizes it.

The lymph or blood plasma is the medium through which the interchanges of gases and fluids is made. It carries oxygen and finishes it to the it to the tissues when they need it. When the lymph needs more, the red blood cells in the capillaries supply it, which they have carried from the lungs. The tissue cells give up their carbon dioxide which is transferred by the lymph to the blood, and by that carried to the lungs where it is exhaled.

Generally defined, respiration is of two kinds: external, which consists in the replacement of gases in the blood, lungs and skin, to gases in the outer air; and internal respiration, which is the change of blood between the capillaries and the tissues of the body. The function of respiration is to supply the body with oxygen and allow the escape of carbon dioxide.

The act of respiration is accomplished by an ingenious mechanism embracing the chest of thoracic cage, the lungs, the diaphragm, and at the abdominal and chest muscles. The lungs lie passive within the chest.   Being very elastic, they follow all the movements of the chest walls.   Alternate contraction and expansion of the lungs, brought about by the contraction and relaxation of the abdominal and thoracic muscles and the diaphragm, constitutes the act of respiration. It is partly voluntary and partly involuntary. The dilatation of the thoracic cage is called **inspiration**; the contraction is called **expiration**. The act is controlled by a brain center in the medulla oblongata, the hind-part of the brain, sometimes called the "vital knot."

17

During inspiration, the diaphragm descends and draws away from the chest wall, while the ribs are elevated and rotate outwardly. Then lengthens the vertical, and increases the transverse diameter of the thoracic cage and the lungs. In expiration, the chest wall contract, the chest muscles relax, the weight of the chest reduces the tension of the abdominal muscles, and the elasticity of the lungs permits them to reduce in size, whence the air is expelled. The central tendon of the diaphragm is drawn up in the thorax by the negative intra-thoracic pressure, which results from the collapse of the lung and the contraction of the abdominal muscles.

As it is important that you understand this act fully, we describe it in another way. When the little air sacs comprising the lungs are filled with air, by a voluntary action of the person, the lungs expand and fill the chest cavity. This is an inspiration. The air quickly becomes rarified, and the pressure outside the chest, due to gravity becomes greater than the pressure within the chest (or which is more correct perhaps but amounts to the same things, the pressure within the chest becomes less than the pressure without). This difference causes the muscles to relax, and the weight of the chest forces it to return to normal size. As a consequence, the air within the lungs is expelled, and the act of respiration is completed.

Inspiration is normally about three times longer than expiration. Both acts follow each other. Inspiration occurs to expiration in the ration of about 5 to 6, i.e., it requires about the same time for five inspiration that it does for six expirations.

Respiratory sounds, or murmurs, heard by the stethoscope over the chest, are produced by the air rushing through the air passages. In normal or vesicular breathing, the sound has been likened to the blowing of the wind over leaves on the ground. It is a swelling rustling sounds. In bronchial or tubular breathing, the sound is quite like that produced by blowing through a tube or over the mouth of a bottle.

Breathing through the nose is the way Nature intended us to breathe. The respiratory tract through the nose, larynx, trachea, bronchial tubes and into the lungs is so constructed as the render the air more fit for use. Bad air and odors are detected, the cilia (hairs) in the nostrils arrest the coarse particles of dirt, the mucus membrane lining the tract aids still further in taking up dust, mucus, etc., and the long distance from the outer air to the lungs, prevents cold air that might chill the delicate lung tissue, from entering.

The healthy adult should have about 18 respirations a minute. The new-born infant averages about 40, and at five years of age, about 25. Respirations are less frequent during sleep, and are increased by muscular exercise, or when there is a deficiency of oxygen in the system. Children use the abdominal muscles chiefly in breathing; men, the lower chest muscles, and women, the upper chest muscles.

Asphyxia is suffocation, and is caused, first, by failure of air to enter the lungs, due to obstruction of the larynx and by a foreign body, or by external contraction, as in strangulation; second, by absence of oxygen in the inspired air; and third, by anything that interferes with the supply of oxygen to the tissues, and edema (fluid within) of the lungs, or other diminution of the respiratory surface, etc. death from asphyxia is caused by deficient oxygen and the consequent accumulation of too much carbon dioxide in the blood. The symptoms of asphyxia by stages are, excessive and difficult breathing, convulsions, and exhaustion and death.

Dyspnea is difficult or rapid breathing due to lack of oxygen or excess of carbon dioxide in the blood. It is characterized by slow, deep, vigorous exhalation. As only about 5% of oxygen is absorbed from the air breathed, it is clear that much air must pass through the lungs, in order to furnish the necessary amount of oxygen.

Certain terms are used to express the normal quantity of air breathed. **Tidal air** is the normal amount breathed during one respiration, about 500 cubic cc. **Reserve air** is the amount that can be forced from the lungs after a normal expiration, about 1500cc.

Vital capacity is the volume of air that can be exhaled after a forced inspiration, i.e., all the lungs can hold about 2500 cc. **Residual** is the amount that remains in the lungs after a forced expiration about 1500 cc.

At birth the lungs contain no air. The lungs and the small bronchi are collapsed. The trachea and the large bronchi are open, but contain fluid instead of air. The first cry of the infant must overcome the adhesions existing in the walls of these collapsed air vessel but when once filled, the lungs are never completely emptied again until after death.

It sometimes becomes necessary to prove that a child is born dead. This is done by removing the lungs from the body, tying the trachea, and placing them in water. If they float, air has entered the lungs; if they sink, the child was still born.

Lesson 1: Introduction

The air exhaled differs from the inhaled air in three particular. The exhaled air is nearly as warm as blood, about 100 deg. Far.; if saturated with moisture, except in cases of severe fever; and it contains about 5% less oxygen and 4$ more carbonic acid gas. It also contains some effete or waste matter that is highly impure. In hours, about 9 ounces of water are given off through the lungs.

Through respiratory movements, certain emotions are expressed. **Sighing** is a deep and long-drawn inspiration, mostly through the nose.

Laughing is an inspiration followed by a series of short, jet expirations with the vocal cords set into vibration the same as when one is speaking.

Yawning is a deep long sigh, drawn through the widely open mouth.

Hiccough is the result of a sudden inspiration that has contracted in the diaphragm, in a sense, a spasm of the diaphragm. The sudden closing of the glottis, cutting off the air entering, gives rise to the characteristic "hic".

Coughing is a double act: a deep, long drawn inspiration, followed by a complete closure of the glottis and a sudden and forcible expiration usually through the mouth.

Sneezing is similar, except that the soft palate drops, the opening into the mouth closes, and the air is forced through the nose.

Sobbing is a series of convulsive inspirations following each other in close succession. Little or no air enters the lungs, as the glottis is closed.

In **crying** the respiratory movements are the same as in laughing.

Lesson 1: Introduction

INSTRUCTIONS FOR TAKING THE EXAMINATION

Do not attempt to answer the questions until you have carefully studied the text for each lesson several times. It is best not to refer to the questions at all until you are ready to write. Be fair with yourself—let the questions be a real and true test of what you know about each lesson. The surer you are of all points in the lesson, the better examination you will be able to write. Bear in mind that the more you know, the better qualified you will be to understand the cases which you will be called upon to handle. Your desire is to acquire knowledge and you can best do this by faithful, persistent study. We are ready to help you become a well-informed and proficient Chiropractor, and you should be willing to follow our instructions carefully. Your success means ours.

1. All questions must be answered without reference to books, papers, or persons.

2. Use light weight, white paper, business letter size, and write with ink or typewriter on one side only—never with pencil.

3. Always write your name and address, page and lesson number, at the top of each sheet. If you change your address from the way you signed the application blank, be sure to notify us at once.

4. Always write the question first, then answer underneath. Begin each question and answer on a separate line.

5. Leave about 1 ½ inch of space on one side of the sheet for corrections, and space the lines wide. Never crowd your answers.

6. Fold your paper carefully and mail in a sealed envelope. It is not necessary to register.

7. Always enclose three two-cent stamps for return of examination papers and forwarding of new lessons.

8. Do not return your lesson books. They belong to you.

9. Allow a week or ten days for the correction and return of your examination. If not returned to you within two weeks, write us the date of mailing, and we will immediately advise you if they have not been received by us.

10. Ask all the questions on a separate sheet of paper.

11. As soon as the questions on one lesson are answered, sealed and mailed to us, go over the questions again and answer them by reference to the text. In this way, you will be able to determine your own mistakes and should make sure then that you know the correct answers. You can then take up the next lesson, while waiting for us to return your examination.

12. An average of 75% must be secured on each lesson in order to obtain your graduation papers.

13. New lessons will be mailed to you separately from the returned corrected examination, and as you need them in study.

14. Remittances may be sent with your examination questions, provided the money order, check or draft is enclosed in a separate envelope and your name and address written on the envelope. Do not send cash or bills unless you register the letter. Make all remittances by P.O. or express money order, bank draft or registered letter payable to American University.

15. Never address mail to any individual member of the faculty, unless of a personal nature. Address all letters to American University, Chicago, Illinois.

QUESTIONS—LESSON 1

1. Give four functions of the blood.

2. Describe Erythrocyte and give function.

3. Describe Leucocyte and give functions.

4. Describe the coagulation of the blood.

5. Tell changes in the blood passing through the kidneys.

6. What is the purpose of respiration?

7. Where is the brain center controlling respiration located?

8. Define asphyxia, dyspnea, residual air, vital capacity.

9. What is the temperature of exhaled air? Why?

10. Describe coughing, sneezing.

EXTENSION COURSE
IN CHIROPRACTIC
AMERICAN UNIVERSITY
CHICAGO, Ill., U.S.A.

LESSON 2

DIGESTION

The student will see that we are telling of the various functions or actions of the different bodily organs, and proceeding upon the assumption that nearly every person is more or less familiar with the organs themselves, at least enough for our present purpose. Later on in Anatomy, we shall take up in detail just how these organs are constructed. By knowing how they act, you will more readily grasp a clear understanding of their construction, which is so important.

Digestion is the process by which ingested food is prepared for absorption in the body. This is accomplished by the action of ferments or digestive juices, after which the food is taken up by the blood and lymph streams and carried to the tissues.

There are four important digestive juices, each secreted in a different part of the alimentary tract. **Saliva** is secreted in the mouth, **gastric juice** in the stomach, **pancreatic juice** in the pancreas which empties into the small intestine (duodenum)

27

through the common bile duct, and **bile** secreted by the liver where it is gathered up by the tiny hepatic ducts and stored in the gall bladder from which it empties into the second part of the duodenum through an entrance into the common bile duct.

FOOD CLASSIFIED

For a moment, we will divert, and classify foodstuffs, so you may know the chemical substances of which they are composed. Five different classes may be named, and all our foods can be placed in some one of these classes. They are:

1. **Carbohydrates**, as starches and sugars.

2. **Nitrogenous proteids and albumens**, as cheese, meats, eggs, beans, peas, etc.

3. **Hydro-carbons**, as fats and oils.

4. **Inorganic**, as oxygen, water, salt.

5. **Condiments**, spices, alcoholic beverages, tea, coffee.

It is essential to know the functions of these different classes. Carbohydrates furnish bodily fuel; proteids repair the tissues; fats supply heat and bodily reserve; water and oxygen are necessaries of life, being constituents of all tissues and fluids, dissolving food, distributing nourishment, and removing waste, tea and coffee are stimulants; while alcohol increases the flow of blood to the stomach, and increases the secretion of gastric juices. In small quantities it is valuable, protecting tissues in sick persons from too rapid consumption, as it easily breaks up into carbon dioxide and water; it replaces fat, stimulates circulation and the nervous system, and supplies food in temporary privation.

Lesson 2: Digestion

A certain amount of adipose tissue or fat is desirable in the body to furnish rotundity, protect the body against cold and mechanical injury, lubricate and prevent friction of muscles and joints, and to act as a reserve store of nutriment and fuel.

The best, all-around results in life seem to be produced by the use of a mixed diet of different food stuffs. An excessive starch diet produces obesity, dyspepsia, etc., which may lead to alimentary glycosuria (sugar in the urine). Green fruits are necessary, because of the fruit acids and salts they contain. A lack of these gives rise to scorbutic conditions, as scurvy.

Milk is considered the one best sustainer of life. Chemical analysis shows it to contain most of the substances needed for sustenance. It will be well to memorize the following comparative table showing the composition of human and cows milk.

Human Milk		Cow Milk
%87.4	Water	%87.4
2.3	Proteids	4.0
2.8	Fats	4.0
6.2	Sugar	4.0
0.3	Salts	0.6

In our later lesson on Dietetics we shall have much more to say on this subject. For the present, it may be sufficient to maintain that the best diet for each individual is that which is most agreeable and give the least amount of work to the digestive organs. Habits, work, climate, seasons, etc., will have their varying effects on the diet of every person.

A calorie is the unit by which heat produced is measured. It is the amount of heat required to raise the temperature of 1 kilogram of water 1 deg. Centigrade. Carbohydrates and proteids have a caloric value of 4 calories per gram; fats 8 to 9.

Much of a man's food requires cooking, the effect of which is considered beneficial. It softens the food and makes it more easily masticated; destroys all parasites and disease germs; develops certain flavors; softens tough fibers, breaks up cellular coats of starch, swells grains and bursts them so that the granules are more easily acted upon by the digestive secretions; it changes some starches into dextrin which is more soluble than starch; and coagulates albumins, proteids, etc.

DIGESTIVE JUICES

Let us now return to a detailed study of the various digestive juices.

Saliva is a clear, sticky, watery, **alkaline,** tasteless odorless fluid containing mucin, inorganic salts, earthy phosphates, and one chemical digestive ferment or enzyme called **Ptyalin,** which acts only on carbohydrates, converting them, if they stay in the mouth long enough, into maltose, a malt-sugar, which is more easily absorbed into the blood stream. Saliva also aids in speaking, dissolves certain articles of food, assists in forming a bolus, and lubricates it so that it is more easily swallowed.

The process of mixing food with saliva is called **insalivation.** **Mastication** is the crushing, grinding, and pulverizing and insalivation of food, by means of the teeth, tongue and cheeks. Anything which excites the taste, causes the salivary glands to secrete saliva, such as the sight of food, the smell, or hearing it prepared, mental emotions, etc. About two or three pints of saliva are secreted in twenty-four hours, the same amount as urine.

Gastric Juice is a clear, colorless fluid, **acid** in reaction, of characteristic odor, containing water, mucin, lactic and hydrochloric acid, pepsin and rennin the two principal ferments, and inorganic salts. It stops fermentation and the action of the saliva on the carbohydrates. The pepsin converts proteids into peptones, which are more easily assimilated; and rennin coagulates the casein of milk. In time, alcoholic stimulants abolish the secretion of gastric juice. From ten to twenty pints are secreted every twenty-four hours; but no secretion takes places without a stimulation, like food, etc., being in the stomach. The time of gastric digestion is from three to five hours; this time may, however, be changed by the quantity and nature of food taken, time since last meal, amount of exercise before and after meals, state of mind and bodily health. Grief retards digestion, tranquility aids it.

Gases formed in the stomach are derived from air swallowed, from regurgitation (flowing back) from the intestines, also from fermentation and putrefactive changes in the food, in dyspepsia.

A very pertinent question may now be asked: why doesn't the stomach digest itself? It cannot be answered positively, but three theories are advanced. 1st. The constant stream of alkaline blood circulating through the inner coats or linings of the stomach may protect it from the action of the acid gastric juices. 2nd. The innermost lining is covered with a thick layer of mucus lining wall that resists the digestive ferments. 3rd. The substance secreted called Pepsin, is really Pepsinogen. It comes from the peptic glands of the stomach. Having a strong affinity for acids it unites with the hydrochloric acid and immediately becomes pepsin. As all the pepsinogen secreted unites with the hydrochloric acid and food, there is nothing left to attack the stomach walls.

It is a known fact, however, that the stomach may, under certain conditions, digest itself. For instance, if a portion of the stomach is deprived of its circulation, it may be attacked by its own secretions and a perforation of the stomach wall result, as in ulceration and cancer of the stomach.

The pancreatic juice is a clear, viscid, odorless, colorless fluid, **alkaline** in reaction like the saliva, but containing five digestive ferments, whose functions are as follows:

Amylopsin converts starch into maltose, dextrin and sugar, continuing the work of the saliva, which has been stopped by the action of the acid gastric juice.

Trypsin acts like pepsin, changing proteids and albuminates to albumoses.

Steapsin breaks up fats into fatty acids and glycerine, from which soap and emulsions are formed.

Rennin, like that in the gastric juice, but this kind requires an alkaline medium instead of an acid.

Invertin converts maltose, a bi-product of starch, into dextrose or grape sugar.

Lesson 2: Digestion

From six to eight ounces of pancreatic juice are secreted every twenty-four hours. It is the one most important digestive secretions in the body.

Bile is a transparent, viscid fluid with a bitter sweetish taste, musk-like odor, and varying in color from reddish yellow to dark green. It is neutral in reaction, and the only digestive juice with NO ferments. It contains mucin, glycol-cholic and tauro-cholic acid which unite with soda and form fats, cholesterin, coloring matter of pigments, and salts. The two most important salts formed from these acids are Sodium Glycocholate and Sodium Taurocholate. Bile is secreted continually, being retarded during fasting and accelerating on taking food. It should be noted that the other digestive fluids are secreted only when the glands are stimulated by the presence of food. From 20 to 40 ounces of bile are secreted daily.

The function of bile are many, but chief of them may be mention the following:

1. Assists in breaking up fats and preparing them for absorption.

2. Prevents putrefactive changes in food while in the intestines because of a certain antiseptic power.

3. Is considered to act as a natural purgative by promoting increased secretion of the intestinal glands and stimulating intestinal peristalsis (the movement by which the intestines carry their contents forward).

4. Stimulate the production of trypsin.

5.   Holds soaps and cholesterin in solution.

6.   Excretes pigments, cholesterin, and harmful compounds containing metals.

7.   Renders the intestinal juices alkaline.

Cholesterin is a fat-like pearly substance, said to have the power of neutralizing snake-venoms and immunizing against them. It appears in minute transparent rhomboid plates which are insoluble in water, but soluble in alcohol, ether and chloroform. It results from the disintegration of the epithelial cells of the biliary passages, and is NOT a secretory product of the liver.

Tests. It sometimes becomes necessary to test feces and stomach contents for biliary acids and biliary pigments or coloring matter. The best test for biliary acids is known as Pettenkofer's. Place a quantity of sulphuric acid on the suspected material, then add a few drops of cane sugar. The result will yield a purple color.

Gmelin's test for biliary pigments is to mix the suspected material with a few drops of nitric acid and add a few drop of nitrous acid. Allow this to flow carefully down the side of the glass without agitation. A play of colors—green, blue, violet, red, and yellow—will result, if there is present any **bilirubin**, the yellow, and **biliverdin**, the green biliary pigment.

Please understand that the substances composing the bile do not exist in the blood. They are the direct result of a true secretive action of the hepatic cells.

Perhaps you may ask, what becomes of the various ferments of the digestive juices? The ptyalin is destroyed by the

34

acid pepsin, and that in turn is destroyed by the alkaline pancreatic and intestinal juices and by trypsin. Acid fermentative changes in the large intestines gradually destroy the ferments of the pancreas. Some bile is discharged with the feces, some is absorbed and eliminated in urine. The salts are mostly absorbed and returned to the blood stream. Cholesterin is eliminated in feces.

It will be well for us to take up here the **function of the liver**, so that a complete idea can be obtained of just how the digested food stuffs are absorbed, assimilated and converted into body tissue.

The liver forms bile, glycogen, fat, urea, uric acid and by-products; destroys certain poisons; and forms a cemetery for red cells and hemoglobin.

Glycogen from the liver originates from the carbo-hydrate food we eat. Albuminous or fatty diets will decrease it, while starch, milk, fruit and cane sugar are said to increase its production. Five or six ounces of it are stored up temporarily in the liver during health, like starch plants. Being an animal starch, it is a carbohydrate, and soluble in water.

The liver converts glucose or cane sugar into glycogen, because of glucose entered directly into the blood, sometimes there would be too much and sometimes too little. Glucose is really the fuel of the body, and must be present in the blood, but only in very small quantity, less than 1/3 ounce in the whole body being sufficient.

Urea is a nitrogenous by-product formed from proteids after the fat and glycogen are eliminated.

Chyme is a grayish, semi-fluid acid substance—a mixture of finely divided food and gastric juice. It contains albuminous matter dissolved or party so, melted fats not dissolved, starch slowly changing to sugar, and digestive fluids.

Chyle is fluid lymph found in the lymphatic vessels of the digestive tract. It is alkaline, and contains fats, proteids in solution, glycerine, lymph cells, and some sugar and salt.

QUESTIONS—LESSON 2

1. Classify foods and give functions of each.

2. Describe the saliva and name its enzyme

3. What effect has gastric juice on saliva?

4. What salts and acids does bile contain?

5. Why doesn't the stomach digest itself?

6. Name the ferments of the pancreatic juice, and give uses.

7. Give the functions of bile.

8. What substances are formed in the liver?

9. What foods increase or decrease the amount of glycogen?

10. Differentiate between chyme and chyle.

EXTENSION COURSE
IN CHIROPRACTIC
AMERICAN UNIVERSITY
CHICAGO, Ill., U.S.A.

LESSON 3

DIGESTION (Continued)

Lymph is the circulating medium in the lymphatic system. It is the fluid by which the process of absorption is effected. It is a clear, transparent, yellowish, albuminous, slightly alkaline liquid containing white blood corpuscles, lymph cells, and some salts. It comes from the blood as a modified blood plasma that has osmosed (escaped) through the capillary walls and form lymph glands that furnish lymphocytes. The quantity formed depends on the arterial blood pressure, the amount of water in the blood, and the permeability of the blood vessel walls.

Lymph is first formed in the lymph spaces surrounding the blood vessels, which unite to form the lymphatic vessels. It is finally emptied into the blood stream at a junction of the jugular and left subclavian veins in the upper thoracic or bronchial region.

Some principal uses of lymph are:

Lesson 3: Digestion (Continued)

1. Nutritive—carries food and digestive products to the tissues.

2. Removes waste products from the tissues.

3. Relieves the blood from excess fluid.

4. Dissolves certain substances.

5. Is a very satisfactory lubricant.

6. Aids in healing wounds.

7. Has a special function of equilibrium in the middle ear.

Now that we know what is going to happen to food, we next proceed to masticate and swallow it—the act of Deglutition.

The first stage of **Deglutition** may be called the buccal stage. After the food has been thoroughly masticated and insalivated ready for swallowing, the mouth is usually closed and the jaws pressed together. The bolus of food is still in the mouth, but thus far the act is entirely controlled by will—voluntary.

The second stage is called the pharyngeal stage. The tip, middle, and root of the tongue successively press against the hard palate, and the food is thrown to the back side of the mouth. At the same time, the soft palate draws up and backward, closing the posterior nares (openings from the pharynx to the nose). The larynx is pulled upward and forward, the glottis is closed by the epiglottis and the approximation of the vocal cords. The bolus is prevented from re-entering the mouth by the closure of the anterior pillars of the fauces, so there is no place for it to go but into the esophagus. Thus far in this stage, the act is considered more reflex than voluntary.

The esophageal stage begins with the successive dilatation and contraction of the tree superior, middle and inferior constricts muscles of the esophagus. This produces a peristaltic or worm-like movement which carries the food downward into the stomach. After this stage begins, the food cannot be voluntarily returned to the mouth, as the muscles are not under the control of the will. Swallowing is purely a muscular act, as it can take place in opposition or gravity.

ABSORPTION

Having learned how food is masticated, insalivated, swallowed and digested, we will next study the process by which free form materials are taken up by the tissues and transformed by them in raw substance, while the refuse or waste is eliminated. This process is called **Absorption**.

It is accomplished, 1st, by osmosis, the passage of fluids through an animal membrane **without** pressure; 2nd, by filtration, which is osmosis **under** pressure; and 3rd, the action of the skin in separation takes place in the alimentary tract, through the skin, and the lungs. The channels of absorption are the capillaries, the lymphatic and the lacteals of the small intestines.

In order to have absorption, the substance to be absorbed must be diffusible in the liquid or gaseous state, for the less dense it is the faster it will be absorbed. Absorption is facilitated by full, tense blood vessels and rapid circulation of blood, also by heat, stimulants (such as condiments), pressure, etc.

You should gain a clear distinction between the following terms: **endosmosis**, the process by which two dissimilar liquids separate by a membrane, effect an interchange until both liquids are alike; **diffusion**, the simple mixing of liquids without the use of a membrane.

We are now ready to learn how the various substances of food eaten are taken into the system and converted into tissue.

The lymphatics or absorbents receive the materials of the digested food not taken directly into the blood stream of the alimentary canal and carry them indirectly to the blood stream, i.e. through the lymphatic system first. Most of this is done in the small intestines where the chyme passes through the epithelial covering of the villi (little projections) in the intestines, by osmosis. In this way, the part of the food taken into the stomach which has become chyme through the digestive processes, is taken up by the blood.

The process by which water, alcohol, salts, carbohydrates and proteids are absorbed is not so complicated because it utilizes organs and mediums of larger size. These substances enter the capillaries of the stomach and are carried directly to the liver by the portal circulation, reaching the blood stream by the hepatic vein.

The Portal Circulation is usually considered by itself. It is the circulation of the liver. The large portal veins (from the spleen, stomach, and intestines), which are filled by the capillaries (little blood vessels) surrounding these organs. When the portal vein enters the liver, it breaks into **inter**-lobular veins running between the lobules of the liver. At the center of the liver, the little capillaries running all through the liver unite to form the **intra**-lobular or central veins. Several of these trunks unite to form the hepatic vein which empties into the inferior vena cava which carries the blood back to the lungs and heart. It will be seen that there is arterial blood in the hepatic artery, portal blood in the portal and inter-lobular veins, and venous blood in the intra-lobular and the hepatic veins.

Fats and fatty acids are absorbed by the lacteals (lymphatics in the intestines), and from there are carried to the Receptaculum Chyli—"receptacle of chyle"—an enlargement of the thoracic duct located near the waist-line just inside the spine. From there it is carried to the left subclavian vein, as before stated.

Absorption by lymphatics and by blood vessels differs in one noticeable particular. The former seem to show a selective action—choosing the materials to be admitted. Blood vessels take any substance capable of permeating their walls.

You will have little difficulty in gaining a clear understand of digestion and absorption, if you do not try to grasp all the details at once. Take up one process at a time. There are many points to be remembered, many different substances to be disposed of, and many organs and means by which the processes are completed. Understand each step, and you will gain a mastery of the whole process.

A **secretion** is a substance manufactured out of material furnished by the blood. An **external secretion** is one discharged on a free surface communication with the exterior, as milk, all digestive juices, sweat, prostatic fluid, etc. An **internal secretion** is one of discharged into the blood stream and lymph (examples later).

An excretion is the elimination of waste products of any organ in the body, as urine, feces, sweat, carbon dioxide, etc.

METABOLISM

This is a name given to the process of building up (Anabolism), and tearing down (Catabolism) of the body. It includes making new tissue, repairing lost tissue, and saving up food material or pabulum for future use.

The best place to study the metabolic processes in the body is in the muscles, glands, etc., because they occupy an intermediate position between the digestion and absorption of food on one hand, and the excretion of waste products on the other.

The chemical changes of metabolism are brought about in different ways: 1st, by combining with water or oxygen; 2nd, by removing water. It should be remembered that the inorganic principles entering into the formation of the body are water, oxygen, and various salts, as sodium, chlorine, calcium, magnesium, potassium, etc.

Certain organs discharge an internal secretion into the circulation which affects metabolism and acts as an antidote to some poisons. These organs are the pituitary bodies, the liver, the kidneys, the testicles, the ovaries, etc.

During the processes of metabolism, the various changes cause the production of animal heat within the body. Muscular and visceral activity, and the circulation of the blood also form a source of animal heat. Age, sex, species, digestion, etc., also affect the production of this heat as well as outside temperature, drugs, etc. Variations of temperature will be effected by exercise, climate, season, time of day (high between 5 and 8 P.M., and low from 2 to 6 A.M.), hemorrhages, poisons, shock, etc.

The blood in the liver is the hottest in the body, due to the heat formed; the coldest part of the body is the tip of the nose. Losing heat is effected by dilatation of the skin cells, by increased sweating, respiration, etc.

When a muscle contracts, it becomes shorter, but its volume remains the same. As more oxygen is used and taken up by the capillaries circulating in the muscles, the myosin (muscle fluid) becomes acid. Carbon dioxide is given off and glycogen is formed.

Muscles are normally always on the stretch, acting as ligaments binding together the whole body. Opposing muscles produce opposite movements. Their elasticity acts as a spring to maintain the tonicity of the limbs and prevent sudden jerks of the body which would result if the muscles contracted quickly.

Muscle fatigue is due to an accumulation of the products and metabolism in the muscular tissues. By washing out these foreign substances, fatigue can be removed. Herein lies the relief of battle.

Soon after death, the muscles stiffen (rigor mortis). It begins with the eye muscles, then those of the jaw, neck, arms, chest, abdomen and lower extremities. By noticing this fact, it can be determined how long a body has been dead. **Rigor mortis** is due to the coagulation of the myosin in the muscle substance, which is caused by the production of heat, lactic acid and the cessation of the circulation.

ELIMINATIVE AND EXCRETORY PROCESSES

It has been shown how each tissue in the body combines with the particular chemic substance in the blood that is required for its own growth and activity. For instance, the liver cells select substances from which bile and glycogen are made; the bones choose lime for hardening them, etc. This selective power of all parts of the body, to choose the proper substances from which to build each particular tissue is most wonderful. The Chiropractor and the drug-less healer can safely depend upon it to right any wrongs found in the body. The great secret of healing is to know how to provide the proper requirements and stimulation for each part.

In the continuous processes of metabolism and catabolism (destructive changes), certain waste products are manufactured. It is the province of the excretory organs to rid the system of these products and thereby prevent their re-absorption. Auto-intoxication (self-poisoning) results from the absorption of waste products that should be eliminated from the body.

Excretion is the process by which cells of the excretory organs separate useless and injurious materials from the blood and discharge them from the body. The principal excretory organs are the lungs, skin, kidneys, and intestines.

From the lungs, carbonic acid and a small quantity of water are discharged; from the skin, uric acid, water and some salts; from the kidneys, more salts, urea, and water; from the intestines, refuse and bulky waste, bacteria, etc.

We have learned how to lungs, with the aid of oxygen from the air, give off carbon dioxide, and the lymphatics take up any excessive water that may not be carried out in the exhaled air.

The skin serves us in many ways: 1st, as an external covering and protection; 2nd, as a sensitive organ of touch; 3rd, as an absorbing, secretory and excretory organ; 4th, as a temperature regulator. Its detailed construction will be treated under the subject of Anatomy, when it extreme value as a covering and organ of sense will become more apparent.

The sebaceous glands in the skin secrete an oily or fatty substance called sebum and keeps the skin soft and pliable, and prevents it from drying and cracking. They are most abundant on the hairy parts of the body.

The sudoriferous glands secrete about two pounds daily, depending on the season, climate, exercise, drink, food, etc., of sweat or perspiration. This consists largely of water, fats, and solids, with a salty taste. Our bodies are sweating continually, but the sweat evaporates without our knowledge. In the whole process of respiration through the skin and the lungs, about 1/67 of the body weight is lost. Sweating is increased by a rise in temperature either internally or externally, by muscular activity, drugs, etc.

As a heat regulator, the skin serves our bodies wonderfully. The average normal temperature of the body is maintained by the equal balance of heat lost and produced. Metabolism and circulation increase heat in the body, and it is lost by radiation from the surface of the skin and the evaporation of the perspiration. Eighty per cent of bodily heat is lost in this way; 3%, by warming the feces and urine; 9%, in exhaled air.

Heat is distributed throughout the body by means of the blood. Where blood vessels are exposed to evaporation, the temperature is lowered; in the inner organs and where oxidation takes place, it is raised. You can easily see, therefore, how the temperature is distributed and regulated.

A fever is an increased-above-normal temperature in some part or the entire body, due to failure of the body to remove and liberate the heat being continually generated. It is also considered Nature's method of burning up refuse matter that has collected and not been fully eliminated. Fevers serve a good purpose in this way. The great danger from them is the possibility of their becoming too great. They are not easy to control. They may burn out some delicate organism in addition to the waste, or exhaust the patient on account of the increased "feverish" activity of the heart and the respiration. The use of baths, sponging, etc., to regulate fevers and increased bodily temperature, will be treated fully in the lesson on Hydrotherapy.

Exposure to cold causes the blood vessels in the skin to contract. Warm blood from the inner body is then sent to the external surface, and the temperature is regulated. Exposure to warmth causes the blood vessels to dilate, and the inner warm blood, which is always warmer than the external heat, is cooled at the surface. It is also probable, that when the blood vessels in the skin contract greater heat is generated, due to the increased friction in forcing the blood through them. When they dilate in warmth, the head decreased, as the friction is less. The skin at all times is cooler than the internal organs, because of the radiation of heat from the skin and the increased heat produced within the body.

Lesson 3: Digestion (Continued)

QUESTIONS—LESSON 3

1. What is the value of lymph?

2. Describe the act of deglutition.

3. How is absorption accomplished?

4. Describe the portal circulation

5. Of what use are the lacteals?

6. Between what hours in the day do most deaths occur? Why?

7. What is the cause of muscle fatigue?

8. Name some uses of the skin.

9. Of what value are fevers?

10. What is the warmest part of the body, and why?

EXTENSION COURSE IN CHIROPRACTIC AMERICAN UNIVERSITY CHICAGO, Ill., U.S.A.

LESSON 4

ELIMINATION (Continued)

THE URINARY ORGANS

The kidneys, the ureters, the bladder, and the urethra are the organs by which the largest amount of waste fluid is eliminated. Urine is the medium of elimination. The function of the kidneys is to remove water, urea, and uric acid from the blood. Both kidneys do no secrete uniformly. One may secrete urine of greater acidity than the other, or containing more salts. Sometimes only one works, the other kidney being inactive, its impaired function being due to any number of causes. It may never have developed, or it may have become diseased.

The amount of urine may be increased by anything that increases the blood supply to the kidneys, such as increased blood pressure or muscular activity, external cold, internal bodily heat, animal foods, etc. From 30 to 50 ounces are normally secreted daily, about 3 pints. It may be decreased by external warmth, constriction of the renal artery (to the kidney) by nerve influence, diminished blood pressure, vegetable foods, etc.

50

Lesson 4: Elimination (Continued)

Healthy urine contains water, urea, uric acid, coloring matter, inorganic salts, gases and some carbon dioxide. It is straw color, has a bitterish taste, characteristic odor, and a slight acid reaction.

The main solid in urine is urea, about 530 grains being excreted daily. It is a crystalline substance, insoluble in ether, but soluble in alcohol and water. It is the final product of all proteid food, therefore a diet rich in proteids will tend to increase the amount of urea in the system. It is found in the liver, intestines, blood and lymph; and has been prescribed as an uric acid solvent. Uric acid is increased by cheese, salt fish, heavy meats, chocolate, cocoa, and some febrile diseases.

After the kidneys have secreted the urine, it is carried by the ureters in the bladder, the reservoir. When the bladder becomes moderately distended, the sensory nerves become irritated and communicate with the vesico-spinal center situated in the spinal cord near the fourth dorsal vertebra. Reflex stimulation is produced through the action of the motor nerves of the bladder. This causes the bladder walls to contract until it becomes so great as to overcome the resistance of the sphincter muscles at the neck of the bladder. When this is done the contents are ejected through the urethra. The respiratory and abdominal muscles also aid by voluntary contraction. This act of voiding urine is called **Micturition**.

THE INTESTINES
We have already considered the use of the upper bowels or intestines in digesting food. Now we will take up its excretory functions. Particularly in the small or upper bowel, also in the stomach is a vermicular or worm-like movement is periodically

51

recurring, which is called peristalsis. It consists of progressive contractions of the walls, beginning in the stomach, at the opening or cardiac end, and terminated at the pyloric end. There is also a rhythmical opening and closing of the latter end. This undulating or contractile waste continues about 20 seconds, succeeded by a rest period of the same time, when another movement recurs. The object of this movement is to move the contents in one direction. In the stomach, another pendulum-like or churning movement sidewise occurs, which thoroughly mixes the food with the gastric juice.

Peristalsis continues throughout the intestines, carrying the feces forward until it is eliminated. Interference with the blood circulation increases peristalsis; but the weight of authority says that is constant, whether awake or asleep.

The discharge of fecal matter from the intestines is called **defecation**. When feces is present in the large intestine, or rectum it irritates the sensory nerves, causing the internal sphincter muscles to dilate. The external sphincter at the same time relaxes. This reflex center of defecation, called Budges-ano-spinal center of defecation, becomes excited. A deep inspiration is taken, an expiration effort it made voluntarily. The abdominal muscles contract, the rectum straightens, and the feces pass out through the anus.

The normal amount of feces in the average man is from 6 to 16 ounces, 75 per cent of which is water. Other ingredients are ingestible food, fruit stones, hair, cellulose, dead tissue cells, albumin, starch, etc.

Sometimes after food has entered the stomach, there is a tendency for it to return to the mouth, causing nausea and vomiting. This is a reflex action due to a stimulation of the vomiting nerve center located in the medulla of the brain. The walls of the stomach contract, the cardia or upper opening of the stomach dilates spemodically, and the ejection of the stomach contents is assisted in the contraction of the abdominal muscles. A reverse peristalsis of the esophagus takes place, the constrictors work upward instead of downward, and the food passes into the mouth and out.

Dr. Albert Abrams, founder of the School of Spondylotherapy, had shown that after food has passed into the stomach, by tapping the person lightly between the 5th and 6th dorsal vertebrae, the stomach will tip over like a bottle. This treatment is said to be the cure for some forms of headache.

FUNCTIONS OF THE NERVOUS SYSTEM

Nerves enable us to sense and act. They carry impressions to the brain, which in turn causes the muscles to act. Nerves must be irritated before they will manifest, as they cannot themselves originate the condition necessary to manifest their own energy.

If a cerebro-spinal nerve fiber in the living body is irritated, a message is conducted to the brain, which is its central termination when there is pain, or to a muscle, which is the peripheral termination when there is movement. It will be seen, therefore, that there seems to be two sets of nerves, viz., **sensory** nerves, which carry sensation to the brain, and motor nerves, which institute motion to the muscles. Whether there really are two sets of nerves, or one set capable of transmitting messages in opposite direction without interference, is not positively known; but certain it is, that the results about mentioned are fully manifested and demonstrated.

Sensory nerve fibers are also knows as **afferent**, or centripetal, carrying impulses from the periphery to the nerve centers; motor nerves are called **efferent**, or centrifugal, from center to periphery. When sensory nerves act, we sense pain, special sensation as in organs of special sense, and reflex action (unconscious or involuntary). When motor nerves act, contraction of muscles may result, also nutrition, secretions, etc., are affected.

Reflex action is action produced quicker than is possible through ordinary nerve stimulation. The message on the sensory nerve is not transmitted directly at first to the brain, but to a center in the spinal cord. Here the need of quick action is noted, and the instructions are immediately sent over the motor nerves to produce the needed movement or function in the peripheral muscle or organ. The reflexes are often used to test the normality of the nervous system. When they do not act quickly, something is wrong.

Reflex action is entirely independent of the will, and is classified, 1st, superficial, as the abdominal or plantar reflexes; 2nd, deep, as the knee-jerk, and chin reflexes; 3rd, visceral, as vomiting, micturition, defecation, etc.

By **irritability** is meant to inherent power of all nerves to act by reason of a stimulus. Good blood supply, bringing nutrition and carrying away waste, perfect connection with the brain without interference of any kind, and normal temperature are necessary to have perfect action of the nerves. When those conditions exist, the nerve force in motor nerves travels about 110 feet per second; in sensory nerves, about 140 feet.

A stimulus to a nerve ending may start within or without the body. When the impulse reaches the brain, it may start up other impulses. This fact is taken advantage of by the Chiropractor or Nerve Specialist, who, by knowing the results to be obtained, can stimulate the nerves that are most closely co-ordinated and correlated, thereby bringing about a condition of perfect health in the entire body.

Generally speaking, nerves are of two kinds—medulated (covered by a medullary substance) in the cerebro-spinal system, and non-medulated in the sympathetic system, we also have inhibitory nerves, whose impulses diminish vitality.

In the great Sympathetic System, we have the vaso-motor and vaso-constrictor nerves, which act on the blood vessels. Irritating the motor or dilator fibers, causes dilatation, and on the constrictor fibers, constriction of the blood vessels.

Stimulation of the vaso-motor nerves, by digestion, exercise, defecation, respiration, etc., causes increased blood pressure.

The sympathetic nerve, called the vagus or pneumogastric, accelerates the heart, decreases the activity of the intestines, and affects other visceral organs, the lungs, etc.

The function of the brain is to act as a center of information of knowledge for all the activity in the body. Whatever goes on in the body is sensed in the brain.

The functions of the spinal cord are two-fold: there is a motor and a sensory tract for carrying messages to and from the periphery, the anterior horn or tract is motor, and posterior, is sensory; also reflex centers are located in the cord, as defecation, micturition, genito-spinal, utero-spinal, etc.

It is quite a difficult matter to separate all the physiology of the nervous system from its anatomy; and inasmuch as the latter is larger and more intricate subject, we will have more to impart when Neurology is taken up later in the course. Let is suffice at this time to say that the whole nervous system is the one agency through which all bodily activities are controlled and regulated. If the nerves are right, the body is all right, and the man is in perfect health.

Sleep is a condition of unconsciousness, a period of rest for nerves and body. It is induced by minimizing the work of the nervous system. Voluntarily we can reduce all sensory manifestations, leaving nothing to be overcome but the involuntary working of the bodily organs.

During sleep, the blood pressure is reduced and the brain is without much blood, in normal health.

Dreams usually appear toward the time of awakening. These are considered psychic activities consisting of hallucinations.

When the muscles are fatigues, we learned they were filled with fatigue poisons (largely carbon dioxide). If there is lack of oxygen in the system, so the brain is not being properly nourished by oxygenated blood, drowsiness is the result. Over-fatigue sometimes causes insomnia (sleeplessness), due to the irritation of the nervous system from the excessive fatigue poisons in the muscles.

Life is the sum total of all activity. It embraces the potential to maintain itself, also to perpetuate its kind. **Death** is the cessation of all bodily functions.

Starvation is not so damaging to the body as loss of sleep, while in Nature's great period of reconstruction. After prolonged loss of sleep, the bodily temperature falls, and the reflexes disappear. The patient seems dull and logy.

ADENOLOGY
FUNCTIONS OF GLANDS

In Lesson 3, we mentioned the fact that certain glandular organs secrete substances into the blood stream, that affect metabolism, etc. there are also other useful purposes served by various glands in the body. The subject of Adenology, though comparatively short, is important and should receive careful study by the student. We shall take up only the most important secreting glandular organs.

All ductless glands, like the suprarenals, the thyroid, tonsils, pituitary bodies, etc., are considered to aid in destroying toxins (poisons) in the body. It is also said of them that their functions are unknown. There are, however, many theories regarding these functions, which we will give hereafter.

The **Thyroid Gland** is considered to secrete a substance rich in iodine which regulate the production of body fat. It also protects and aids the circulation of the blood to the head and brain. Some authorities say it has something to do with destroying

57

red blood cells. Its removal usually leads to tremors, convulsions, myxedema, emaciation, atrophy, and finally death.

The **Suprarenal Capsules** increase the blood pressure by increasing the contraction of the blood vessels. They are thought to stop the excessive formation of skin pigments or coloring matter, because, when removed, Addison's Disease is the usual result. In this disease the patient turns copper color.

The **Mammary Glands** are always undeveloped in the male and the female during childhood. As the girl approaches puberty, they enlarge in size, the veins become prominent, and the lobules can be easily felt. During pregnancy, they increase still more, the areola (circular area of dark colored skin around the nipple) darkens, and the veins become more prominent. After the nursing period, they diminish in size and return to normal, non-secreting condition.

The **Liver**, as we have seen, forms bile, urea, produces glycogen, and other waste products.

The **Gall Bladder** acts as a reservoir for bile, furnishing it to the intestines during digestion as needed. It holds about one or two ounces. If the bile ducts become occluded (stopped up), the bile is thrown back into the system, and Icterus (Jaundice) results.

The **Spleen** forms and destroys red blood cells, stores up and elaborates the albuminous food for nutrition, and serves as a reservoir for blood when the portal circulation is obstructed. It enlarges during digestion, also when filled to capacity, and during all diseases including fevers, blood diseases, etc.

Lesson 4: Elimination (Continued)

The **Lachrymal Glands** furnish moisture for the eyes to bathe in, which is called tears when it overflows. The secretion is a saline fluid that escapes through the nasal ducts into the nose.

The **Lymphatic Glands** are merely enlarged continuations of the lymphatics. They are most numerous in the intestines and near the great organs of the abdomen, chest, and neck, also under the arms and in the groin. They are believed to change the material and passes through them, having no secretion of their own. When become enlarged, it indicated a poisoned system, a toxic condition. Sometimes they collect so much toxin that pus forms and they break open. In this way the foreign substances are expelled.

The **Salivary Glands**, three in number, are called the Parotid, Submaxillary, and the Sublingual. The first secretes pure saliva containing ptyalin; the second secretes a mixed mucus and salivary substance. The third, a mucus substance.

The **Prostate Gland** has from 10 to 30 openings into the prostatic urethra, and furnishes a lubricating fluid which forms a part of the semen and assists in keeping up the vitality of the spermatozoa.

Serous and Synovial Membranes are considered in the same with secreting organs. The former line closed or visceral cavity as the arachnoid, a delicate membrane between the pia mater and dura mater of the brain and spinal cord; the **pericardium**, the sac around the heart; the **pleura**, the investment of the lungs, etc.

The synovial membranes line the joints, sheath the tendons and ligaments, furnishing smooth, moist surfaces to facilitate movement and prevent injurious effects of friction.

QUESTIONS—LESSON 4

1. How much urine is normally secreted daily?

2. Describe micturition.

3. What is peristalsis?

4. Name the kinds of nerves in the cerebro-spinal system.

5. Describe reflex action.

6. What is necessary to have perfect working nerves?

7. Give the functions of the spinal cord.

8. Name as many glands of the body as you can think of.

9. What are the functions of the thyroid gland?

10. What are the excretions of the body?

Chiropractic The Science of Spinal Adjustment

STUDENT NOTES

CHIROPRACTIC

The Science of Spinal Adjustment

———

A SERIES OF LESSONS CORRELATING AND
SYSTEMATIZING THE KNOWLEDGE NECESSARY TO
PRACTICE CHIROPRACTIC

Nature's Greatest Ally

IN RESTORING DISEASED CONDITIONS OF THE
BODY TO PERFECT HEALTH, WITHOUT THE AID OF
DRUGS OR SURGERY

———

BOOK 2

OSTEOLOGY AND ARTHROLOGY

Lessons 5, 6, 7 and 8

———

ORIGINALLY PUBLISHED BY
AMERICAN UNIVERSITY
CHICAGO, ILLINOIS, U.S.A.
COPYRIGHT 1913, 1916

Disclaimer

We are proud to republish this series of books on chiropractic medicine.

Originally published as a home-study course in 1913 by American University in Chicago, the 16 volumes give us an historical look at the theory and practice of chiropractic medicine in the early part of the 20th century.

This series is republished for historical interest only. The modern practice of chiropractic has advanced significantly in the century since these books were published. If you want to actually learn modern chiropractic techniques, please consult one of the many fine schools in this country.

The materials in these books are not intended to diagnose or treat disease. If you believe you are ill consult a licensed practitioner for care immediately. The publishers assume no liability for the use, misuse or nonuse of the materials in these books.

Thank you

EXTENSION COURSE
IN CHIROPRACTIC
AMERICAN UNIVERSITY
CHICAGO, Ill., U.S.A.

LESSON 5

INTRODUCTION

In the preceding four lessons you have been given briefly the structure of the body as a whole and of some of the important organs as well as the functions of the various organs and systems. In the next sixteen lessons the various parts of the body will be described in greater detail.

That science that deals with the form and structure of living bodies is called Anatomy. In this course only human anatomy will be considered.

Before any method of treatment can be used it is necessary that the practitioner know the condition of the various organs and systems of the patient's body. Diseases make themselves known to the patient or to the examiner by the failure of certain organs or parts to perform the functions required of them. This failure of the part may be due to some change in the form or structure of the part, or to merely some disturbance of its function.

These unnatural changes in the form or structure are considered in that division of practice known as **Pathology**. The pathology present in the body makes itself known to the patient and to the practitioner by Symptoms. Some of these changes can be detected only by careful examination of the patient. The process of determining the condition of the patient is called **Diagnosis**.

Disease is a condition in which there has been sufficient pathological changes in the structure (Anatomy) or function (Physiology) of the body as a whole or of any of its parts to interfere with vital functions. In other words, the conditions known as diseases are the result of, or are accompanied by, some unusual anatomical or physiological condition.

No one can treat any patient or any disease intelligently unless he thoroughly understands the fundamentals of Pathology and Symptomatology, and the student must have a thorough understanding of Anatomy and Physiology before he can understand Pathology or Symptomatology.

ANATOMY

The term Anatomy is derived from two Greek words, meaning dissection; but it has come to be applied to the science which treats of the structure of organized bodies.

The subject is divided into many smaller parts, each dealing with specific structures, as: Osteology, the anatomy of the bones; Arthrology, of the joints; Myology, of the muscles; Neurology, of the nerves; Angiology, of the vessels, usually blood and lymph; Splanchnology, of the internal viscera, etc. All of these and other subdivisions will be treated in due order.

Throughout the study of Anatomy, the student should have the Anatomical and Physiological Charts continually before him. Reference is not always made to the charts; but with the illustrations in the text matter, all the important facts about the anatomy of the human body are fully shown. If further explanation is needed at any time, it may be found in the complete manual accompanying the charts.

Much that is taught in the standard text books on Anatomy and in medical schools is of no real value to the Drugless Practitioner. In this course we will give you sufficient instruction in this branch to enable you to diagnose and treat all conditions that can be helped by drugless methods. No unnecessary details will be given.

When you have finished this course, if you desire for your personal satisfaction to know more about the Anatomy of some parts, you may secure additional information from any standard text book. We would advise you, however, not to do much additional reading while studying the part of the course devoted to Anatomy.

OSTEOLOGY

There are 200 bones in the adult human body, not counting the teeth, the six bones of the middle ear, the Wormian Bones in the skull, and the Sesamoid Bones in the ligaments. The bones not counted do not enter into the formation of the skeleton proper.

In Book 2 you will find the divisions of the skeleton together with the names of the bones that make up each division. In this lesson the more important of the bones of the skeleton will be described.

Lesson 5: Introduction

Bones are divided according to their shape into four different classes: long, short, flat and irregular. There are 90 long bones, 30 short bones, 40 flat bones and 40 irregular bones.

The Long Bones act as supports or levers. They all have a shaft, two large extremities, and the internal canal for the bone marrow. The long bones are the Humerus, Femur, Tibia, Fibula, Radius, Ulna and the bones of the hand, foot, fingers and toes.

The Flat Bones are the Scapula, Innominate, Rib and some of the skull bones.

The Short Bones are usually cuboidal in shape and are located where considerable strength, but limited motion, is needed. The bones of the wrist and of the ankle are short bones.

The Irregular Bones are the Vertebrae, Sacrum, Coccyx and some of the bones of the skull.

The principal portion of a bone is called the Body or Shaft. On the body or shaft are elevations, depressions and grooves. The large elevations or prominences may contain smaller elevations, depressions or openings. The elevations are for the attachment of muscles and ligaments or for formation of joints. The depressions may aid in the formation of joints or may be for the passage of vessels, nerves or ligaments. The openings are for the passage of vessels and nerves. (See Figure 6 of Plate I of Charts.)

The elevations are called Heads, Condyles, Trochanters, Tuberosities, Tubercles and Spines according to their size and shape. The depressions are known as Cavities, Fossae, Fissures, Grooves, and Notches. The openings are named, according to their situation and nature, Foramen, Notches, Canals or Sinuses.

69

Each of the above points will be described in greater detail when the individual bones are considered.

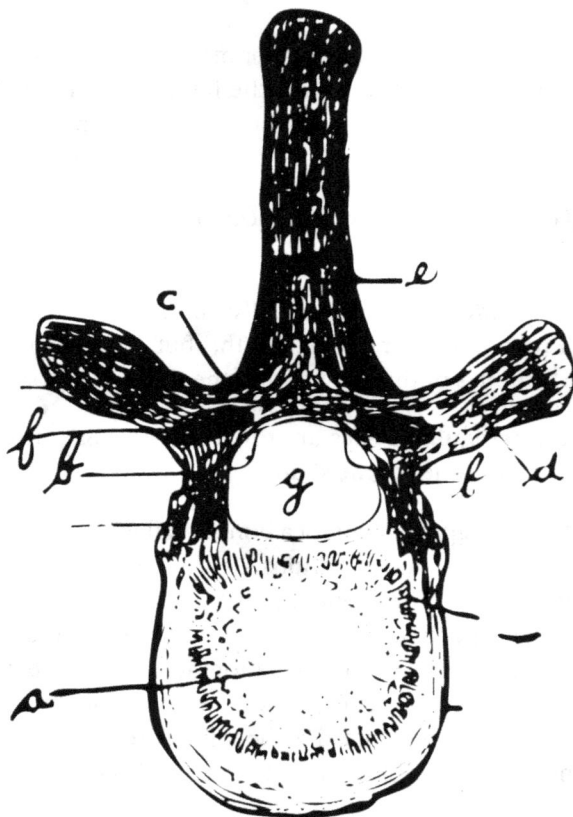

Figure 1. Top View. Third Dorsal Vertebra.

THE SPINE

The Vertebral Column consists of 33 segments or vertebrae. The lowermost of these in the adult, have become fused together. The vertebrae that have undergone the fusion, form one bone and are called fixed or false vertebrae; while those in which the fusion has not taken place are called movable or true vertebrae.

For descriptive purposes, the vertebral column is subdivided and named according to the region through which it passes. Thus the vertebrae of the neck are called **Cervical**; those of the upper back, **Dorsal** or **Thoracic**; those of the loins, **Lumbar**; those of the pelvis, **Sacral**; and those of the tail, **Coccygeal Vertebrae**.

There are 24 true vertebrae and nine false vertebrae. The true vertebrae are: The 7 Cervical, 12 Dorsal and 5 Lumbar. The false vertebrae are: 5 Sacral (fused to form the Sacrum) and 4 Coccygeal (fused to form the Coccyx). The vertebrae differ in size and shape according to their location, but all of them have many points of similarity.

One of the upper Dorsal Vertebra may be taken as the typical or average vertebra. This will be described first and then the differences between this vertebra and other vertebrae of the spine will be pointed out. See Figures 1 and 2.

A Typical Vertebra consists of a body, two pedicles, two laminae, two transverse processes, one spinous process and four articular processes.

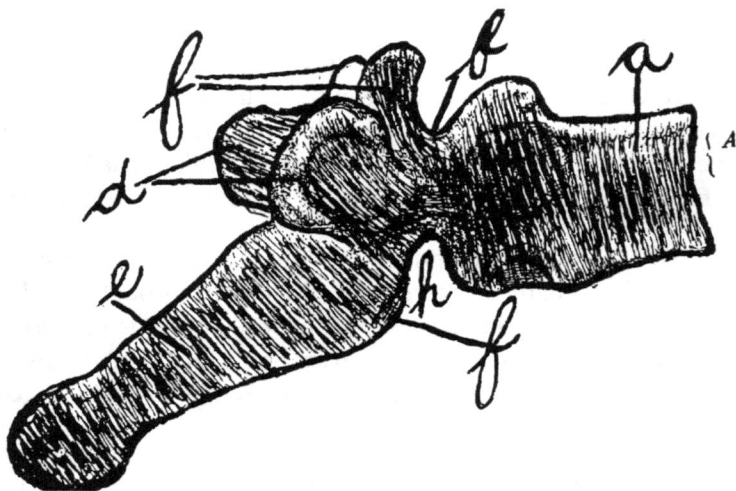

Figure 2. Side View. Third Dorsal Vertebra.

The Body forms the anterior part of the vertebrae and is composed of a circular mass of spongy bone. See (a) Figures 1 and 2.

The Pedicles are two cylindrical masses projecting backwards and outwards from the posterior surface of the body. See (b) Figures 1 and 2.

The Laminae are two flat plates of bone projecting backward and inward from the posterior extremities of the pedicles. The laminae are joined together behind. See (c) Figures 1 and 3.

Lesson 5: Introduction

The Vertebral Foramen is the nearly circular opening surrounded by the body, two pedicles and the two laminae. See (g) Fig. 1.

The Transverse Processes are two masses of bone projecting laterally and slightly backward from the junction of the pedicles and laminae. See (d) Figures 1 and 2.

The Spinous Processes project backward and slightly downward from the junction of the two laminae behind. See (e) Figures 1 and 2.

The Articular Processes project upward and downwards from the junction of the transverse processes, the laminae, and the pedicles. Two of the articular processes are on the upper side of the vertebra and two on the lower side. The upper articular processes of one vertebra articulate (form a joint) with the lower articular processes of the vertebra above. The articular surfaces of the uppermost processes face upward and backward and outward which allows the vertebrae to rotate around the Spinal Cord. See (f) Fig. 1 and 2.

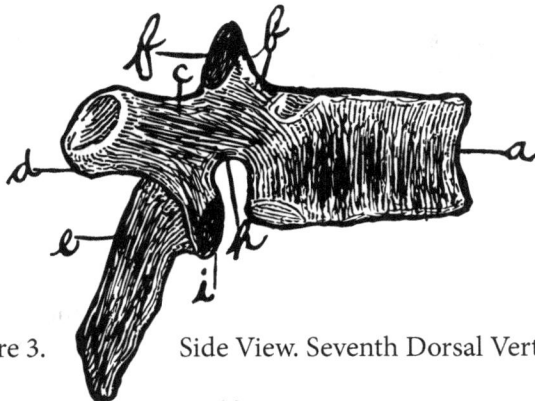

Figure 3.   Side View. Seventh Dorsal Vertebra .

73

Between the pedicles of the two adjacent vertebrae are two openings (one on either side of the Vertebral Foramen) called the Intervertebral Foramen. See (h) Fig. 2 and 3.

When the 26 vertebrae are joined together to form the spinal column, a spinal canal is formed by the vertebral foramen of the different vertebrae.

The spinal cord is contained within this vertebral canal. The spinal nerves pass out through the intervertebral foramina between the vertebrae.

The vertebrae are held together by ligaments which will be described in Lesson 8.

The Middle Dorsal Vertebrae differ from the upper dorsal (or typical) vertebrae in the following respects: The Spinous Process is longer and more slender and is bent more towards the feet, and the Transverse Processes are shorter. (See Figure 3.)

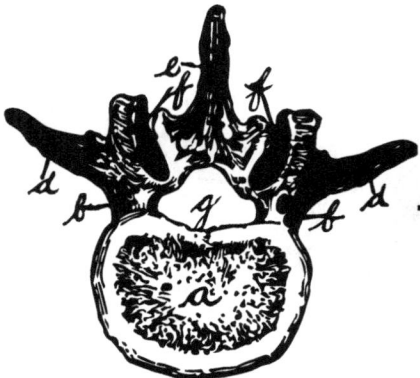

Figure 4. Top View Second
Lumbar Vertebra

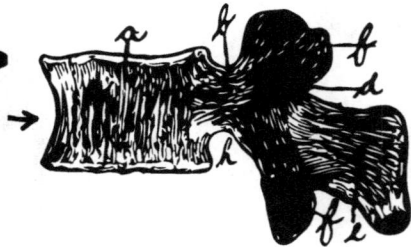

Figure 5. Side View. Second
Lumbar Vertebra

Lesson 5: Introduction

The **Lumbar Vertebrae** differ from the typical vertebra in that the Body is proportionately larger; the spinous process is shorter and thicker and the Transverse Processes are longer and more slender. The articular surfaces of the uppermost Articular Process face backward and inward, preventing the vertebrae from rotating around the spinal cord. (See Figures 4 and 5.)

The **Lower Dorsal Vertebrae** have some of the characteristics of the Middle Dorsal and some of the Lumbar Vertebrae. For this reason they are called Transitional Vertebrae.

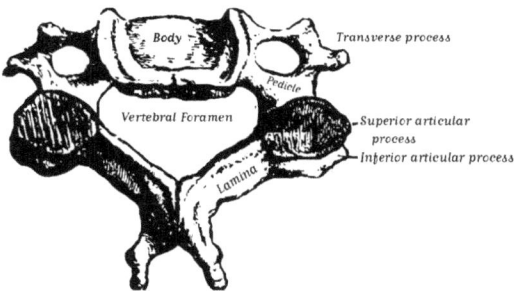

Figure 6.
Fourth Cervical Vertebra

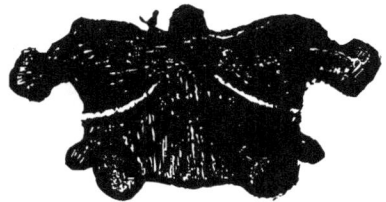

Figure 7.
Front View of Atlas and Axis

The **Cervical Vertebrae** differ much in appearance from the typical vertebra. The Transverse Processes project from the body of the vertebra instead of from the junction of the pedicles and laminae. The Transverse Processes are pierced by an opening or foramen through which passes the vertebral artery. The Spinous Processes are short and end in two projections. The Articular Processes are proportionately much larger. The articular surfaces of these processes face upward, backward and slightly outward. (See Figure 6.)

75

On either side of the Upper Surface of the body of the vertebrae there is a Flange projecting upward. The lower surface of the body of the upper vertebrae fits in between these two flanges. This prevents the vertebrae from rotating around the spinal canal as they do in the dorsal region.

The Second Cervical or Axis has a tooth-like projection on the upper surface of its body. This is called the Odontoid Process and it forms a pivot around which the First Cervical Vertebra turns when the head is turned from side to side. The Spinous Process of the second cervical is much larger than that of the third which it very nearly covers. (See Figure 7.)

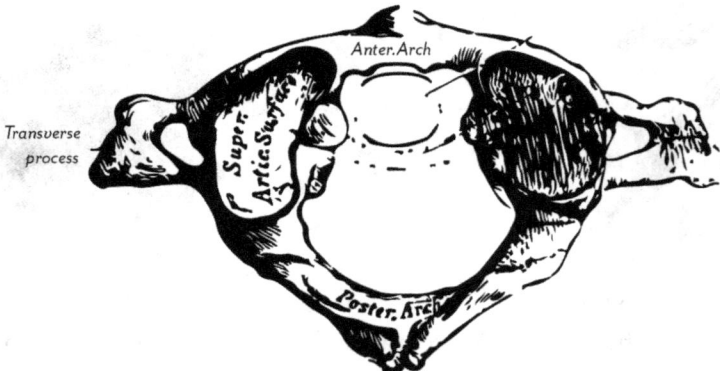

Figure 8. The Atlas

The **First Cervical or Atlas** has very little resemblance to the other cervicals or to the typical vertebra. It has no body and no spinous process. It may be described as a Bony Ring, which is thicker on either side than it is in front or behind, and having a long Transverse Process projecting laterally from either side of these Lateral Masses. The front part of the ring is called the Anterior Arch and the posterior portion of the ring is called the Posterior Arch. The posterior surface of the anterior arch articulates with the anterior surface of the odontoid process of the axis. The odontoid process being held in that position by a ligament passing behind it and across the vertebral foramen of the atlas. (See Figure 8 on Plate II of the Anatomical Charts.)

The Lower Articular Processes of the atlas resemble those of the cervical vertebrae. The articular surfaces of the Upper Articular Processes are concave and face inward and upward. They articulate with the articular processes (Condyles) of the lowermost bone of the skull (the Occiput).

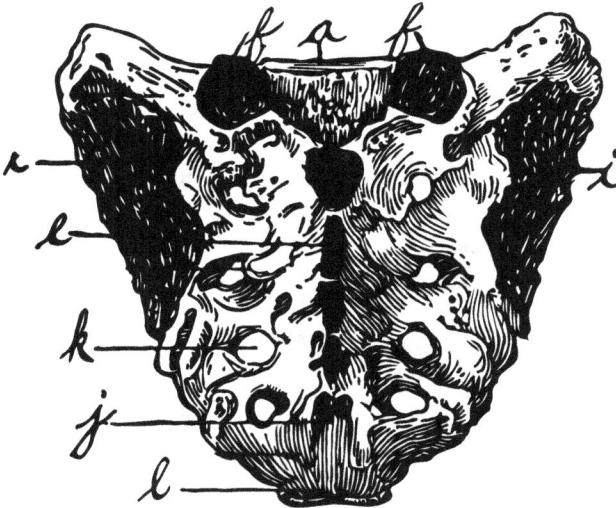

Figure 9. The Sacrum as seen from Behind

FALSE VERTEBRAE

The Sacrum is a wedge-shaped bone formed by the fusion of the Five Sacral Vertebrae. It is situated between the two innominate bones and it supports the true or movable vertebrae above it. It may also be considered as part of the Pelvis of which it forms the posterior wall. (See Figure 9.)

The Base or upper part of the sacrum is larger than the lower part (or Apex) (a). Its upper surface resembles the under surface of the 5th Lumbar Vertebrae with which it articulates in the same way that the lumbar vertebrae articulate with each other. It has Five Spinous Processes projecting from its posterior surface (e). Its Laminae resembles those of the vertebrae except for the openings between them for the posterior divisions of the Spinal Nerves (k).

The Anterior Surface is concave and smooth except for the openings for the Sacral Nerves. On either side of the Sacrum is a large, rough, irregular surface which articulates with the inner surfaces of the two innominates which support the sacrum. (See (i) of Figure 9 and Plate I of the Chart.) The Vertebral Canal passes down through the center of the Sacrum.

The **Coccyx** is another wedge-shaped bone formed by the fusion of the Four Coccygeal Vertebrae. Its Base articulates with the apex of the sacrum. (See Figure 14, Lesson 6.) The Fifth Sacral Nerve passes out between the Coccyx and the Sacrum.

Lesson 5: Introduction

QUESTIONS—LESSON 5

1.   What is Anatomy and why is it necessary to have a knowledge of this subject?

2.   Give the Divisions of the Skeleton and the Number of Bones in each division.

3.   Name the Principle Points used in the description of Bones.

4.   Name the Divisions of the Spinal Column and give the Number of Vertebrae in each division.

5.   Describe the Parts of the Typical Vertebra except the Processes.

6.   Name and describe the Processes on the Typical Vertebra.

7.   How do the Lumbar Vertebrae differ from the Upper Dorsal or Typical Vertebra?

8.   How do the Cervical Vertebrae differ from the Middle Dorsal Vertebrae?

9.   Briefly describe the Atlas.

10. Briefly describe the Sacrum.

EXTENSION COURSE
IN CHIROPRACTIC
AMERICAN UNIVERSITY
CHICAGO, Ill., U.S.A.

_____

LESSON 6

_____

THE VERTEBRATE ON THE WHOLE

When all of the vertebrae are articulated together they form the spine or Spinal Column. (See Figures 10 and 11.) In addition to the Ligaments which hold the vertebrae together there is a circular disk of soft spongy material between the bodies of the adjacent vertebrae. These cushions are called the Intervertebral Disks.

In the Lumbar and Cervical Regions these disks are thicker in front than they are behind producing curves with their concave side facing backward. In the Dorsal Region these disks are thicker behind than before, producing a curve with its convex side directed backward. The shape of the vertebrae and manner in which they are joined together makes the spinal column a very strong yet a very flexible structure. (See Figure 6 on Plate I of the Chart.)

All regions of the spine may be bent forward or backward, the spinous process separating when it is Flexed (bent forward)

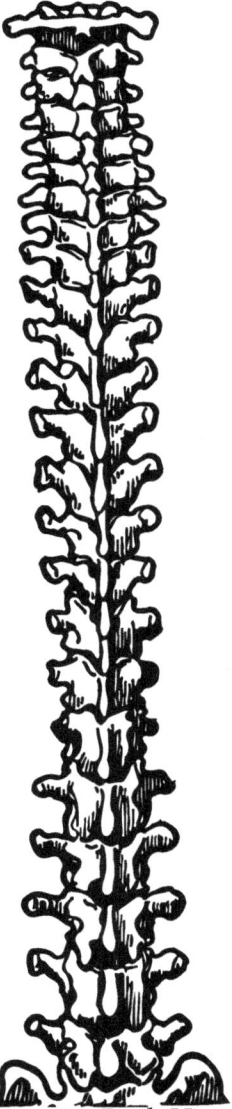

Figure 10. Back View.
Spinal Column

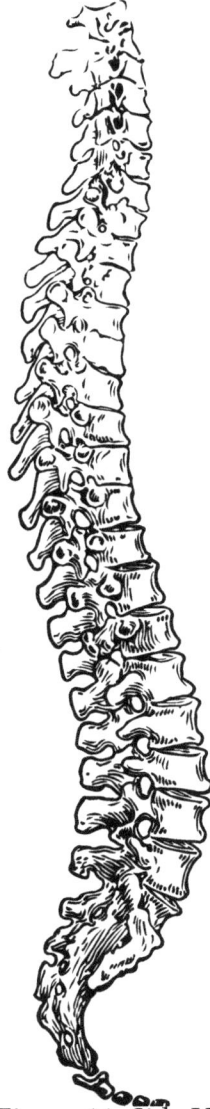

Figure 11. Side View.
Spinal Column

and approaching one another when the spine is Extended (bent backward).

There is Rotation in all regions of the spine, but it is greatest in the cervical region and diminishes from above downward. Owing to the differences in the shapes of the articular processes, the centers of rotation of the vertebrae are not the same in all regions of the spine.

When the spine is bent sideways the vertebrae rotates in addition to a slight amount of flexion or extension. The movements of the individual vertebra will be considered in greater detail in a later lesson when subluxations are discussed.

The Vertebral (or Neural) Canal is the largest in the cervical region and smallest in the dorsal region. In the cervical and lumbar regions it is triangular in shape, while it is nearly circular in the dorsal region.

The Intervertebral Foramina increases in size from above downward, being the largest in the lumbar region.

The Length of the Spinal Column varies with the height of the individual and with the relative length of his trunk. It averages from 24 to 28 inches in the adult.

The Function of the Spinal Column is to support the chest and head and to allow movement between them and the pelvis as well as to protect the spinal cord. For spinal diagnosis and treatment the movements of the spine must be thoroughly understood. They will be considered in greater detail in subsequent lessons. The ligaments and muscles of the spine will be considered in Lessons 8 and 9.

Lesson 6: Vertebrae

THE SKULL

The Skull consists of 22 bones and it is divided for description into the Cranium and the Face. (See Figures 12 and 13 and Plate I of the Anatomical Charts.)

THE CRANIUM

The cranium is the upper-posterior portion of the skull and is composed of the following eight bones:

The Frontal Bone is the flat, curved bone that forms the front part of the cranium (forehead). It has two curved horizontal plates which form the upper part of the orbits which contain the eyes. (See Figure 13 and the Chart.)

The Parietal Bones are quadrilateral, curved plates forming the upper and lateral portions of the cranium (between the frontal and the occipital bones). There is one on either side of the skull above and behind the ears. (Figure 13 and the Chart.)

The Occipital Bone is the flat, trapezoidal, curved plate forming the posterior-inferior portion of the skull. It separates the Cranial Cavity from the neck and the pharynx. It has a large rounded opening called the Foramen Magnum for the passage of the spinal cord. On either side of this opening is a rounded projection (Condyle) which articulates with one of the superior articular processes of the atlas. (Figures 12 and 13.)

The Temporal Bone is an irregular bone containing the Organs of Hearing and Equilibrium and forming the inferior lateral portion of the cranium (between occipital, parietal and sphenoid bones). There is one on either side surrounding the external ear. The Mastoid Process is a large pointed prominence

83

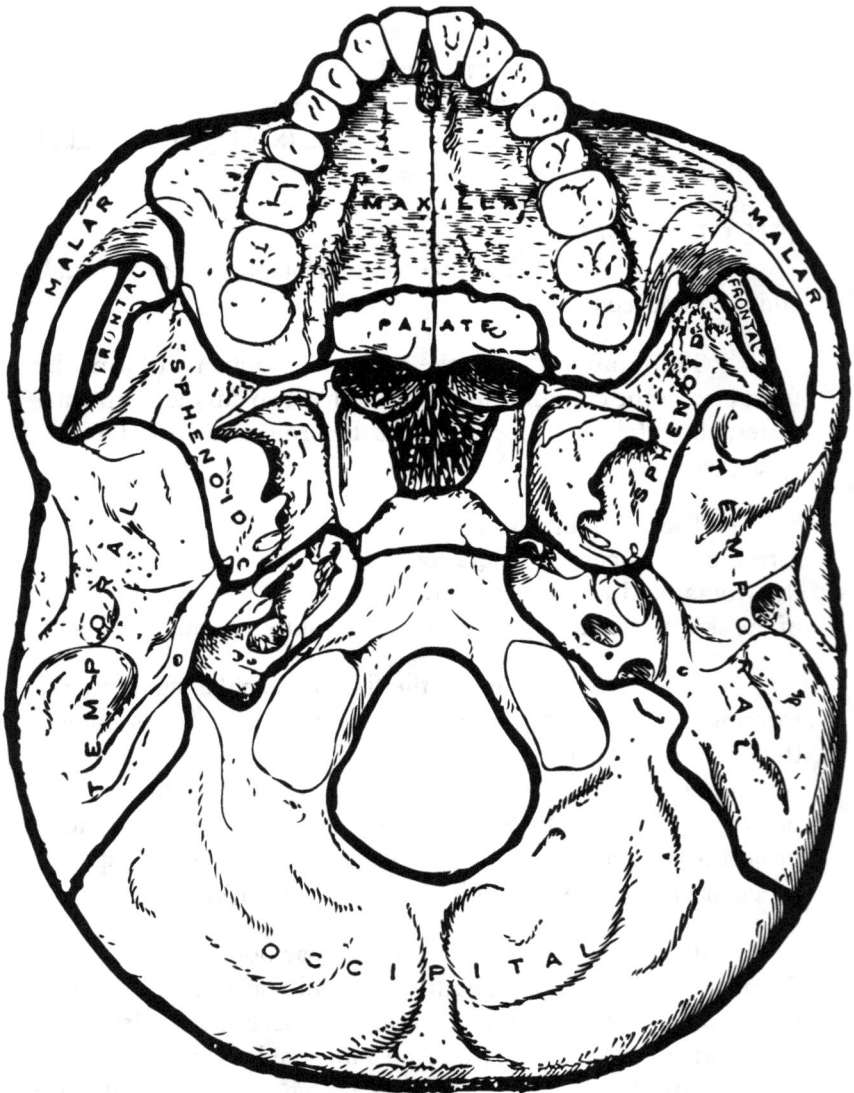

Figure 12. The Skull. The Bases as seen from Below.

projecting downward from behind the ear. The Glenoid Cavity is a depression in the outer surface of the bone in front of the ear for the reception of the condyle of the mandible. (Figures 12 and 13.)

The Sphenoid Bone is a bat-shaped bone forming the anterior portion of the inferior surface of the Cranium (between the occipital, parietal and frontal bones). It, together with the ethmoid, separates the cranial cavity from the nasal cavity. (Figures 12 and 13.)

The Ethmoid is an irregular bone lying between the orbital plates of the frontal bone and in front of the sphenoid bone. It has two Lateral Masses which project downward and form part of the lateral walls of the nasal cavities. It also has a Vertical Plate extending downward between the two lateral masses and forming the anterior- superior portion of the nasal septum. (Figure 12.)

THE FACE

The Face is the anterior-inferior portion of the skull and consists of the following 14 bones: (See Figures 12 and 13 and the Chart.)

The Maxillary Bones are two large, hollow, cuboidal bones that form the greater part of the anterior and lateral portion of the face (upper jaw). Their Lower Surfaces form the roof of the mouth; their Inner Surfaces assist in forming the lateral walls of the nasal cavities; their Upper Surfaces form the floors of the orbits. (Figures 12, 13 and Chart.)

The Mandible is a bent-horseshoe-shaped bone forming the lower jaw. The vertical posterior portion is called the Ramus. The Angle is a projection behind the junction of the ramus and the Body of the Mandible. The rounded knobs projecting from the posterior part of the upper extremity of the ramus are called Condyles. They articulate with the glenoid cavities of the temporal bones. (Figure 13.)

The **Malar Bones** are two irregular bones forming the upper, outer portion of the face (cheek), and the inferior, outer portion of the orbits. The Zygoma is the arch formed on the side of the head behind the orbit by processes connecting the malar and the temporal bones. (Figure 1213.)

The **Palate Bones** are two L-shaped bones in the outer and lower walls of the nasal cavities and in the roof of the mouth (between the maxillary bones). (Figures 12 and 13.)

The **Vomer** is a thin, flat plate forming the posterior, inferior portion of the nasal septum (behind and below the vertical plate of the ethmoid). (Figure 13.)

The **Lachrymal Bones** are two small plates in the anterior-inner walls of the orbits. (Chart.)

The **Nasal Bones** are two small, flat bones forming the bridge of the nose. (Figure 13.)

The **Turbinate Bones** are two thin, curled plates on the inside of the outer walls of the nasal cavity. (Chart.)

The **Orbits** are the two pyramidal cavities in the upper, anterior and outer portion of the face. They contain the organs of vision. Each orbit is formed principally by the frontal, sphenoid, malar and maxillary bones; small portions of the lachrymal, palate

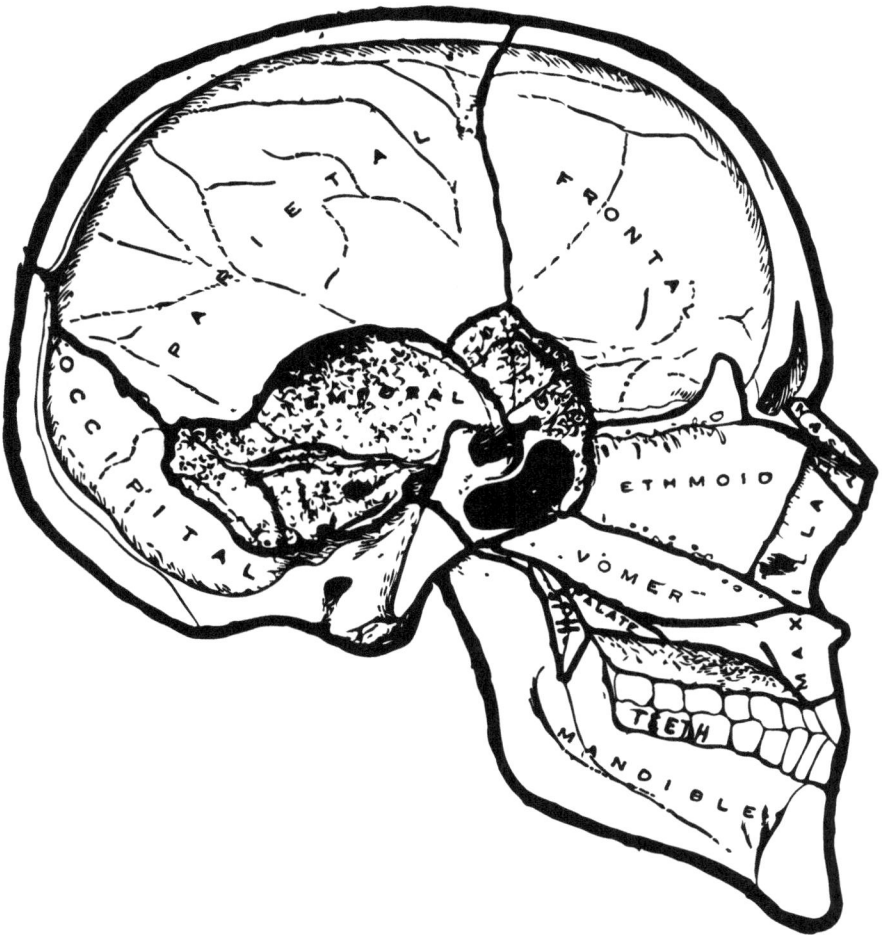

Figure 13. The Skull. Side View from the Inside

and ethmoid bones assist in forming the inner wall. (See Plate I of Charts.)

The Nasal Cavities are the two large cavities in the center of the face, above the mouth, below the base of the cranium and between the nose and the throat. The two cavities are separated by a vertical plate called the Septum, which is formed by the vomer and the vertical plate of the ethmoid, assisted by a flat plate of cartilage (anterior portion). The Lateral Walls are formed by the inner walls of the maxillary bones and the lateral masses of ethmoid, and the vertical portion of the palate bones. (Figure 13 and Chart.)

Two Turbinate Processes and the Turbinate Bone form the Nasal Turbinates (three on each lateral wall). The Roof of the nasal cavities is formed by the ethmoid and sphenoid bone; the Floor is formed by the horizontal plates of the maxillary and palate bones. (Figure 13.)

THE PELVIS
The Pelvis is formed by the articulation of the two innominate bones with the sacrum behind, and their union with each other at the joint called Symphysis Pubis, in front. It is divided into false pelvis, comprising the upper and expanded portion— and the true pelvis, below the Ileo-pectineal line. The male pelvis is narrower and stronger than the female. (See Chart.)

The False Pelvis supports the abdominal contents; while the True Pelvis contains the pelvic viscera; and in the female forms the bony canal through which, at full term, the foetus is expelled. (See Figure 14.)

The Innominates are the largest of the flat bones and consist of three parts—the Ilium, the Ischium, and the Pubis. These three bones are fused together in the process of growth to form one large bone. At the junction of the Ilium, the Ischium and the Pubis, a deep cup-shaped cavity is located called the Acetabulum or Cotyloid Cavity. The Ilium forms 2/5, the Ischium 2/5, and the

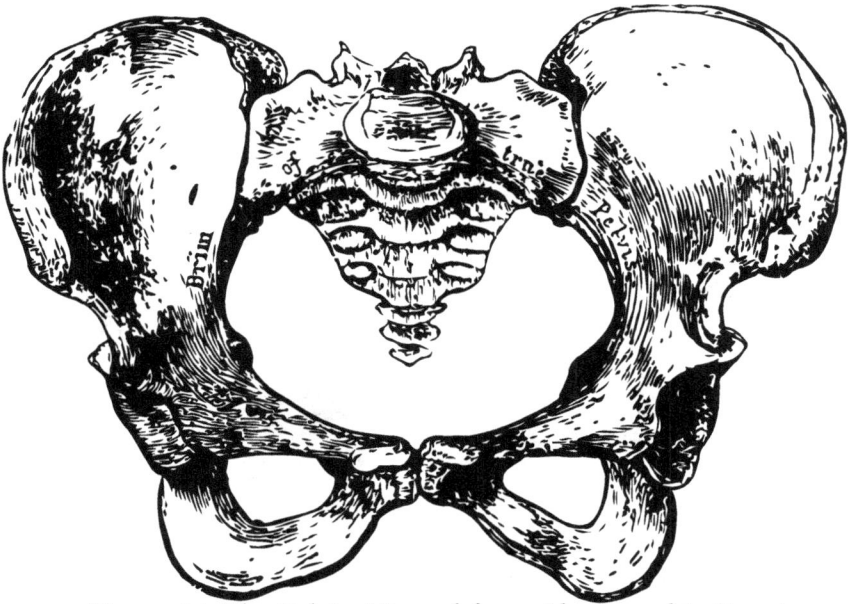

Figure 14. The Pelvis. Viewed from Above and in Front
Pubis 1/5 of this cavity which receives the head of the femur. (See Figures 15 and 16.)

Between the Ischium and the Pubis is a large foramen called the Obturator Foramen. In the male, it is large and oval; in the female, it is small and triangular. The foramen is entirely closed by the Obturator Membrane except where the nerves and blood vessels pass through it.

The Ilium is the superior part of the Innominate bone, and together with its fellow forms the false pelvis. The Ilium has two Surfaces—External (or lateral) and Internal (or medial)—and two Borders, Anterior and Posterior. The medial surface is smooth and concave and extends from the Crest of the Ilium to the ileopectineal line, and from the anterior to the posterior border. The

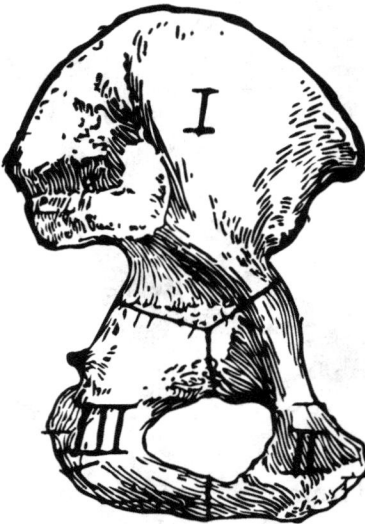 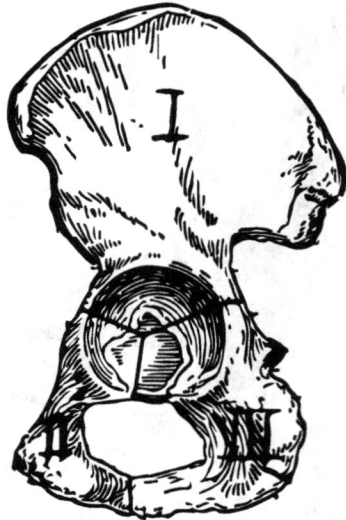

Figure 15. Figure 16.
Inner Surface, Left Innominate Outer Surface, Left Innominate

posterior 1/3 of the medial surface is rough for articulation with the sacrum; the anterior 2/3 of the medial surface is called the Iliac Fossa.

Lesson 6: Vertebrae

The upper edge of the Ilium is called the Crest. It ends in front at a point or projection called the Anterior Superior Spine; below this spine is another one less prominent called the Anterior Inferior Spine of the Ilium. Posteriorly the crest terminates in the Posterior Superior Spine, below which is also a Posterior Inferior Spine. Below the posterior inferior spine is the Great Sacro-Sciatic Notch bounded below by the Spine of the Ischium. This notch is closed behind by the sciatic ligaments, and through it pass the nerves and blood vessels to the back of the thigh and hip.

The Ischium forms the lower and posterior part of the Innominate bone, and has: a Body which is the most superior portion of the ischium and forms the inferior 2/5 of the Acetabulum; a spine, called the Spine of the Ischium, below which is the Lesser Sciatic Notch, which transmits several nerves, ligaments, and muscles; a Tuberosity which is the lowest and most prominent part of the Ischium, and the Ascending Ramus which bounds the obturator foramen inferiorly and joins with the descending ramus of the pubis.

The Pubis forms the anterior part of the true pelvis. It is by means of the union of this bone with its fellow of the opposite side that the pelvic girdle (pelvis) is completed in front. The pubis consists of a Superior (or Ascending) Ramus and an Inferior (or Descending) Ramus. The broad part of the bone formed by the fusion of the two rami is called the Body, which, with its fellow, forms the Symphysis Pubis; the body of the pubis is quadrilateral in shape.

The Spine of the Pubis is the most anterior part and gives attachment to the very important ligament called Poupart's Ligament, which extends from it to the anterior superior spine

91

of the ilium. Posteriorly from the spine of the pubis runs the Ileopectineal Line, which forms the dividing line between the true and the false pelvis.

The Descending Ramus of the pubis passes downwards and backwards from the lower part of the body of the pubis and unites with the ascending ramus of the ischium and in that way encloses the Obturator Foramen.

The Sacrum and Coccyx form the posterior wall of the pelvis and may be considered as part of the pelvis or as the lowermost portion of the spine. They have been described in Lesson 5. (See Chart.)

The Two Innominates may also be considered as a part of the lower extremities corresponding to the clavicle and scapula which form the shoulder girdle. (See Chart.)

QUESTIONS—LESSON 6

1. What is the Spinal Column and How is it Formed?

2. Describe the Intervertebral Disk.

3. What Movements are possible between the Vertebrae?

4. Describe the Vertebral Canal and the Intervertebral Foramen.

5. What is the Skull and what are the Divisions of the Skull? 6. How many Bones in each Division?

7. Describe the Occipital Bone.

8. Describe the Temporal Bone.

9. Describe the Maxillary Bone.

10. Describe the Orbits.

11. Describe the Nasal Cavities.

EXTENSION COURSE
IN CHIROPRACTIC
AMERICAN UNIVERSITY
CHICAGO, Ill., U.S.A.

LESSON 7

THE THORAX

The chest (or Thorax) is the bony cage of the upper trunk formed by the 24 Ribs, Sternum, and the Bodies of the 12 Dorsal Vertebrae. The 12 dorsal vertebrae have been described in Lesson 5. The remaining bones of the Thorax will be described below. (See Plate I of the Anatomy Charts.)

The Sternum is the flat bone to which the anterior extremities of the ribs are attached. It extends from the base of the neck to the upper boundary of the abdomen in the middle line of the front part of the body. It is commonly known as the breastbone. This bone is composed of three parts, which have the following names from above downward: Manubrium, Gladiolus, and Ensiform. The upper extremity of the Sternum is connected to the outer angle of the scapula by the clavicle.

The Ribs are narrow, flat, curved bones forming the lateral walls of the thorax as well as the greater portion of the posterior and anterior walls. They are 24 in number (12 on each side).

94

Lesson 7: Thorax and Extremities

The Anterior Extremities of the ribs are composed of cartilages which are known as Costal Cartilages. The first seven ribs articulate with the sternum by means of their cartilages and are called True Ribs; the lower five do not connect directly with the sternum and are called False Ribs.

The 8th, 9th and 10th ribs are connected through their cartilages with the 7th Costal Cartilage, which is connected to the sternum. The 11th and 12th ribs are free at their anterior extremities, and for this reason are called Floating Ribs. The 1st, 2nd, 11th and 12th ribs differ slightly in their shape from the other ribs and consequently are called Peculiar Ribs; all of the other ribs are called Typical Ribs.

A Typical Rib consists of a Shaft, Head, Neck and Tuberosity. (See Figure 18.)

The body or a greater portion of the rib is called the Shaft (a—Figure 18). It resembles in appearance a widened barrel hoop except that it is curved in two directions. The Shaft makes a rather sharp bend at the point where the lateral chest wall joins the posterior wall; this bend is called the Angle of the Rib (b). The shafts of the upper and lower ribs are shorter than those of the middle ribs.

The rib ends posteriorly in a rounded knob which is called the Head (c). It articulates with the bodies of two adjacent vertebrae. Between the head and the shaft is a constricted portion called the Neck (d). On the posterior portion of the shaft near the neck is an irregular projection which is known as the Tuberosity (e). It articulates with the anterior surface of the transverse process of the vertebrae.

95

The lower border of the shaft contains a groove (Costal Groove) for the intercostal nerves and arteries. The anterior extremity has an oval depression into which fits the articular costal cartilage.

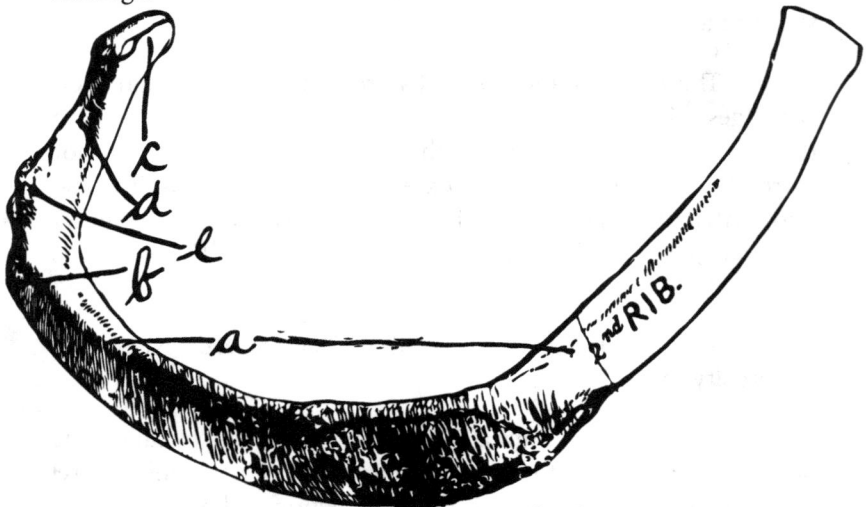

Figure 18. The Second Rib.
Viewed from Above

The Costal Cartilages are bands of hyaline cartilage shaped very much like the shaft of the ribs. The costal cartilages increase in length from above downward.

The First Rib is shorter and broader than the typical ribs; it has no angle and its curves are not so great as those of the typical ribs.

The Second Rib resembles the first rib somewhat, but is more nearly like the typical ribs.

The 11th and 12th Ribs are very short and have no neck and no tuberosity. The 12th rib has no angle or groove.

The Thorax as a Whole is conical in shape. The Apex is upward and the Base forms the upper wall of the abdominal cavity. The apex is open for the passage of the trachea, esophagus and the large vessels and nerves passing between the head and the trunk. The lower opening of the thorax is closed by a large umbrella-like muscle called the Diaphragm.

The changes in the shape of the Thorax that take place in respiration are described in Lesson 3.

THE UPPER EXTREMITIES

Each upper extremity is composed of one Arm, two Forearm, eight Wrist and nineteen Hand bones, in addition to the Clavicle and the Scapula which form the Shoulder Girdle.

The Scapula (shoulder blade) is a triangular, flat bone situated posteriorly and laterally to the upper thorax. It does not articulate directly with any of the bones of the thorax. (See Figure 19.)

Its Anterior (under) Surface is smooth and concave. Extending across the superior-posterior portion is a large ridge called the Spine of the Scapula (a). This Spine terminates in a large, bent projection which extends behind and above the shoulder joint and is called the Acromion Process (b). The inferior end of the vertebral border of the scapula is called the Angle (c).

At the junction of the superior and outer border is the Glenoid Cavity (d) for the head of the humerus. The clavicle

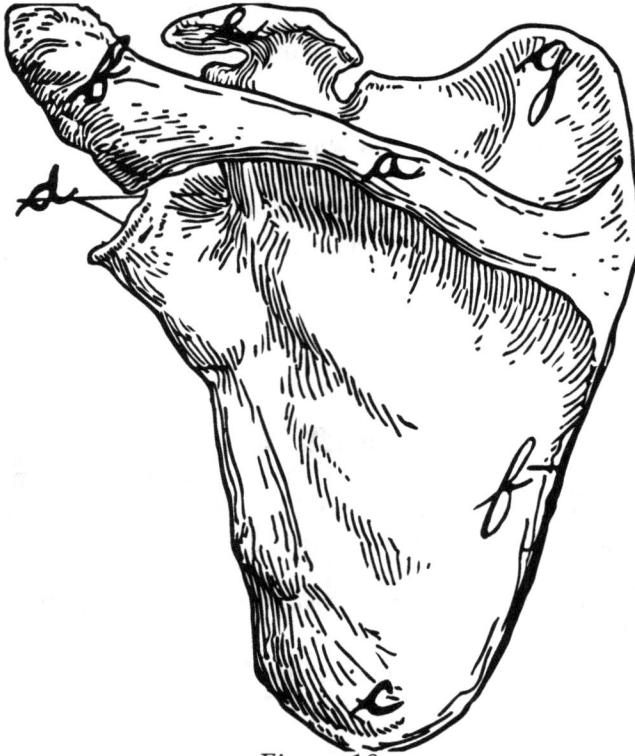

Figure 19.
Posterior View of Left Scapula

articulates with the anterior superior surface of the acromion process. Below the clavicle is the Coracoid Process (e) which extends outward above and in front of the glenoid cavity.

The Clavicle is a long curved bone connecting the upper end of the sternum with the outer upper part of the scapula (Acromion Process). It is placed horizontally across the upper chest and is shaped like the letter f. (See Figure 20 and Plate I of Charts.)

The Humerus is the long, cylindrical bone of the upper arm. (See Plate I.) Its body or principle portion is called the Shaft. On the inner side of its upper extremity is a large rounded mass called the Head, which articulates with the glenoid cavity of the scapula. Projecting upward and outward from just below the head is the Greater Tuberosity. Projecting forward from below the head is the Lesser Tuberosity.

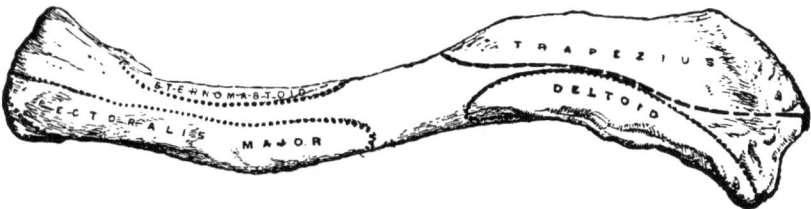

Figure 20. Top View of Left Clavicle

At the Lower Extremity are two large, rounded prominences called the Condyles. Between these Condyles is a large, smooth surface called the Trochlear Surface for the reception of the upper extremities of the ulna and the radius.

The Ulna is the largest bone in the forearm and is situated at the inner side. (See Plate I.) The Upper Extremity contains a large curved cavity called the Greater Sigmoid Cavity which articulates with the trochlear surface of the humerus. The Olecranon Process projects upward from the posterior portion of the upper extremity and assists in forming the sigmoid cavity.

Projecting forward from the lower part of the sigmoid cavity is the Coronoid Process. The lower extremity is called the Head, which articulates with the inner surface of the lower extremity of the radius. It does not articulate directly with the bones of the wrist; a triangular disk of cartilage lies between them.

The Radius is the small prismatic bone of the forearm (outside). (See Plate I.) Its upper extremity is smooth and cup-shaped and is called the Head. It articulates with the outer condyle of the humerus and with the outer surface of the ulna. Projecting inward from below the head is the Bicipital Tuberosity. The Lower Extremity presents a large, quadrilateral, smooth surface for the reception of the bones of the wrist. On the outer edge of the lower surface is the Styloid Process which projects outward and downward.

The Hand is composed of 27 bones divided into three groups: the Carpal (wrist); the Metacarpal (palm), and the Phalanges (fingers). (See Plate I.)

The Carpal Bones are arranged in two rows; the one nearest the forearm is called the Proximal Row, the one nearest the hand is called the Distal Row. In the Proximal Row are: Scaphoid, Semilunar, Cuneiform and Pisiform, and in Distal Row are: Trapezium, Trapezoid, Os Magnum and Unciform. All carpal bones are small, cuboidal-shaped, and all have six surfaces with the exception of the pisiform, which has five.

The Metacarpal Bones are five in number and form the connection between the wrist and the fingers. They are long bones. They are named, 1st, 2nd, 3rd, 4th and 5th Metacarpal, the 1st, being on the thumb side of the hand and the 5th on the little finger side.

The Phalanges are fourteen in number, three in each of the four fingers and two in the thumb. They are long bones with shaft, base and head.

THE LOWER EXTREMITY

Each lower extremity contains one Thigh, two Leg, seven Ankle, nineteen Foot and one Knee bones in addition to the two innominates which also aid in forming the pelvis.

The Femur is the long cylindrical bone of the thigh, being the largest bone of the skeleton. (See Plate I.) The upper extremity is spherical and is called the Head. Between the Head and the Shaft of the bone is a constriction called the Neck. Projecting upward and outward from the point where the Neck joins the shaft is a large quadrilateral prominence called the Greater Trochanter. Projecting from the inner side of the shaft just below the neck is a small rounded prominence called the Lesser Trochanter.

The lower extremity of the shaft terminates in two rounded projections called Condyles. Their lower surfaces and the space between them is smooth for the articulation of the upper extremity of the tibia and the patella.

The Tibia is the large prismatic bone in the inner part of the leg. (Plate I.) On its upper extremity are two large cup-shaped processes called the Tuberosities for the reception of the condyles of the femur.

The Inferior Surface of its Lower Extremity is flat and smooth for the reception of the astragulas. Projecting downward from the inner edge of this lower surface is the pointed process called the Internal Maleolus (ankle bone).

The Fibula is a slender bone external to the tibia. (Plate I.) The upper extremity is called the Head. It articulates with the lower and outer surface of the external tuberosity of the tibia.

Its lower extremity is called the External Maleolus (outer ankle bone). The internal surface of the shaft just above the maleolus articulates with the external surface of the lower extremity of the tibia. The internal surface of the maleolus articulates with the astragulas of the ankle bone.

The Foot is composed of 26 bones, one less than in the hand, divided into the 7 Tarsals, 5 Metatarsals, and the 14 Phalanges.

The Tarsals are short bones, arranged in two rows side by side; in the internal row are five bones: Astragulas; Scaphoid; External, Middle, and Internal Cuneiform; in the external, are two: Os Calcis and Cuboid.

The Metatarsals are five long bones. Their heads articulate with the first row of phalanges; their bases articulate with the tarsal bones and with each other.

The Phalanges are long bones, fourteen in number, the great toe having two and the other four toes three each. The anterior extremities of the distal phalanges broaden for the support of the nails.

QUESTIONS—LESSON 7

1. What is the Thorax and of What Bones is it Composed?

2. Describe the Typical Rib.

3. Describe the Sternum.

4. Briefly describe the Shoulder Girdle.

5. Briefly describe the Humerus.

6. Name and briefly describe the Bones of the Forearm.

7. Briefly describe the Femur.

8. Briefly describe the Tibia.

10. Briefly describe the Fibula.

11. How does the Hand differ from the Foot in Number, Shape and Arrangement of the Bones?

EXTENSION COURSE IN CHIROPRACTIC AMERICAN UNIVERSITY CHICAGO, Ill., U.S.A.

LESSON 8

ARTHROLOGY

When two bones are joined together the connection is called an articulation or joint. Articulations are divided into three general classes: Synarthroses, Amphiarthroses and Diarthroses.

A **Synarthrosis** is an immovable joint such as those between the bones of the Cranium.

An **Amphiarthrosis** is a joint in which there is a limited amount of movement as in the joints between the bodies of the vertebrae and between the innominates and sacrum.

An **Amphiarthrosis** is a joint in which there is a limited amount as in the joints between the bodies of the vertebrae and between the innominates and sacrum.

A **Diarthrosis** is a freely moveable joint. These joints are subdivided, according to the kind of movement they have, into six classes.

104

Those having a hinge movement like the knee and elbow are called Ginglymus joints. Those having a gliding movement as the joints between the bones of the wrist and ankle are called Arthrodial joints. Ball-and-socket joints like the hip and shoulder are known as Enarthrodial.

Joints composed of an ovoid head fitting into an elliptical cavity are called Condyloid (like the joint between the radius and the carpal bones). When each of the articular surfaces are both concave and convex, as the articulation between the 1st phalanx of the thumb, and the trapezium, it is called a Reciprocal or Saddle Joint.

If one bone turns around another as around a pivot, the joint is called Trochoid. The articulation between the atlas and the axis as well as those between the radius and the ulna are Trochoid.

Four varieties of movement are possible in joints, but all varieties are possible only in the enarthrodial joints.

Gliding movement takes place in the Arthrodial, Enarthrodial, Condyloid and Reciprocal Joints. The Ginglymus, Condyloid, Reciprocal and Enarthrodial have an angular movement. Rotation is possible only in Trochoid and Enarthrodial joints. Circumduction takes place in Reciprocal, Condyloid and Enarthrodial joints.

All true joints contain the following structures: Articular Surfaces of the Bones, Hyaline Cartilage, Ligaments, and Synovial Membrane. Some joints contain in addition to the above, masses of Fibrous Cartilage. The Synarthroses are not usually considered as true joints; the adjacent surfaces of the bones are firmly fixed together. (Figures 4 and 5 of Plate II of the Charts show the structure of typical joints.)

The Articular Surfaces of the bone (of true joints) are smooth and the bone tissue is more dense and compact than the other portions of the bone.

The Hyaline Cartilage is a layer of dense, firm cartilage covering the articular surfaces of the bones.

Ligaments are bands of white fibrous tissue which serve to hold the bones together and to prevent excessive movement in the joints.

Synovial Membrane is a thin serous membrane lining the ligaments and covering the articular cartilages. It secretes a colorless sticky fluid which lubricates the surfaces of the joints.

Practically all joints have a capsular ligament which surrounds and encloses the joint. In many joints the other ligaments are merely a part of this capsular ligament, the fibrous tissue being thicker in certain regions. In some joints the other ligaments are separate and distinct bands named according to their positions (anterior, posterior, internal, external, intertransverse, etc.), and according to the bones or process which they connect (Sacro-Iliac, Sterno-Clavicular and Coraco-Humoral, etc.).

THE ARTICULATIONS OF THE SPINE

Between the Bodies of the Vertebrae are Amphiarthrodial Joints. There is a ligament in front and another one behind the bodies as well as a spongy disk of white fibrous cartilage between them which is called the Intervertebral Cartilage or Disk. (See Figures 21 and 22.)22.)

Between the Articular Processes of the Vertebrae are Arthrodial Joints. In addition to the Capsular Ligaments there are ligaments between the Transverse Processes, between the Spinous Processes and over the tips of the Spinous Processes as well as a yellow elastic ligament between the Laminae. (See Figures 21 and 22 and Plate II.)

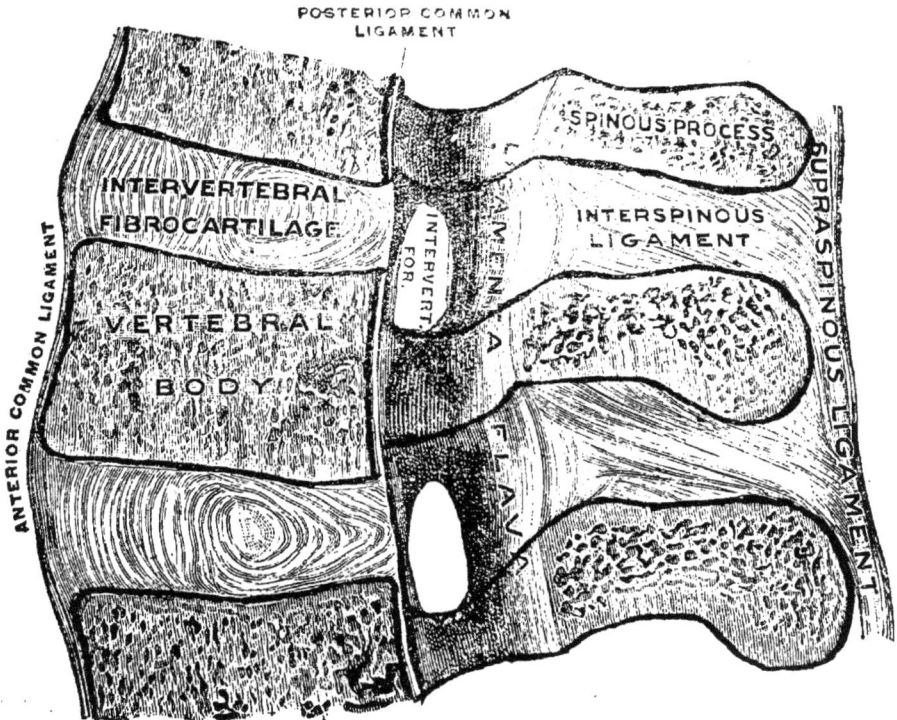

Figure 21. Inside Lateral View of Lumbar Ligaments.

The Atlantal-Axal Joint is a Pivot Joint (Trochoid) between the Odontoid Process of the Axis and the Anterior Arch of the Atlas, in addition to the Arthrodial Joints between the Articular Processes of the two bones. There is a Transverse Ligament extending from one side of the atlas to the other behind the Odontoid Process. There are also Anterior and Posterior ligaments connecting the anterior and posterior parts of the two bones. (See Figures 3 and 8 of Plate II.)

The Occipital-Atlantal is a Condyloid joint between the Condyles of the Occiput and the Articular Processes of the Atlas. There is a Capsular ligament on each side as well as an Anterior ligament connecting the anterior arch of the atlas with the occiput

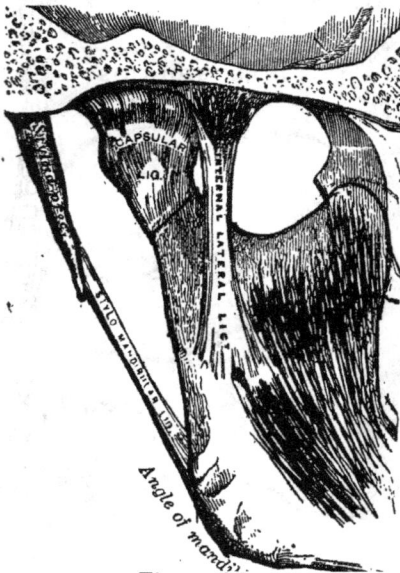

Figure 25.
Temporo-Mandibular Articulation

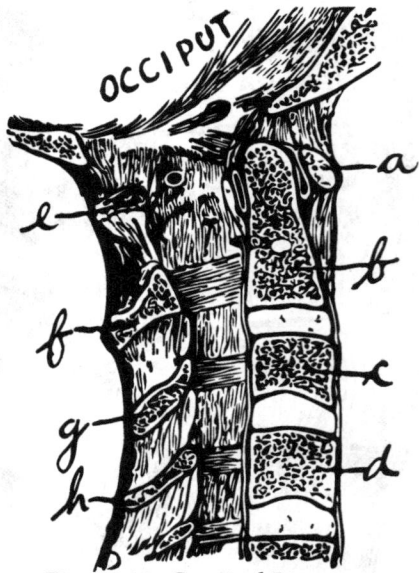

Figure 22. Cervical Ligaments
Inside Lateral View

108

and a Posterior ligament connecting the posterior arch with the occiput. (See Figure 22.)

The Occiput and the **Axis** are connected by ligaments but the bones are not in contact with each other.

ARTICULATIONS OF THE THORAX

The Costal-Vertebral Articulations are Arthrodial Joints between the Heads of the Ribs and the Bodies of the Two Adjacent Vertebrae. They have a Capsular ligament surrounding the head, of the rib and Interarticular Ligament connecting the head of the rib with the intervertebral disk and an Anterior ligament which is really a part of the capsular ligament. (See Figure 23.)

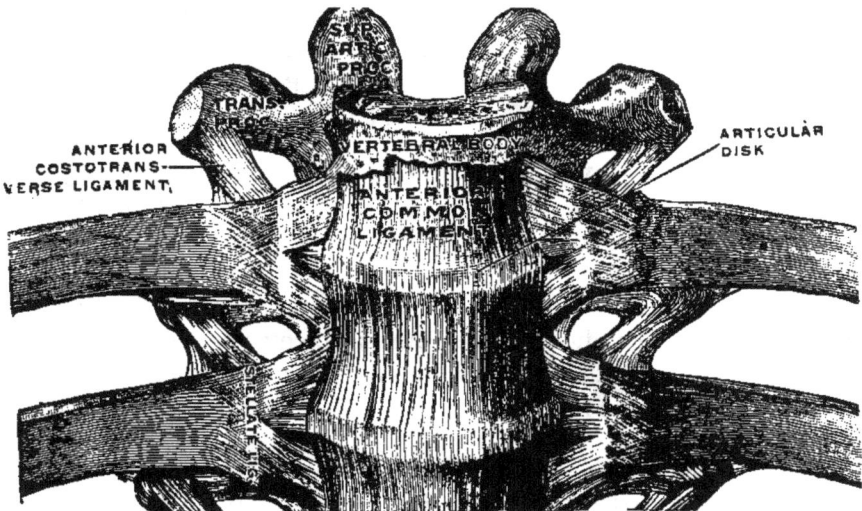

Figure 23.
Front View of Rib Articulations

109

The Costal-Transverse Articulation is an Arthrodial Joint between the Tuberosity of the Rib and the Anterior Surface of the Transverse Process of the vertebrae. There is a capsular ligament between the tip of the transverse process and the tuberosity and Three Bands connecting other parts of the transverse process with adjacent parts of the rib. (Figure 23.)

The Chondro - Sternal Articulation is an arthrodial joint between the Anterior Extremities of the Costal Cartilages and the Lateral Surfaces of the Sternum. The Capsular ligament is the only important ligament. (Plate II.)

ARTICULATIONS OF THE PELVIS

The Sacro-Iliac Articulation is an Amphiarthrosis between the Lateral Surfaces of the Sacrum and the Internal Lateral Surfaces of the Ilium. There is an Anterior and a, Posterior Sacro-Iliac Ligament on each side. (See Figure 24 and Plate II.)

The Sacro-Ischiatic Articulation is an Amphiarthrosis. The bones are not in direct contact, but are connected by Two Sacro-Ischiatic ligaments on each side. (Figure 24.)

The Pubic Symphysis is the connection between the Two Pubic Bones. In addition to the Four Ligaments Surrounding the joint there is a Disk of White Fibrous tissue between the Articular Surfaces. (See Plate II.)

The Sacro-Vertebral Articulations resemble those between the vertebrae except that there are Two Additional Ligaments on each side which connect the Transverse Processes of the 5th Lumbar Vertebrae with the Ilium and with the Sacrum. (See Plate I and Figure 24.)

110

The Sacro-Coccygeal Articulation is an amphiarthrodial joint between the Apex of the Sacrum and the Base of the Coccyx. It has two ligaments, one in front and one behind.

The Temporo-Mandibular Articulations are the only true joints in the skull. They are formed by the Condyles of the Mandible articulating with the Glenoid Cavities of the Temporal Bones. The two articular surfaces are separated by a thin oval

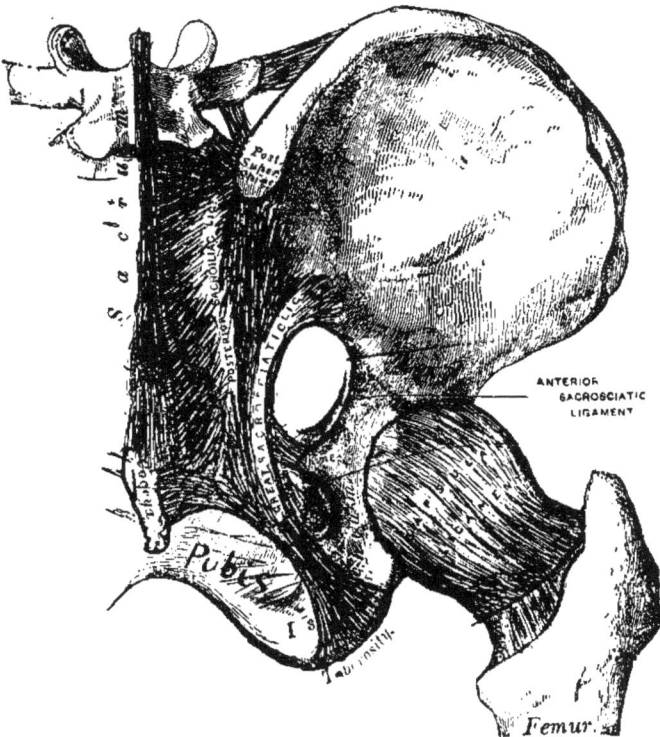

Figure 24. Back View.
Articulations of the Sacrum, Innominate and Femur

mass of yellow, elastic cartilage making practically two joints of each articulation. In addition to the Capsular ligament there is an Internal and an External Lateral and a small ligament extending from the temporal bone to the angle of the Mandible. (See Figure 25.)

ARTICULATIONS OF THE UPPER EXTREMITY

The Sterno-Clavicular Articulation is an Arthrodial joint between the Upper Extremity of the Sternum and the Inner Extremity of the Clavicle. There is a small ligament connecting one Clavicle with the other and a wide band connecting the lower surface of the clavicle with the upper surface of the 1st rib in addition to the capsular ligament between the sternum and clavicle. (See Plate II.)

The Acromio-Clavicular Articulation is an Arthrodial joint be-tween the Acromion of the Scapula and the Outer Extremity of the Clavicle. There is a superior and inferior ligament between these two parts as well as a band between the clavicle and the corcoid process of the scapula.

The Shoulder Joint is an Enarthrodial joint between the Head of the Humerus and the Glenoid Cavity of the Scapula. The Capsular ligament is very large and thick. The Other Two Ligaments of this joint are really parts of the capsular ligament. The Glenoid Cavity is surrounded by a Circular Piece of white fibrous Cartilage which serves to enlarge and deepen the cavity. (See Plate II.)

The Elbow Joint is a Ginglymus joint between the Trochlear Surface of the Humerus and the Greater Sigmoid Cavity

112

of the Ulna. Its ligaments are Capsular and Anterior, Posterior and Internal Lateral and External Lateral. The head of the radius also articulates with the external condyle of the humerus.

The Radio-Ulna Articulations are formed by the Head of the Radius and the Lesser Sigmoid Cavity of the Ulna above and the Head of the Ulna and the Sigmoid Cavity of the Radius below. The Upper Articulation is a trochoid joint, the radius being held in contact with the Ulna by a Ligament Passing Around it. The Lower Joint is also trochoid. It has a Capsular and an Anterior and Posterior ligament. There is also a Fibrous Membrane connecting the shaft of the radius with the shaft of the ulna. (See Plate II.)

The Wrist Joint is a Condyloid joint formed by the Lower End of the Radius and a Triangular piece of Cartilage on the Lower End of the Ulna articulating with the Upper Row of Carpal Bones. It has Capsular, Anterior, Posterior, Internal and External Lateral ligaments.

The Articulations between the Carpal Bones and between the Carpal and Metacarpal Bones are Arthrodial joints and are connected together by a large number of ligaments. The Finger Joints are Hinge Joints, the capsular ligament being the principal ligament.

ARTICULATIONS OF THE LOWER EXTREMITY

The Hip Joint is an Enarthrodial joint between the Head of the Femur and the Acetabulum of the Innominate. The Capsular ligament is very large and thick and is re-enforced in front by the Iliofemoral ligament. There is a Round ligament between the Head of the Femur and the lower portion of the Acetabulum which is called the Teres ligament. The cavity of the innominate is surrounded by a Circular mass of Fibrous Cartilage which enlarges and deepens it. (See Figure 24 and Plate II.)

The Knee Joint is a very complicated one. It is a Condyloid, articulation between the Condyles of the Femur and the Tuberosities of the Tibia. In addition to a very large Capsular Ligament which surrounds the entire joint and is re-enforced in front and behind and on each side by Additional ligaments, there are some Smaller ligaments Inside of the joint. (See Figures 1 and 5 of Plate II.)

Surrounding the Tuberosities of the Tibia are the Semi-Lunar Fibro Cartilages, one external and one internal. The Anterior Ligament also serves as the tendon in the large muscles on the front of the thigh. In this ligament there is a flat triangular bone (patella) which glides over the anterior and lower surface of the femur when the knee is bent.

The Ankle Joint is a Ginglymus joint between the Lower Extremities of the Tibia and Fibula and the Upper Surface of the Astragulus. The ligaments are Anterior, Posterior, Internal and External Lateral.

The Tarsal and Metatarsal Articulations and those between the Phalanges of the Foot resemble those of the wrist and hand.

QUESTIONS—LESSON 8

1. What is an Articulation? Name Three Main Classes of Articulations.

3. What is an Enarthrosis? What is a Ginglymus Joint?

4. What Structures enter into the Formation of Joints?

5. Describe the Articulations between the Vertebrae.

6. Briefly describe the Sacro-Iliac Articulation and the Atlantal-Axial Joint.

7. Describe the Articulations between the Ribs and the

Vertebrae.

9. Describe the Shoulder Joint.

10. Describe the Elbow Joint.

11. Describe the Hip Joint.

12. Describe the Knee Joint.

CHIROPRACTIC

The Science of Spinal Adjustment

———

A SERIES OF LESSONS CORRELATING AND
SYSTEMATIZING THE KNOWLEDGE NECESSARY
TO PRACTICE CHIROPRACTIC

Nature's Greatest Ally

IN RESTORING DISEASED CONDITIONS OF THE
BODY TO PERFECT HEALTH, WITHOUT THE AID
OF DRUGS OR SURGERY

———

BOOK 3

MYOLOGY AND ANGIOLOGY

Lessons 9-11

———

ORIGINALLY PUBLISHED BY
AMERICAN UNIVERSITY
CHICAGO, ILLINOIS, U.S.A.

Disclaimer

We are proud to republish this series of books on chiropractic medicine.
Originally published as a home-study course in 1913 by American University in Chicago, the 16 volumes give us an historical look at the theory and practice of chiropractic medicine in the early part of the 20th century.

This series is republished for historical interest only. The modern practice of chiropractic has advanced significantly in the century since these books were published. If you want to actually learn modern chiropractic techniques, please consult one of the many fine schools in this country.

The materials in these books are not intended to diagnose or treat disease. If you believe you are ill consult a licensed practitioner for care immediately. The publishers assume no liability for the use, misuse or nonuse of the materials in these books.

Thank you

EXTENSION COURSE
IN CHIROPRACTIC
AMERICAN UNIVERSITY
CHICAGO, Ill., U.S.A.

LESSON 9 A

MYOLOGY

In this lesson we will describe the principal voluntary muscles, giving their names, locations and functions. The involuntary muscles will be described with the organs or structure of which they form a part. The microscopic structure of muscles is given in Lesson 20.

There are 682 voluntary muscles in the body; most of them are arranged in pairs, one on either side of the median line. This lesson will deal with only those muscles of which a knowledge is necessary to successfully practice Chiropractic.

Voluntary muscles are attached to and connect two or more movable bones and their principal function or action is to change the position or relationship of these bones. The end, or part, of the muscle that usually remains stationary when the muscle is contracted, is called the Origin of the muscle; the extremity that changes its position when a muscle is used, is called the Insertion of the muscle.

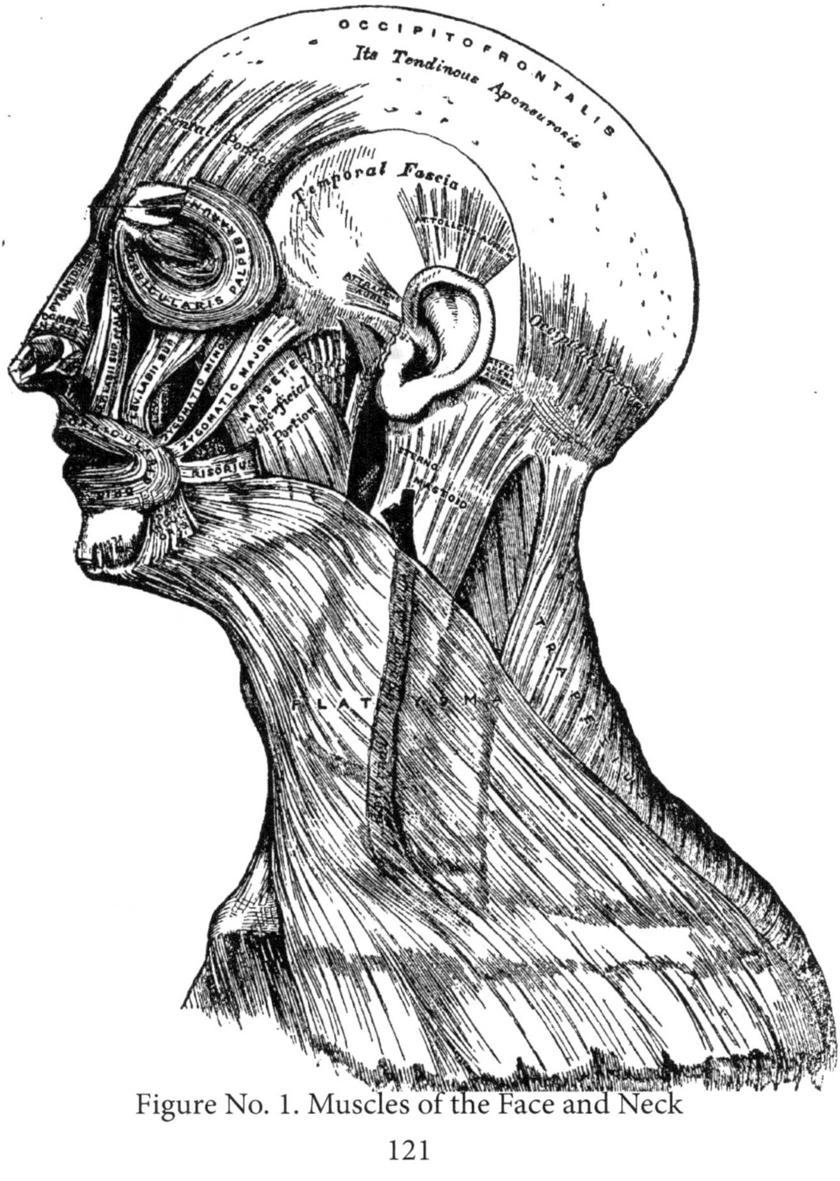

Figure No. 1. Muscles of the Face and Neck

Muscles are surrounded by a fibrous sheath of connective tissue which is called the Fascia of the muscle. This fascia also serves to connect the muscles to the bones.

When the connective tissue between the muscle mass and its attachment to the bone is in the form of a rounded cord, or a flat band, it is known as a Tendon. Occasionally, the attachment is by means of a fan-like fibrous membrane which is called an Aponeurosis.

Muscles are generally named from their size, shape, location, or attachments.

Plate 3 of the Charts should be studied with this lesson.

MUSCLES OF THE HEAD

Lessons 5, 6 and 7 should be reviewed before studying this lesson, in order that you may thoroughly understand the origin, insertion and action of the muscles.

The Orbicularis Palpebrarum is the circular muscle which forms the greater portion of the eyelids. It has its origin from the borders of the Bony Orbit and its inner edge forms the free margin of the Eyelids. Its action is to close the eyelids. It is supplied by the Facial Nerve.

The Levator Palpebrae Superioris is a long, flat muscle in the upper portion of the orbit. It has its origin from the Sphenoid Bone, and is inserted through the Upper Eyelid. Its action is to raise the upper lid and it is supplied by the third Cranial Nerve.

The Orbicularis Oris is a circular muscle surrounding the mouth and forming the lips. Its origin is from the anterior surfaces of the Mandible and the Superior Maxillary bones. Its inner edge forms the free margin of the Lips. Its action is to close the lips and it is supplied by the facial nerve.

The Masseter is situated in front of the ear and is one of the principal muscles of mastication. Its origin is from the Zygoma and Superior Maxilla and it is inserted into the Ramus of the Mandible. When it contracts, it brings the posterior teeth together. It is supplied by the facial nerve.

The Temporal is a large, fan-shaped muscle in front of the ear. It has its origin from the Parietal bone and is inserted into the Coronoid Process of the Mandible. Its action is to close the anterior teeth, and it is supplied by the facial nerve.

The Pterygoid Muscles (Internal and External) are placed behind and inside of the ramus of the mandible. Their origin is from the Sphenoid bone and they are inserted into the Ramus and Coronoid Process of the Mandible. Their action is to move the lower jaw laterally, and they are supplied by the facial nerve.

MUSCLES OF THE NECK

The Sterno-cleido-mastoid is a long, thin, flat muscle at the side and the front of the neck. Its origin is from the inner end of the Clavicle and upper portion of the Sternum and it is inserted into the Mastoid Process of the Temporal bone. One muscle, acting by itself, will rotate the face to the opposite side; both acting together will extend the head on the neck. It is supplied by the 11th Cranial and upper cervical nerves.

The Platysma Myoides forms the thin, flat sheet covering the front of the neck. Its origin is from the Clavicle and the Acromion Process of the Scapula and it is inserted into the Angle of the Mouth and the body of the Mandible. Its action is to flex the head on the neck and chest. It is supplied by the 7th cranial and the upper cervical nerves.

The Scleni Muscles (three) lie in front and at either side of the cervical vertebrae. Their origin is from the Transverse Processes of the 2nd to 7th Cervical Vertebrae and they are inserted in the 1st and 2nd Ribs. Their action is to raise the upper ribs or to flex the head laterally. When both sets contract together the head is flexed on the chest. They are supplied by the lower cervical nerves.

MUSCLES OF THE BACK

The muscles of the back are divided into five layers. The first three layers contain muscles that extend from the spine to other parts of the body; in the fourth and fifth layers are the muscles that have both their origin and insertion on the vertebrae.

The Trapezius (First layer) is the large, flat, triangular muscle of the upper back and neck. Its origin is from the Spinous Processes of the Cervical and Dorsal Vertebrae and from the Occiput. It is inserted into the Spine and Acromion Process of the Scapula and the Outer End of the Clavicle. One muscle acting by itself will flex the head laterally; both acting together will extend the head on the neck. It is supplied by the 11th cranial and the upper cervical nerves.

The Latissimus Dorsi (First layer) is the large flat muscle of the lower back. Its origin is from the Crest of the Ilium, the Spinous Processes of All of the Vertebrae from the 5th Sacral to

124

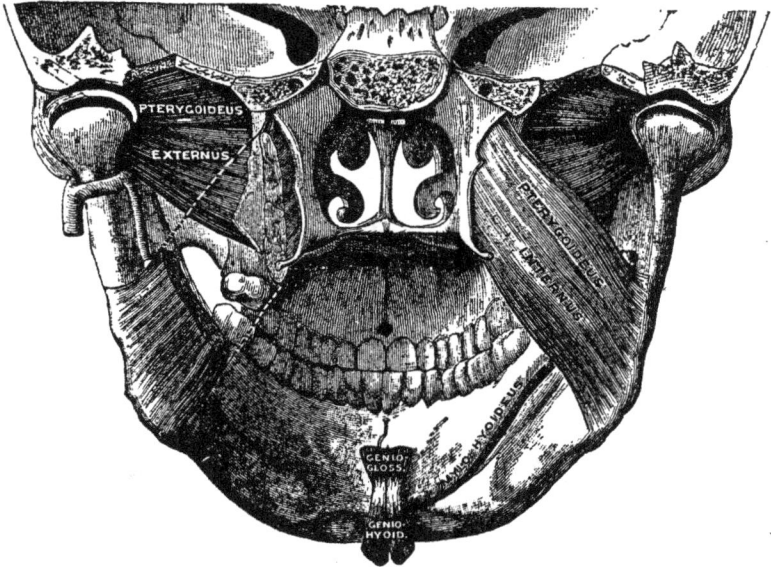

Figure No. 2. The Ptyregoid Muscles

the 7th Dorsal and the four lower ribs. It is inserted into the Upper Internal Surface of the Humerus. Its action is to draw the arm downward and backward or, when the arm is held stationary, to raise the lower ribs. It is supplied by the brachial plexus.

Rhomboids (Second layer) are small, flat muscles between the shoulder blades. They originate from the Spines of the 7th Cervical to the 5th Dorsal Vertebrae and are inserted into the Vertebral Border of the Scapula. Their action is to draw the scapula backward and upward. They are supplied by the brachial plexus.

The Splenius (Third layer) is a large, thick muscle forming the greater portion of the muscle mass at the back of the neck. Its origin is from the 7th Cervical and the 1st to 6th Dorsal Spines and

125

the Supra-spinous Ligament. It is inserted into the Upper Cervical Vertebrae, the Occiput, and the Mastoid Process of the Temporal bone. One muscle acting alone flexes the head laterally and rotates the cervical vertebrae; both muscles acting together extend the head upon the neck. The nerve supply is from the brachial plexus.

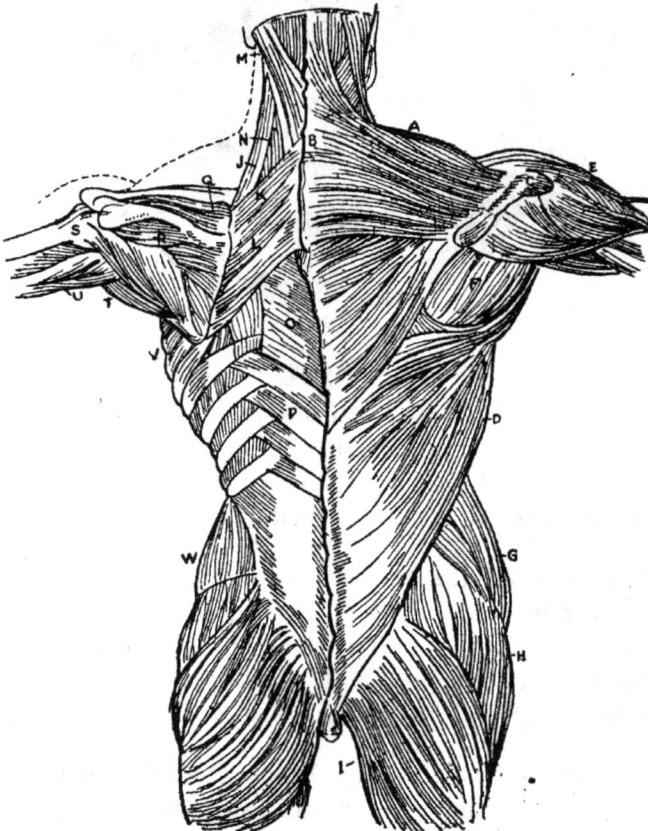

Figure No. 3. Muscles of the Back and Shoulder

126

Lesson 9 A: Myology

Serratus Posticus Superior and Inferior (Third layer) are two small, flat muscles extending from the spine to the ribs.

A - Trapezius	C - Scapula	D - Latissimus Dorsi
E - Deltoid	K & L - Rhomoboids	M & N - Splenius
P - Serratus Posticus	R - Infraspinatus	V - Serratus Magnus

Erector Spinae (Fourth layer). This name is applied to a mass of muscles that cover the posterior surfaces of the vertebrae from the sacrum to the occiput. They are divided into three main groups; one at the side of the spinous processes, one behind the transverse processes and one behind the angles of the ribs. They may be said to originate from the Sacrum, Ilium and Lumbar Vertebrae and to insert into the Spinous and Transverse Processes of the Dorsal and Cervical vertebrae, the Occiput, and the Angles of the Ribs. Their action is to extend the spine and to bend the head, neck, and trunk backwards. If the muscles on one side act independently of those on the other side, the spine will be flexed towards the side of the muscles that are acting. These muscles are supplied by the posterior primary divisions of the spinal nerves from the related regions of the spine.

Multifidus Spinae (Fifth layer). This name is applied to a large number of small muscles which are placed transversely behind the laminae of the vertebrae. They originate from the Sacrum and from the Transverse Processes of All of the Vertebrae from the 5th Lumbar to the 6th Cervical and are inserted into the Spinous Processes and Laminae of the Vertebrae just above those

127

from which they have their origin. Their action is to rotate and to extend the spine. They are supplied by the posterior primary divisions of the corresponding spinal nerves.

MUSCLES OF THE THORAX

External Intercostals. These muscles are placed between the ribs, originating from the lower border of the rib above and inserting into the upper border of the rib below. Their action is to raise the ribs during inspiration and they are supplied by the intercostal nerves.

The Internal Intercostals also lie between the ribs (internal to the external intercostals). Their origin is from the upper border of the rib below and their insertion is into the lower border of the rib above. Their action is to depress the ribs in expiration and they are also supplied by the intercostal nerves.

The Diaphragm is a large, umbrella-like muscle between the thoracic and abdominal cavities. It originates from the Inner Surfaces of the Six Lower Ribs, the Lower Portion of the Sternum and the Bodies of the Lumbar Vertebrae. The Central Portion of the diaphragm is composed of fibrous tissue and the muscle fibres are said to insert into this Tendon. It is the principal muscle of respiration; when it contracts the central portion is lowered, thus deepening the thoracic cavity. It is supplied by the phrenic nerve.

MUSCLES OF THE ABDOMEN

The External Oblique is a large, flat muscle forming the outer layer of the lateral abdominal wall. It originates from the Eight Lower Ribs, and its fibres pass obliquely downward and forward to be inserted into the Anterior Portion of the Crest of the Ilium and to unite in the Median Line of the Abdomen with

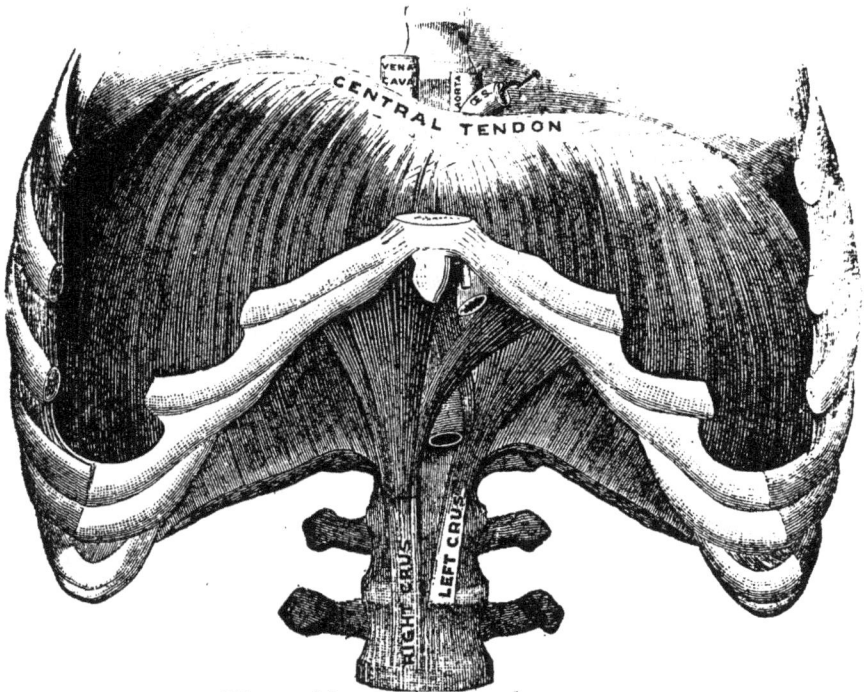

Figure No. 4. The Diaphragm

the corresponding muscle from the opposite side. The line of union between the two muscles is called the Linea Alba. The lower edge of the aponeurosis of this muscle extends from the anterior superior of the ilium to the pubic spine and is known as Poupart's Ligament.

The Internal Oblique is also a large, flat muscle of the lateral abdominal wall placed just underneath the external oblique, its fibres running upward and forward. It originates from the Transverse Processes of the Lumbar Vertebrae and the Crest

129

of the Ilium and is inserted into the Four Lower Ribs, Linea Alba and the Pubic crest. Its lower edge assists the external oblique in forming the Poupart's Ligament.

The Transversalis is the innermost muscle of the abdominal wall. Its fibres extend horizontally around the abdomen. Its origin is from the Lumbar Vertebrae, the Six Lower Ribs, the Crest of the Ilium, and Poupart's Ligament. It is inserted into the Linea Alba and the Pubic Crest.

The Rectus Abdominus is the large, thick muscle forming the anterior portion of the abdominal wall. It originates from the Pubic Crest and is inserted into the 5th, 6th and 7th Ribs.

The Quadratus Lumborum is a thick, quadrilateral muscle in the posterior abdominal wall. Its origin is from the Ilio-Lumbar Ligament and the Posterior Crest of the Ilium and it is inserted into the 12th Rib and the Transverse Processes of the Lumbar Vertebrae.

The Psoas Magnus is a long, spindle-shaped muscle in the lower posterior portion of the abdomen. Its origin is from the Transverse processes of the Lumbar Vertebrae and it is inserted into the Lesser Trocanter of the Femur.

The Iliacus is a flat, triangular muscle that fills up the whole of the Iliac Fossa. It passes outward and forward over the horizontal ramus of the pubic bone and is inserted with the psoas magnus into the Lesser Trocanter of the Femur.

The action of the External and Internal Oblique and Transversalis Muscles is to compress and support the abdominal contents. The Rectus Abdominus aids the above named muscles

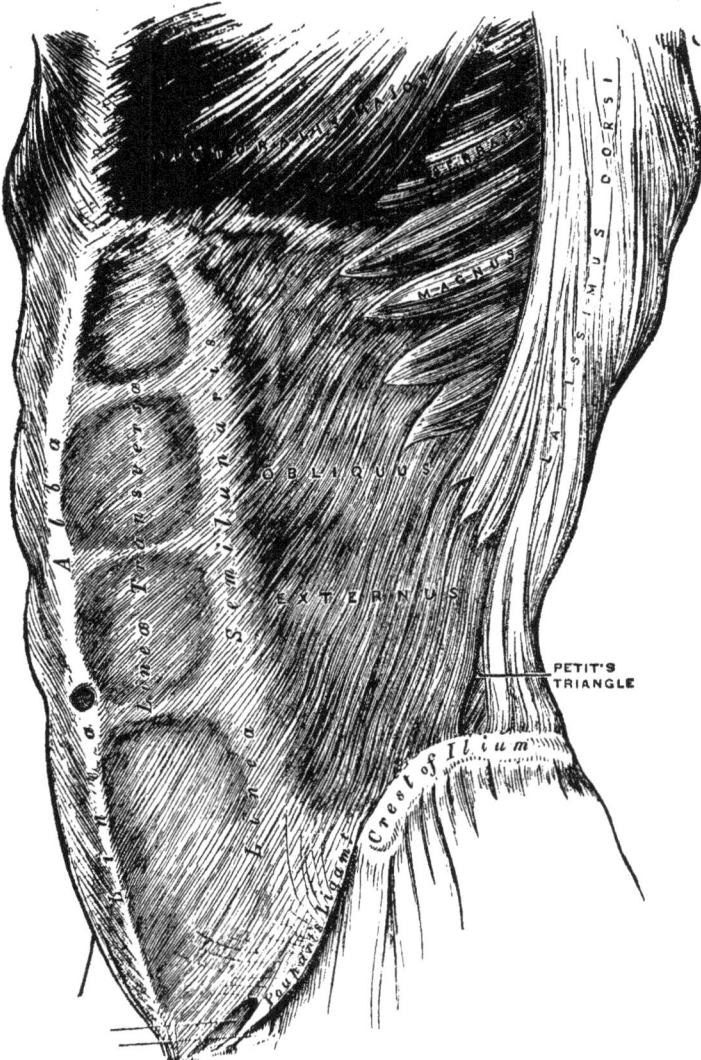

Figure No. 5. Muscles of the Trunk

and also acts with the Psoas and Iliacus in flexing the chest on the pelvis. The last two muscles are used when the thigh is flexed on the abdomen. The Quadratus Lumborum flexes the chest laterally on the pelvis. All of the abdominal muscles are supplied by the lower dorsal and upper lumbar spinal nerves.

QUESTIONS—LESSON 9 A

1. What is the difference between a Tendon and an Aponeurosis?

2. Describe the Orbicularis Palpebrarum.

3. Describe the Temporal Muscles.

4. Describe the Scleni Muscles.

5. Describe the Trapezius Muscle.

6. Describe the Erector Spinae Muscles.

7. Describe the Diaphragm.

8. Describe the Rectus Abdominus Muscle.

9. Describe the Psoas Magnus.

10. Describe the External Oblique.

EXTENSION COURSE
IN CHIROPRACTIC
AMERICAN UNIVERSITY
CHICAGO, Ill., U.S.A.

LESSON 9 B

MUSCLES OF THE PELVIC OUTLET

The Levator Ani forms the anterior and lateral portions of the pelvic floor. It is said to originate from the Spine of the Ischium and the Body and Descending Ramus of the Pubis. It is inserted into the Apex of the Coccyx and joins the corresponding muscle from the opposite side in the Median line forming the Central Tendon of the Perineum. It is supplied by the pubic nerve.

The Coccygeous forms the upper part of the posterior pelvic floor. Its origin is from the Spine of the Ischium and the Lesser Sacro-sciatic ligament, and it is inserted into the Side of the Coccyx and the Apex of the Sacrum. It is supplied by the pubic nerve.

MUSCLES OF THE SHOULDER

The Pectoralis Major is a large, fan-shaped muscle on the upper portion of the anterior chest wall. Its origin is from the Clavicle, Sternum and Upper Six Ribs and it is inserted into the Anterior Upper Surface of the Humerus. Its action is to draw the arm forward and downward and to raise the ribs. It is supplied by the brachial plexus.

The Pectoralis Minor is a thin, flat, triangular muscle situated at the upper part of the thorax beneath the pectoralis major. Its origin is from the 3rd, 4th and 5th ribs and it is inserted into the Coracoid Process of the Scapula. Its action is to depress the point of the shoulder or to raise the ribs. It is supplied by the brachial plexus.

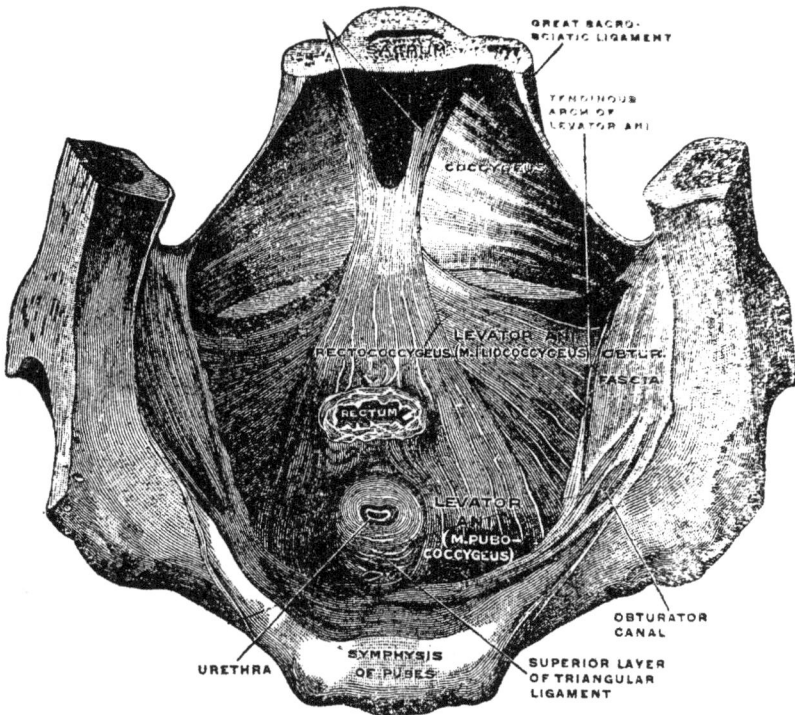

Figure No. 6. Muscles of the Pelvic Outlet

135

The Subscapularis is a large triangular muscle filling up the subscapular fossa. Its origin is from the Anterior Surface of the Scapula and it is inserted into the Lesser Tuberosity of the Humerus. Its action is to rotate the arm inward and it is supplied by the brachial plexus.

The Infraspinatus is a thick, triangular muscle occupying the greater portion of the infraspinatus fossa. It arises from the Posterior Surface of the Scapula Below the Spine and it is inserted into the Greater Tuberosity of the Humerus. Its action is to rotate the arm outward and it is supplied by the brachial plexus.

MUSCLES OF THE ARM

The Biceps is a long, spindle-shaped muscle occupying the whole of the anterior surface of the arm. It arises above by two heads from the Outer Angle of the Scapula and is inserted into the Tuberosity on the Inner, Upper Surface of the Radius. Its action is to flex the forearm and to turn the palm forward and its nerve supply is from the brachial plexus.

The Triceps is situated on the back of the arm, extending the entire length of the posterior surface of the humerus. Its origin is by three heads, two from the Outer Angle of the Scapula, and one from the Upper Posterior Surface of the Humerus, and it is inserted into Upper Posterior Surface of the Ulna. Its action is to extend the forearm and to draw the humerus backwards and toward the thorax, and it is supplied by the brachial plexus.

MUSCLES OF THE FOREARM

There are twenty muscles of the forearm, and they are divided for description into four groups.

Lesson 9 B: Muscles

The **Flexor Muscles** occupy nearly the entire anterior portion of the forearm. Their origin is from the Inner Condyle of the Humerus and they are inserted into the Anterior Surfaces of the Bones of the Hand and Wrist. Their action is to flex the wrist and fingers, and they are supplied by the brachial plexus.

The **Extensor Muscles** occupy the outer and posterior portions of the forearm. Their origin is from the Outer Condyle of the Humerus and they are inserted into the Posterior Surfaces of the Bones of the Hand and Wrist. Their action is to extend the fingers and wrist and they are supplied by the brachial plexus.

The **Pronator Muscles** are situated beneath the flexor muscles. Their origin is from the Anterior Surface of the ulna and they are inserted into the anterior surface of the Radius. Their action is to turn the palm backwards and they are supplied by the brachial plexus.

The **Supinator Longus** is a long, flat muscle on the outer side of the forearm. It originates from the External Condyle of the Humerus and is inserted into the Styloid Process of the Radius. Its action is to turn the palm forward and it is supplied by the brachial plexus.

MUSCLES OF THE HAND

There are twelve muscles in the hand. They are situated on the anterior (palmar) surface and are divided into three groups: Those of the thumb, which occupy the Radial side and form the thenar eminence, those of the little finger which occupy the Ulnar Side and form the hypothenar eminence, and those of the middle of the Palm and Between the Fingers.

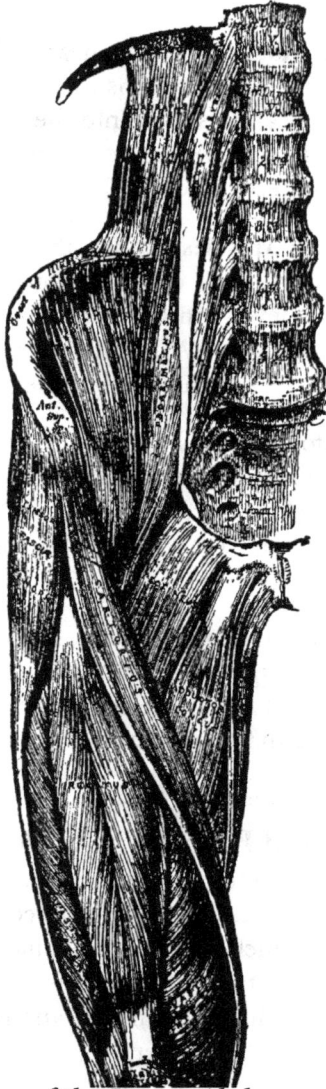

Figure No. 7. Muscles of the Lower Abdomen and Anterior Thigh

MUSCLES OF THE HIP

The Gluteus Maximus is a broad, thick muscle which forms the greater part of the buttock; it covers the greater portion of the posterior surface of the innominate. Its origin is from the Posterior Surface of the Ilium and Sacrum, and it is inserted into the Greater Trochanter of the Femur. Its action is to extend and abduct the thigh and to rotate it outward, and it is supplied by the fifth lumbar and the first and second sacral nerves.

The Gluteus Medius and Minimus lie in front and beneath the Gluteus Maximus. Their origin is from the Crest and Outer Surface of the Ilium (anterior portion) and they are inserted into the Greater Trochanter of the Femur. Their action is to abduct the thigh and rotate it inward. They are supplied by the fourth and fifth lumbar and the first sacral nerves.

MUSCLES OF THE THIGH

The Quadriceps Extensor is the large muscle mass on the front of the thigh, covering the greater portion of the anterior and lateral surfaces of the femur. It is composed of four separate muscles, but may be considered as one muscle. Its origin is from the Upper Portion of the Femur (internal, external and anterior surfaces) and the Anterior Surface of the Ilium, and it is inserted into the Upper Surface of the Tibia Between the Tuberosities. The ligament of insertion passes over the front of the knee joint and contains the patella. Its action is to extend the leg upon the thigh and it is supplied by the second, third and fourth lumbar nerves.

The Hamstring Muscles are composed of three separate muscles on the posterior surface of the femur; they may be considered together. Their origin is from the Upper Portion of the Posterior Surface of the Femur and from the Tuberosity of the

139

Ischium and they are inserted by two tendons into the Tuberosities of the Tibia, forming the Internal and External Hamstring Tendons. Their action is to flex the leg on the thigh and they are supplied by the great sciatic nerve.

The Adductor Muscles are situated on the inner side of the thigh. There are three separate muscles, but they may be described as one. Their origin is from the Inferior and Anterior Surfaces of the Innominates and they are inserted into the Posterior Surface of the Femur. Their action is to adduct the thigh and they are supplied by the third and fourth lumbar and first sacral nerves.

MUSCLES OF THE LEG

There are thirteen leg muscles. These can be divided for description into three groups.

The Flexor Muscles lie on the anterior surfaces of the tibia and fibula. Their origin is from the Upper Outer Surface of the Tibia and the Anterior Surface of the Fibula, and they are inserted into the Bones of the Ankle and Foot. Their action is to flex the foot forward, to raise its inner border, and to extend the toes (forward), and they are supplied by the fourth and fifth lumbar and the first sacral nerves.

The Extensor Muscles are on the back of the leg. Their origin is from the Condyles of the Femur and the Upper Posterior Surfaces of the Tibia and Fibula and they are inserted into the Bones of the Ankle and Foot. Their action is to extend the foot (backward), and to raise its outer border and to flex the toes (backward). They are supplied by the fourth and fifth lumbar and the first and second sacral nerves.

140

The Peroneal Muscles lie on the outside of the leg. Their origin is from the Outer and Anterior Surfaces of the Fibula and they are inserted into the Bones of the Foot. They extend, invert or evert the foot, depending upon which of the three muscles is contracted. They are supplied by the fourth and fifth lumbar and first and second sacral nerves.

MUSCLES OF THE FOOT

There is One Muscle on the Upper Surface of the Foot, Four Muscles between the Metatarsal Bones, and Fifteen Muscles on the Lower Surface of the Foot, the latter being divided into four layers.

QUESTIONS—LESSON 9 B

1. Describe the Levator Ani.

2. Describe the Pectoralis Major.

3. Describe the Deltoid.

4. Describe the Triceps.

5. Describe the Flexor Muscles of the Forearm.

6. Describe the Gluteus Maximus.

7. Describe the Quadriceps Extensor.

8. Describe the Hamstring Muscles.

9. Describe the Peroneal Muscles.

10. Describe the Muscles of the Foot.

EXTENSION COURSE IN CHIROPRACTIC AMERICAN UNIVERSITY CHICAGO, Ill., U.S.A.

LESSON 10

THE CIRCULATORY SYSTEM

The organs of circulation are the Heart and the Blood Vessels. There are two distinct systems of blood vessels in the body, both connected with the heart. One system carries the blood to, through, and from the lungs; the other carries the blood through all of the remaining parts of the body. The vessels that carry the blood from the heart are called Arteries; those carrying the blood towards the heart are called Veins. The Capillaries are very small vessels connecting the arteries with the veins.

The entire system of Arteries, Capillaries and Veins form a series of closed tubes. The Lymphatics are an independent set of vessels which assist the veins by carrying back to the heart some of the liquid portion of the blood which passes through the capillary walls. (The Physiology of the Circulation is given in Lesson 3.)

Plate 4 of the Charts should be studied with this lesson.

THE HEART

The Heart is the central organ of the blood vascular system. It consists of a conoidal mass of hollow muscular tissue. It is situated in the middle mediastinum between the two lungs, behind the sternum, in front of the bodies of the dorsal vertebrae and above the diaphragm. It is five inches long (left to right), three and one-half inches wide (superior-inferiorly), and two and one-half inches deep (anterior-posteriorly.)

The heart occupies approximately the center of the chest. The right border is one-half inch to the right of the right border of the sternum, the lower border is in contact with the liver at the junction of the middle, and lower portions of the sternum, the upper border is just above the third rib and the apex of the heart lies between the fifth and sixth ribs about one inch inside of the nipple.

The interior of the heart is divided by muscular partitions into four cavities, arranged in pairs; one pair on each side of the heart. The Right Auricle is the posterior-superior portion, the Right Ventricle, the anterior- inferior portion; the Left Auricle, the anterior-superior portion, and the Left Ventricle the posterior-inferior portion. The right auricle and the right ventricle together are usually spoken of as the right side of the heart, and the left auricle and the left ventricle as the left side of the heart.

The venous blood is carried into the right auricle by the superior and the inferior vena cavae. The blood passes from the right auricle to the right ventricle through the Tricuspid Valve. When the right ventricle contracts the blood is forced through the Pulmonary Valve into the pulmonary arteries and through the lungs. The pulmonary veins carry the purified blood from

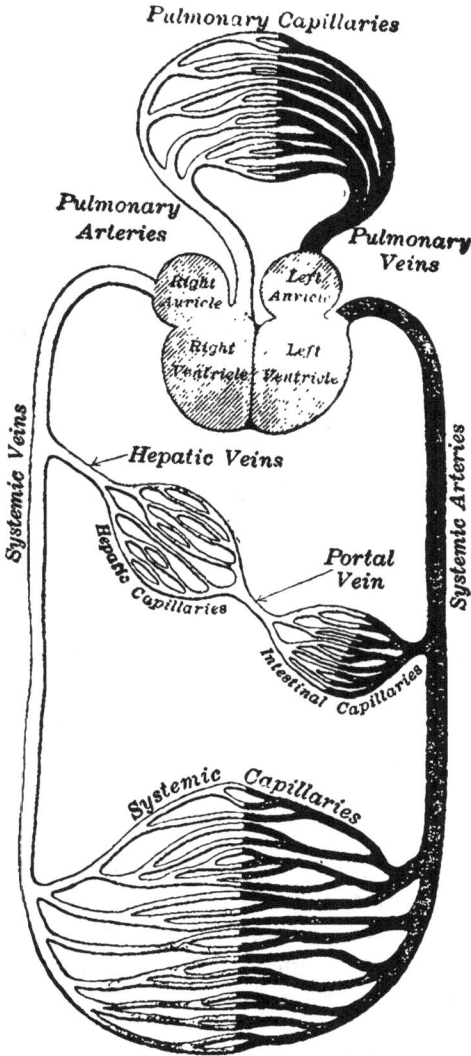

Figure No. 8. Diagram of the Circulation.

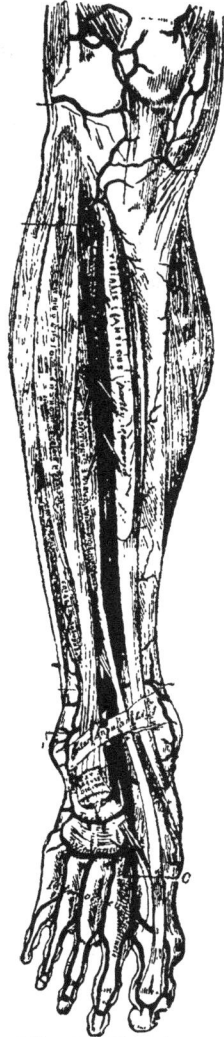

Figure No. 9. The Anterior Tibial Artery.

the lungs to the left auricle. From the left auricle the blood passes through the Mitral Valve into the left ventricle. Contraction of the left ventricle forces the blood through the Aortic Valve into the aorta and the general circulation.

The heart is composed of a special form of muscle tissue, which will be described in Lesson 20. The Cavities are lined by endothelial tissue (see Lesson 1). The Valves of the heart are formed by folds of connective tissue which are covered by the endothelium.

Surrounding the heart is a double sac which forms the covering of the heart and lines the cavity in which it lies. It is called the Pericardium and is composed of an outer layer of fibrous tissue and an inner layer of endothelial tissue.

The Arterial System has four principal divisions. The Aorta is the large main trunk, extending from the heart to the pelvis. The Pulmonary Arteries connect the heart with the lungs. The Visceral Arteries are from the aorta and common iliacs to the viscera. The Peripheral Arteries supply the extremities, the walls of the trunk, and the face and neck.

PULMONARY ARTERIES

The Pulmonary Artery begins at the external opening of the right ventricle and passes upward for about two inches when it divides into two branches of nearly equal size; one passing to the right and the other to the left. Each branch subdivides into two smaller branches and which enter the lungs with the bronchi.

AORTA AND ITS BRANCHES

The Aorta begins at the external opening of the left ventricle, and arches upward and backward to the fourth dorsal vertebrae (Arch of the Aorta). It then passes downward on the left side of the spinal column to the diaphragm forming the Thoracic Aorta. The Abdominal Aorta is a continuation of the thoracic aorta and it lies in front of the bodies of the lumbar vertebrae. At the level of the fourth vertebrae the abdominal aorta divides and forms the two Common Iliacs which pass downward and forward through the pelvis.

In addition to the two Coronary Arteries, the Innominate is given off on the right side and the Left Common Carotid and Left Sub-clavian are given off on the left side of the arch of the aorta. From the thoracic aorta branches are given off to supply the Pericardium, Bronchi, Esophagus, and the Chest Walls. The abdominal aorta gives off branches to supply the Diaphragm, Stomach, Liver, Pancreas, Spleen, Kidneys, Intestines, Ovaries, Testes, and Abdominal Walls.

ARTERIES OF THE HEAD AND NECK

The Common Carotids (right and left) begin at the arch of the aorta (left) or innominate (right) and pass upward beneath the sterno-cleido-mastoid muscles to the upper border of the thyroid cartilage where they divide into external and internal carotids.

The External Carotid begins at the termination of the common carotid and passes upward behind the angle of the jaw and in front of the ear where it divides into the superficial temporal and the internal maxillary.

147

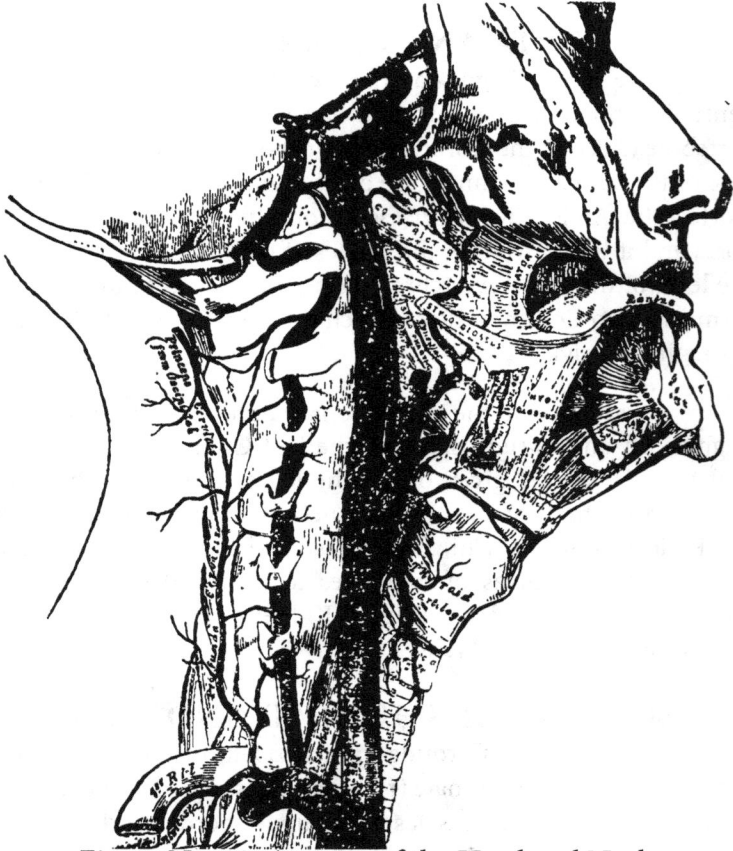

Figure No. 10. Arteries of the Head and Neck

The Internal Carotid begins at the termination of the common carotid and passes upward in front of the transverse processes of the upper cervical vertebrae and into the cranium to the temporal bone. It terminates in a network of arteries known as the Circle of Willis, which supplies the brain.

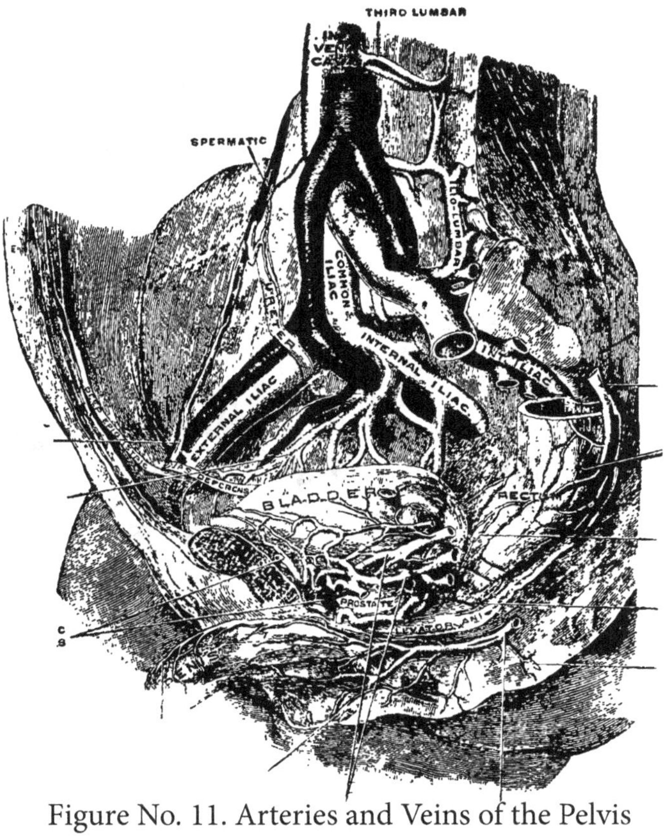

Figure No. 11. Arteries and Veins of the Pelvis

The Vertebral Artery begins at the subclavian and passes upward through the canals in the transverse processes of the cervical vertebrae to the cranium where it terminates in the Circle of Willis.

ARTERIES OF UPPER EXTREMITIES

The Subclavian begins at the arch of the aorta (left) or innominate (right) and passes beneath the clavicle to the outer

149

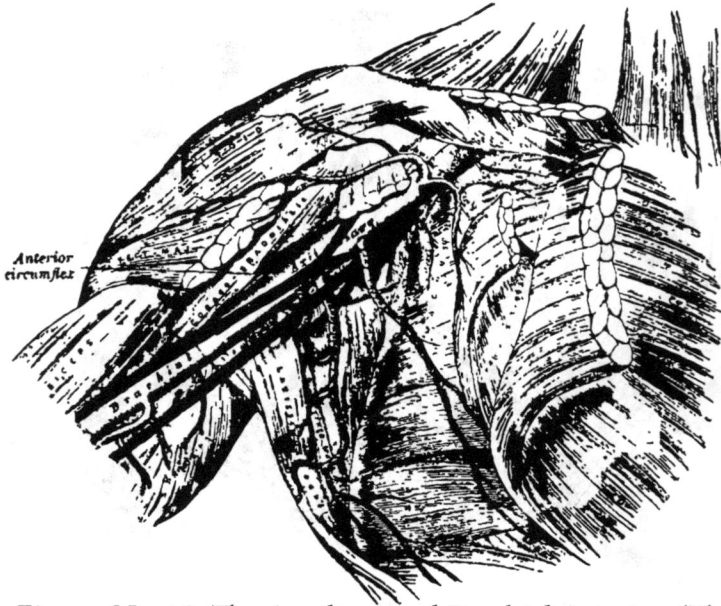

Figure. No. 12. The Auxiliary and Brachial Arteries. (The black cords are nerves.)

border of the first rib where it terminates in the axillary. It is three inches long.

The Axillary begins at the termination of the subclavian and passes between the arm and the chest to the lower border of the pectoralis major muscle, where it terminates in the brachial. It is nine inches long.

The Brachial begins at the termination of the axillary and passes down the inner side of the arm, gradually approaching the front to a point one-half inch below the bend of the elbow where it divides into the radial and ulna arteries.

150

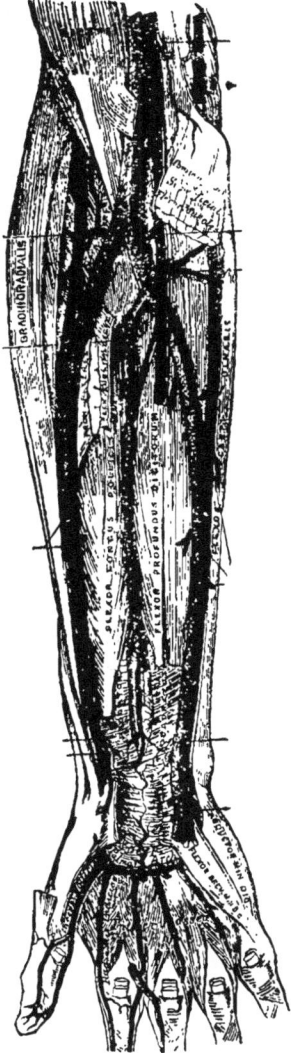

Figure No. 13. Arteries of the
Forearm

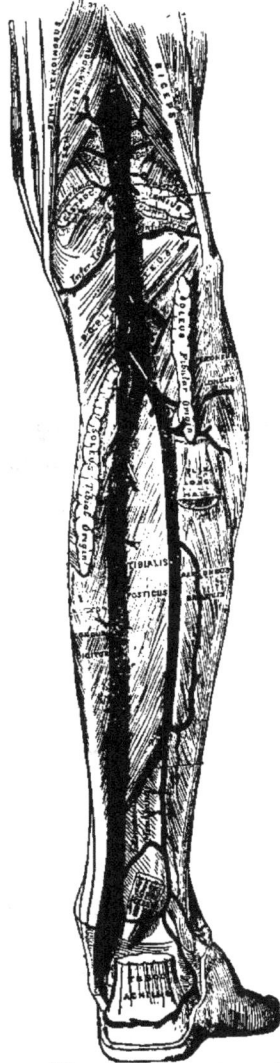

Figure No. 14. Arteries of the
Thigh and Leg.

151

The Radial begins at the division of the brachial and passes down on the outer side of the forearm to the hand where with the ulnar it forms the palmar arches.

The Ulnar begins at the division of the brachial and passes down the middle and inner side of the forearm to the hand where it joins the radial.

The Palmar Arches are situated in the hand and serve to connect the radial and ulnar arteries. Branches from these arches supply the hand and fingers.

ARTERIES OF LOWER ABDOMEN AND PELVIS
The Common Iliacs (right and left) begin at the termination of the abdominal aorta (fourth lumbar vertebrae) and pass downward and forward to the sacro-iliac articulations where they divide into the internal and external iliacs. Each one is two inches long.

The Internal Iliac begins at the division of the common iliac and extends downward and backward to the greater sciatic ligament, where it divides into a posterior and an anterior division which supply the hip and walls of the abdomen and pelvis, and the pelvic organs.

The External Iliac begins at the division of the common iliac and passes downward, outward and forward to Poupart's Ligament, where it terminates in the femoral.

ARTERIES OF LOWER EXTREMITY
The Femoral begins at a point midway between the anterior iliac spine and the pubic symphysis and passes down the

inner anterior thigh to the inner condyle of the femur where it terminates in the popliteal.

The Popliteal begins at the termination of the femoral and passes down behind the knee for six inches, where it divides into the anterior and posterior tibial arteries.

The Anterior Tibial begins at the division of the popliteal and passes forward and downward along the outer surface of the tibia to the front of the ankle joint where it becomes the dorsalis pedis which supplies the upper surface of the foot.

The Posterior Tibial begins at the division of the popliteal and passes downward behind the tibia to a point below the internal malleolus where it divides into the internal and external plantar arteries which supply the sole of the foot.

QUESTIONS—LESSON 10

1. Draw a diagram showing the course of the Blood through the Systemic,

2. Pulmonary and Hepatic Systems.

3. Briefly describe the Heart.

4. Describe the Pulmonary Artery.

5. Describe the Aorta.

6. Describe the Internal Carotid Artery.

7. Describe the Brachial Artery.

8. Describe the Radial Artery.

9. Describe the Internal Iliac Artery.

10. Describe the Femoral Artery.

11. Describe the Anterior Tibial Artery.

EXTENSION COURSE IN CHIROPRACTIC AMERICAN UNIVERSITY CHICAGO, Ill., U.S.A.

LESSON 11

THE CIRCULATORY ORGANS (Continued)
THE VEINS

The Veins are the vessels carrying the blood from the tissues and organs to the heart. Their structure is similar to that of the arteries except that the middle coat contains less muscle tissue. Veins also differ from the arteries in that they are larger, are more numerous, less regular in their course, and many of them contain valves.

The Veins from the Viscera and the Trunk generally accompany the arteries and have the same name. The arteries of the Extremities are also accompanied by Veins which are usually in pairs, two to each artery. In addition to these Deep Veins of the extremities there are Superficial Veins just beneath the skin. These are not usually accompanied by arteries.

The Pulmonary Veins drain the lungs and empty into the left auricle of the heart. The Portal Vein is formed by smaller veins from the stomach, spleen, pancreas and intestines. It passes

155

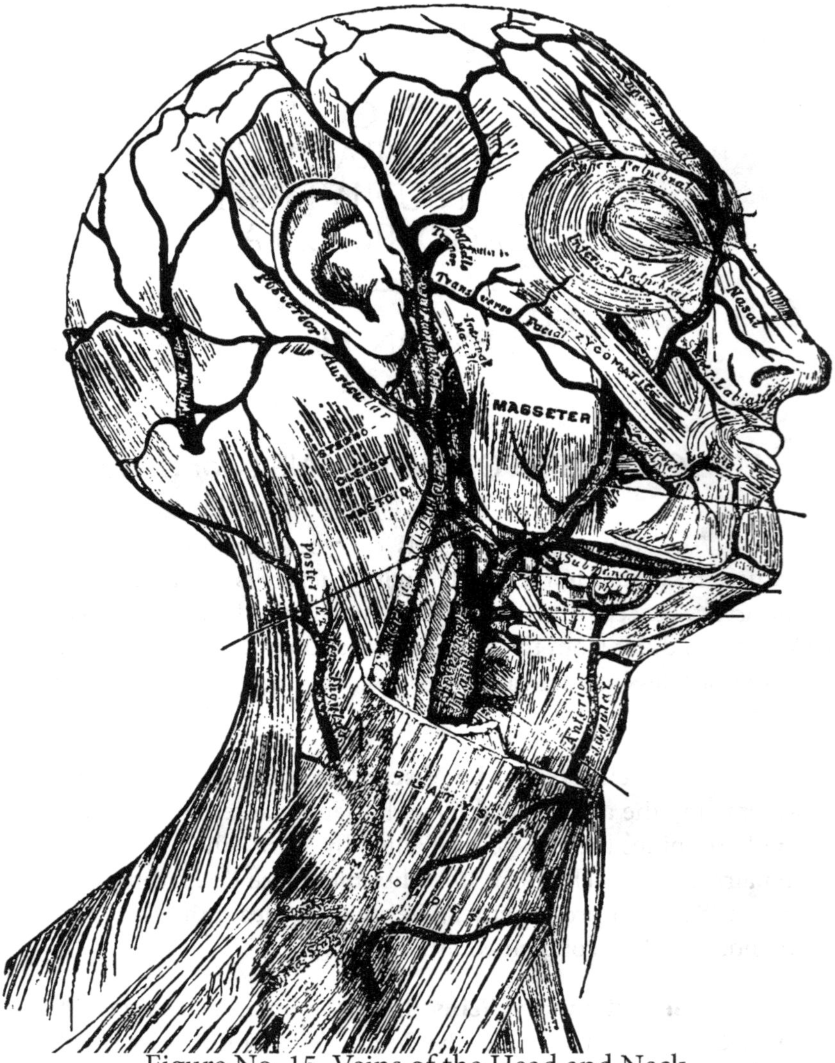

Figure No. 15. Veins of the Head and Neck

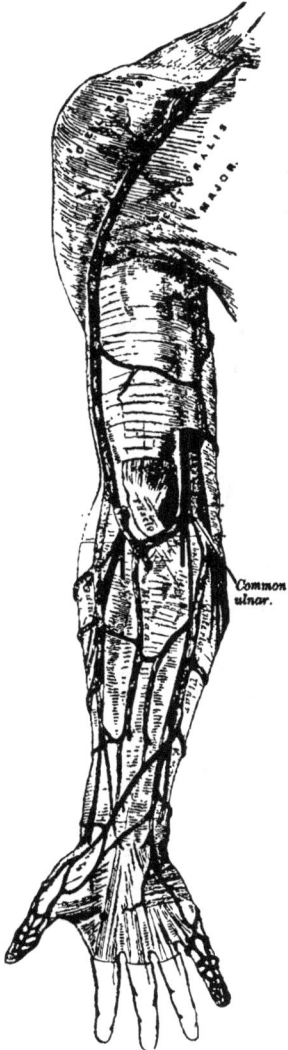

Figure No. 16. Superficial Veins of the Arm and Forearm.

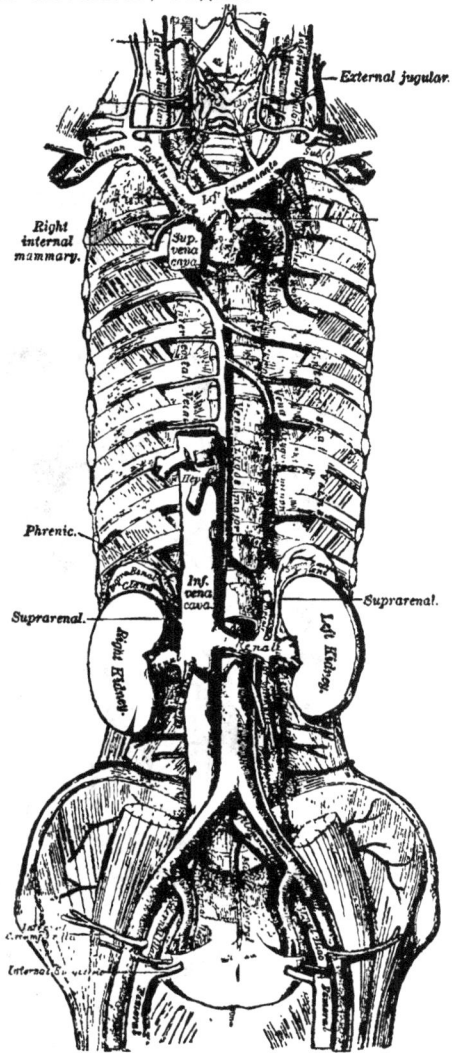

Figure No. 17. Inferior Vena Cava and Abdominal Veins

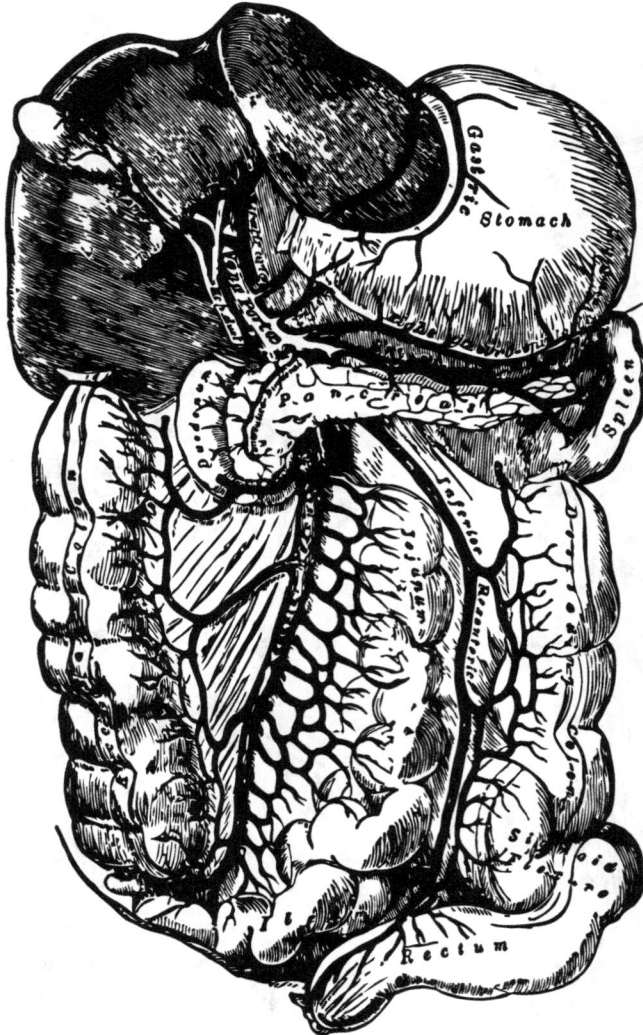

Figure No. 18. The Portal System of Veins

into the liver where it breaks up into small veins and capillaries. The large Veins of the Cranium Veins of the Cranium lie between and are formed by the two layers of the dura mater and are called Sinuses.

VEINS OF THE HEAD AND NECK

The External Jugular is formed by the union of the veins from the face and scalp. It passes downward on the external surface of the sterno-cleido- mastoid muscle and empties into the subclavian at the base of the neck.

The Internal Jugular is formed by the union of the sinuses of the brain. It passes downward beneath the sterno-cleido mastoid muscle in the same sheath with the carotid artery and the vagus nerve. It joins the subclavian at the base of the neck to form the innominate.

The Vertebral is formed by the union of the veins of the neck and of the posterior scalp. It passes downward through the transverse processes of the cervical vertebrae and empties into the innominate.

VEINS OF THE UPPER EXTREMITIES

The Deep Veins accompany the arteries and bear the same names.

The Superficial Veins of the forearm (Radial, Ulnar, and Median) pass up the anterior surface of the forearm to the bend of the elbow where they unite to form the Cephalic and Basilic veins, which pass up the anterior surface of the arm to the axilla where they join to form the axillary.

The Axillary Vein is formed by the cephalic, basilic and the deep brachial veins. It extends to a point beneath the clavicle where it becomes a Subclavian Vein.

The Subclavian unites with the Internal Jugular Vein to form the in-nominate veins.

The Two Innominate Veins (right and left) unite to form the Superior Vena Cava which empties into the right auricle of the heart.

VEINS OF THE THORAX

The External Veins of the Thorax accompany the arteries and have the same names.

The Azygos Veins drain the internal surfaces of the walls of the thorax and empty into the superior vena cava.

VEINS OF THE ABDOMEN AND PELVIS

Portal System. The Superior and Inferior Mesenteric (from intestines) unite with the Splenic and Gastric (from spleen and stomach) to form the Portal Vein which also receives the veins from the Pancreas and Gall Bladder. The portal vein passes into the liver through the transverse fissure dividing into right and left branches which accompany the corresponding branches of the hepatic artery into the substance of the liver. After passing through the liver the blood is carried to the inferior vena cava by the Hepatic Vein.

The remaining abdominal and pelvic organs and the walls of the abdomen and pelvis are drained by veins which accompany the corresponding arteries and are given the same names. They empty into the Inferior Vena Cava.

VEINS OF THE LOWER EXTREMITIES

The Deep Veins are similar to and accompany the arteries and are given the same names. They are connected with the Inferior Vena Cava by the Iliac Veins.

The Internal Saphenous is the long, superficial vein of the lower extremity. It begins in front of the internal malleolus and passes up the inner side of the leg and thigh to a point one and one-half inches below Poupart's Ligament where it empties into the deep femoral vein.

The External Saphenous is the short, superficial vein of the leg. It begins behind the external malleolus and passes up the back of the leg to a point behind the knee where it empties into the deep popliteal vein.

LYMPHATICS

Lymphatic Vessels. The lymphatic vessels are similar to the veins in structure. They carry the lymph from the tissues and organs to the heart.

The Thoracic Duct is the main lymph vessel of the body. It begins in a pouch at the level of the second lumbar vertebrae and passes upward in front of the spinal column to the seventh cervical vertebrae, where it arches forward and outward to empty into the left subclavian vein. It drains all of the trunk of the body except the right upper half.

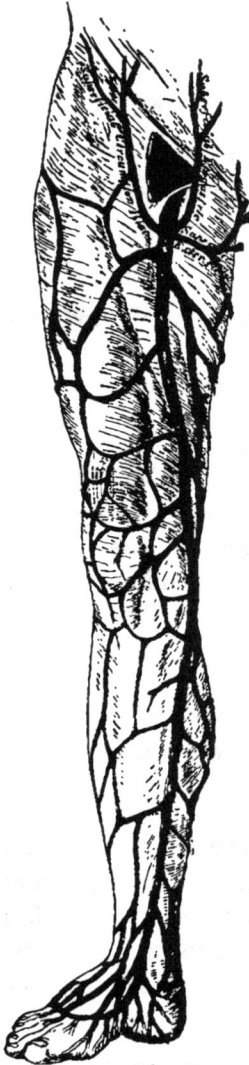

Figure No. 19. The Internal
Saphenous Vein.

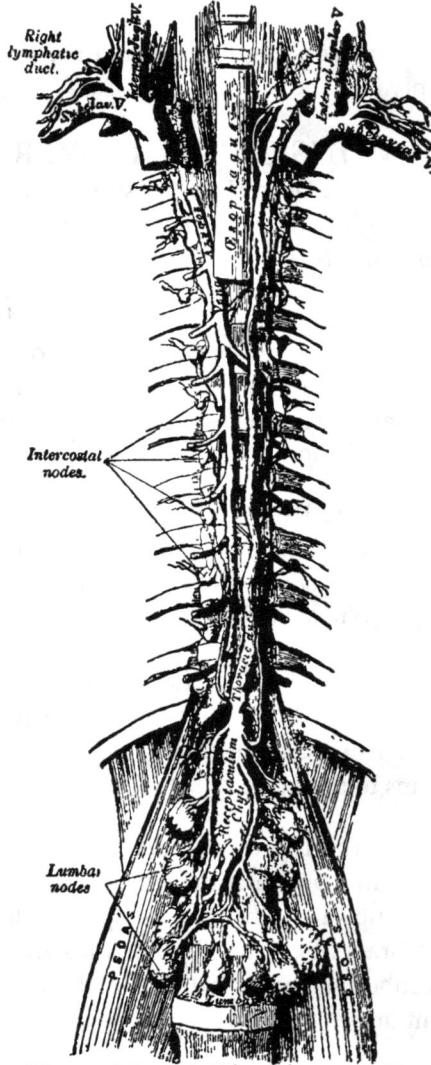

Figure No. 20. The Thoracic Duct

Lesson 11: The Circulatory Organs

The Right Lymphatic Duct is a short Vessel (one-half inch long), draining the right half of the thorax and the right half of the face and neck. It empties into the right subclavian vein.

The Peripheral Lymphatics accompany the veins and arteries and are given the same names.

Lymphatic Glands. These are rounded bodies occurring along the course of the lymphatic vessels. They are not true glands. The more important groups are described below.

Neck. There are many lymphatic glands in the neck. The principal groups follow the course of the sterno-cleido-mastoid muscles.

Axilla and Groin. There are ten or twelve large glands in each axilla, and eight or ten large glands in each groin. There is a group along the middle third of the femoral artery and another group accompanying the popliteal artery.

Chest, Abdomen and Pelvis. There is a large number in the pelvis along the course of the iliac arteries, in the mesentery of the small intestines and in the mediastinal space between the lungs.

QUESTIONS—LESSON 11

1. Give the difference between the Veins and the Arteries.

2. What are the Sinuses?

3. Describe the Internal Jugular.

4. Describe the Axillary Vein.

5. Describe the Portal System.

6. Describe the Internal Saphenous Vein.

7. Describe the Thoracic Duct.

8. Locate the Lymphatic Glands of the Chest, Abdomen and Pelvis.

9. Describe the Superficial Veins of the Forearm.

10. Describe the Inferior Vena Cava.

CHIROPRACTIC

The Science of Spinal Adjustment

———

A SERIES OF LESSONS CORRELATING AND
SYSTEMATIZING THE KNOWLEDGE NECESSARY
TO PRACTICE CHIROPRACTIC

Nature's Greatest Ally

IN RESTORING DISEASED CONDITIONS OF THE
BODY TO PERFECT HEALTH, WITHOUT THE AID
OF DRUGS OR SURGERY

———

BOOK 4

NEUROLOGY: Spine etc.

Lessons 12, 13, 14 and 15

———

ORIGINALLY PUBLISHED BY
AMERICAN UNIVERSITY
CHICAGO, ILLINOIS, U.S.A.

Disclaimer

We are proud to republish this series of books on chiropractic medicine.
Originally published as a home-study course in 1913 by American University in Chicago, the 16 volumes give us an historical look at the theory and practice of chiropractic medicine in the early part of the 20th century.

This series is republished for historical interest only. The modern practice of chiropractic has advanced significantly in the century since these books were published. If you want to actually learn modern chiropractic techniques, please consult one of the many fine schools in this country.

The materials in these books are not intended to diagnose or treat disease. If you believe you are ill consult a licensed practitioner for care immediately. The publishers assume no liability for the use, misuse or nonuse of the materials in these books.

Thank you

EXTENSION COURSE IN CHIROPRACTIC AMERICAN UNIVERSITY CHICAGO, Ill., U.S.A.

LESSON 12

GENERAL NERVOUS PHYSIOLOGY

The function of the Nervous System as a whole is to adjust the body to its surroundings and to make the individual organs and parts work in harmony with each other and for the good of the body as a whole. The functions of the separate parts of the Nervous System will be given when that part is described.

The nervous system is made up of a large number of individual units called "Neurones," each of which consists of a rounded nerve cell and two fibres (Axone and Dendrite) projecting from it. The work of the Nervous System is carried on by "nerve impulses" which pass over the nerve fibres and through the nerve cells.

The nerve fibres carry the impulses like telegraph wires; the nerve cells nourish the nerve fibres as well as store the nervous energy. The exact nature of nervous energy or "Vital Force" is not known, but it is assumed to be similar to electricity.

Anything that will increase the number or strength of the impulses passing over motor or sensory nerves is called a "Stimulant" and the process is called "Stimulation." When the number or strength of the impulses is decreased the process is called "Inhibition."

THE NERVOUS SYSTEM

The Nervous System is divided anatomically into two divisions: The Cerebro-Spinal System, and the Sympathetic System.

The Cerebro-Spinal System consists of Brain, Spinal Cord, Cranial Nerves, and Spinal Nerves. The brain nearly fills the cranial cavity, and the spinal cord is located in the neural canal which it but partially fills. These are connected with each other at the junction of the occipital bone with the atlas. The twelve pairs of cranial nerves are given off from the brain, and the 31 pairs of spinal nerves are given off from the spinal cord. See plate 7 of the Anatomy and Physiology Charts.

The Sympathetic Nervous System consists of the following four divisions:

1. Two rows of ganglions connected together by intervening cords. These gangliated cords are located one on each side of the vertebral column, along the whole length of it.

2. Three large gangliated plexus, which are called: (a) Cardiac, (b) Solar, (c) Hypo-Gastric, and are located in the chest, abdomen and pelvis.

3. Many small Plexuses located in or near the

individual organs and surrounding the principal blood vessels.

4. Numerous nerve fibres connecting the above three divisions with each other and with the various organs.

THE CEREBROSPINAL SYSTEM
THE BRAIN

The Brain is the largest mass of nerve tissue in the body. It is located in the cranial cavity and divided into the following parts: Cerebrum, Isthmus, Cerebellum, Medulla Oblongata, and Pons Varolii. See plate 7 of the charts.

The Brain is composed of the following structures:

1. Gray matter (Cells), which makes up the Cortex of the Cerebrum and of the Cerebellum and the solid bodies within the brain, and various nerve centers.

2. White matter (Fibres), which makes the inner

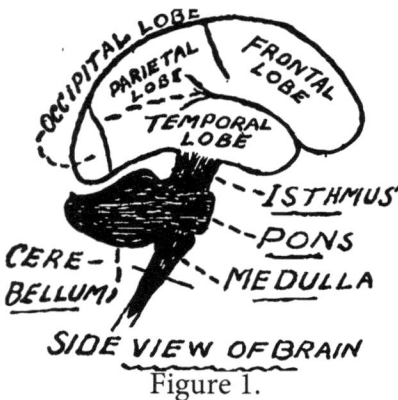

Figure 1.

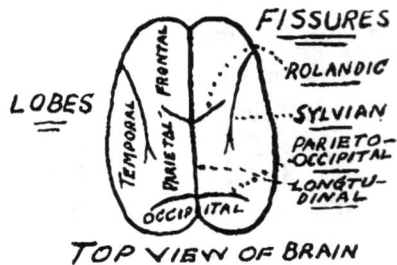

Figure 2.

portion of the Cerebrum and Cerebellum (except the solid bodies), and the greater part of the Isthmus, Pons, and Medulla.

3.   Ventricles, which are cavities within the brain substance.

The Cerebrum, or Fore-Brain, is the largest portion of the human brain. When viewed from above, it forms an ovoid mass with a deep cleft in the center running antero-posteriorly. This cleft is called the Great Longitudinal Fissure, and it separates the two hemispheres completely with the exception of a white band, (Corpus Callosum) which forms a floor for the Great Longitudinal Fissure and connects the two hemispheres. A fold of the Dura Mater, the Faux Cerebri, is located in this fissure. Each hemisphere is divided into five lobes by fissures. (See Figures 1 and 2.) The five lobes are:

1.   The Frontal Lobe, the largest of the Cerebral Lobes, is bounded behind by the fissure of Rolando, below by the fissure of Sylvius, and internally by the longitudinal fissure.

2.   Parietal Lobe forms a large part of the external surface of the hemisphere, and in front is separated from the frontal lobe by the fissure of Rolando. Behind it is separated from the Occipital lobe by the parieto-occipital fissure. Below it is bounded by the temporal lobe.

3.   Occipital Lobe, which forms the posterior

pyramidal portion of the hemisphere, is separated in front from the parietal lobe by the parieto-occipital fissure.

4. Temporal Lobe, which lies in the middle fossa of the skull, is bounded in front by the Sylvian fissure.

5. Central Lobe or **Island of Reil**, also called the Insula, is tri-angular shaped, and lies in the fissure of Sylvia.

Each Cerebral Hemisphere is composed of gray matter which forms an outside coating called the Cerebral Cortex, and the white matter lying internally called the Medullary Center. In addition to the gray matter on the outside there are large deposits of gray matter in the base of each hemisphere, which are called Corpus Striata and Optic Thalami.

The white medullary center of the cerebral hemisphere lies subjacent to the gray cortex, and is composed of medullated nerve fibres which are classified into three groups: Commissural Fibres, Association Fibres, and Protection Fibres.

The Commissural Fibres connect the various parts of the gray cortex with the corresponding parts of the opposite hemisphere.

The Association Fibres connect different parts of the same hemisphere. They are arranged in bundles which, on account of their length are called the long and the short association fibres.

Lesson 12: Nervous Physiology

The Projection Fibres connect the Cerebrum with the Medulla Oblongata and the Spinal Cord (through the Isthmus and Pons).

The Optic Thalami are two ovoid masses of gray matter situated on either side of the 3rd ventricle. They form the most important portion of the Interbrain. Each Optic Thalamus connects with the optic tract, and also sends out cortical fibres to all parts of the cortex. (See Figure 5.)

The Corpora Striata are two Biconvex masses of gray matter situated above and external to the Optic Thalami (one on either side of the brain).

The Isthmus (Crura Cerebri) are composed of large bundles of Nerve Fibres which pass downward from the Cortex of the brain to the Pons and Medulla.

The Pons Varolii or Bridge forms the union between the Cerebrum, Cerebellum, and the Medulla Oblongata. It is composed of bundles of nerve-fibres which pass transversely through it, and at either side come together and form a strand, which is termed the Middle Peduncle of the Cerebellum.

The Cerebellum lies behind the Pons Varolii and the Medulla Oblongata, and below the posterior portion of the cerebral hemispheres. It consists of gray matter on the surface and white matter internally, and its surface is not convoluted like the Cerebrum, but is filled with curved fissures and furrows. It is subdivided into a central portion called the Vermis and two larger parts called the lateral hemispheres; these parts are again subdivided into many lobes. The gray matter is on the surface,

173

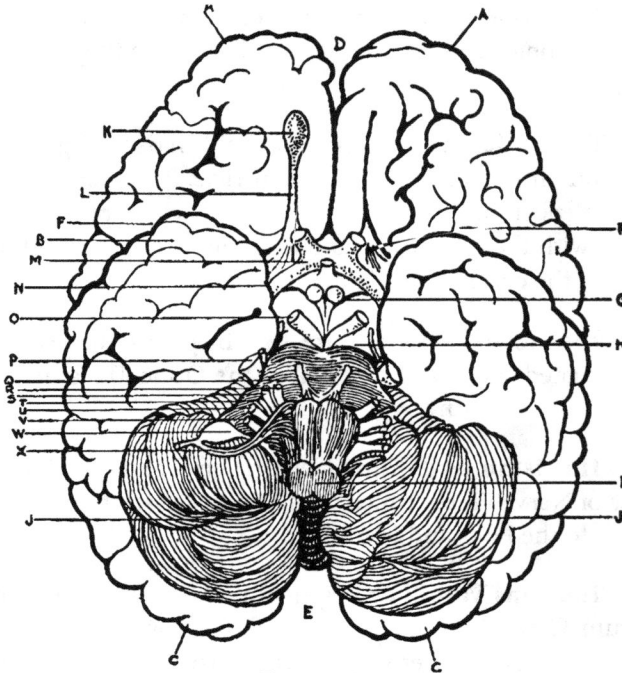

Figure 3.

A-A, frontal lobe of cerebrum; B, temporal pole; C-C, occipital pole; D, median fissure; E, posterior extremity of median fissure; F-F, Sylvian fissure; G, corpora albicanti; H, cruri cerebri or cerebral peduncle; I, medulla oblongata; J-J. hemispheres of cerebellum; K, olfactory bulb or ganglion of olfactory nerve; L, olfactory nerve or tract; M, optic chiasm or commissure; N, optic nerve or tract; O, third cranial or motoroculi nerve; P, fifth cranial or trifacial nerve; Q, sixth cranial or abducens nerve ; R, facial nerve; S, auditory nerve; T, glossopharyngeal nerve; U pneumogastric or vagus nerve; V, spinal accessory nerve; W, spinal ganglion; X, anterior roots of spinal nerve.

174

forming the cortex, and is spread out in a uniform layer. The white matter forms a compact mass in the interior. (See Figures 1, 3 and 5.)

The Medulla Oblongata is that part of the brain which connects the whole Brain and the Spinal Cord, being an enlarged continuation of the Spinal Cord upwards. It is one inch in length, extending from the lower margin of the Pons to the lower margin of the Foramen Magnus. Its surface presents two fissures; the anterior median, and the posterior median fissure.

The Floor of the 4th Ventricle is formed by the posterior surface of the Pons, and by the Medulla Oblongata. It contains eminences for the origin of a number of cranial nerves.

There are four Ventricles (Cavities). The two Lateral Ventricles are situated on either side of the Cerebrum (one in each hemisphere). These are connected to each other and to the third ventricle, which is a narrow cleft between the Optic Thalami.

The fourth Ventricle connects the third ventricle with the central canal of the Spinal Cord. It lies behind the Pons and Medulla and is covered over behind by the Cerebellum.

The Cranial Ventricles, the Central Canal of the Cord, and the space between the meninges are filled with a fluid.

The Brain is covered by three membranes called Meninges, the Dura Mater, the Arachnoid, and the Pia Mater, found in the order named from without inward.

The Dura Mater is a fibrous membrane which lines the skull and forms the internal periosteum. It is called the protective membrane, as its function is protection. It is very dense, thick, and strong. Strong fibrous partitions or septa are given off from it and pass into the cranial cavity thereby subdividing it.

The Arachnoid is the middle coat. It is a very thin, delicate, and transparent membrane.

The Pia Mater is a delicate and very vascular membrane which covers the brain and dips down into all of the fissures. It carries the arteries that nourish the outer surface of the brain.

FUNCTIONS OF THE BRAIN

The Cerebrum is the seat of sensation, memory, reasoning, volition, and emotion. These functions are located in the Cortex of

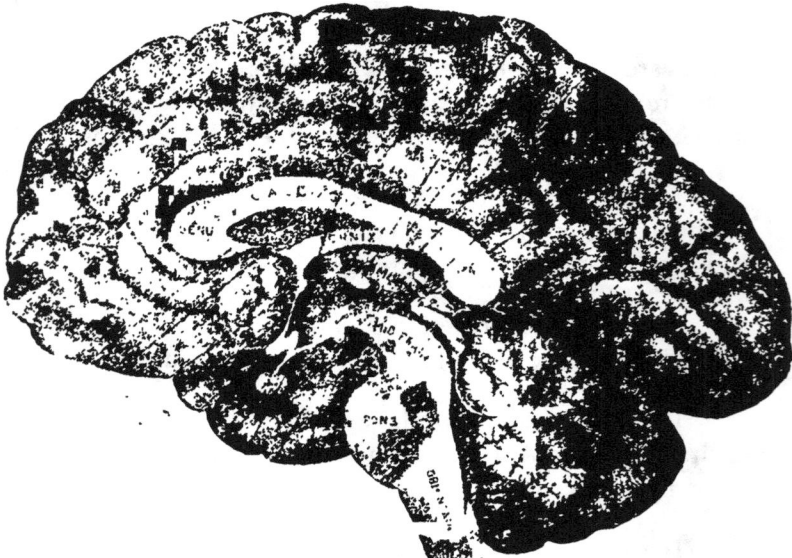

Figure 5. Internal View of Brain

Lesson 12: Nervous Physiology

The Cerebellum maintains the normal muscle tone of the body, co-ordinates complicated muscular movements (such as walking), and maintains the equilibrium or balance of the body.

The Medulla is really the upper portion of the cord, and has practically the same functions as the Spinal Cord, in addition to connecting the cord proper with the Pons (and other parts above it). It also contains the origins and terminations of the ninth, tenth, eleventh and twelfth Cranial Nerves. The most important of the vital reflex centers are located in the Medulla. Among these may be named the general Vasomotor Center, the Cardiac Center, the Respiration Center, the Centers of Mastication, Deglutition and Articulation.

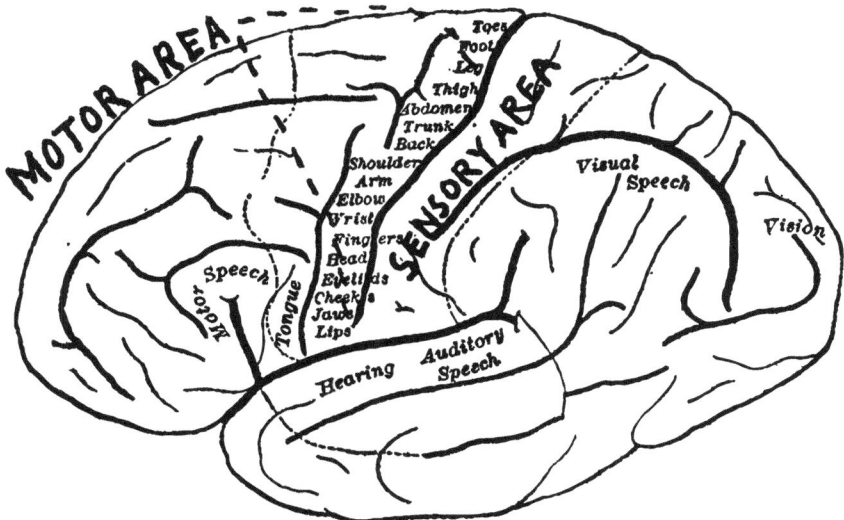

Figure 6. Side View of External Surface Showing Location of the Functional Areas of Cerebrum

The brain as a whole has complete control of all of the voluntary activities of the body, but only partial control over the involuntary activities (respiration, digestion, etc.) The functional processes of the body are controlled very largely through the spinal cord and the sympathetic system.

QUESTIONS—LESSON 12

1. Describe briefly the main divisions of the nervous system.

2. Give location of each of the five lobes of the cerebrum.

3. Describe the white matter of the cerebrum.

4. Describe the gray matter of the cerebrum.

5. Describe the medulla and pons.

6. Describe the coverings of the brain.

7. Locate and describe the 4th ventricle.

8. Give functions of the cerebrum.

9. What is the function of the Medulla?

10. If the patient had difficulty in walking or maintaining his balance, what part of the brain would you suspect as being diseased?

EXTENSION COURSE IN CHIROPRACTIC AMERICAN UNIVERSITY CHICAGO, Ill., U.S.A.

LESSON 13

THE SPINAL CORD

The Spinal Cord is that part of the Cerebro-Spinal axis which is situated in the upper two-thirds of the neural canal of the vertebral column. It is 17 to 18 inches long, cylindrical in shape, with two enlargements, one in the cervical region, the other in the lumbar.

It extends from the upper border of the axis to the lower border of the 1st lumbar vertebra, where it forms a conical extremity termed cornus medullaris, from which a slender thread continues downward within the spinal canal. This slender thread, called filum terminates, together with the lower lumbar and sacral nerve roots, forms the cauda equina or horse's tail. (See Figure 7.)

The spinal cord is not nearly as large as the neural canal so there is ample room for the motion of the spine without injury to the delicate structure.

180

Lesson 13: The Spinal Cord

The spinal cord is composed of white and gray matter, which is arranged directly opposite to that of the brain, the white being outside and the gray inside. The gray matter consists of nerve-cells, and nerve-fibres. The gray matter increases in volume relatively to the white, from above downward.

On cross-section of the cord, the gray matter will be found to resemble a letter H. The projections are called cornua or horns, and according to position they are named Anterior Horn and Posterior Horn. The anterior horn is short and broad, the posterior horn is long, narrow and pointed, and almost reaches the surface of the cord behind. (See Figure 8.)

The white matter consists of medullated nerve-fibres, blood vessels, and fibrous tissue (neuroglia). The neuroglia supports the nerve-fibres of the white substance as well as the gray matter.

The white matter has the following nerve tracts, arranged as in the accompanying illustration:

Crossed pyramidal tract, consisting of descending fibres from the Rolandic area of the cerebral cortex of the other side. It transmits 90% of motor impulses.

Direct pyramidal tract is a small nerve strand which conducts 10% of the motor impulses through descending fibres from the Rolandic area of the cerebral cortex of the same side.

Tract of Lissaur is a small tract consisting of fibres of the posterior nerve roots, and passes upward in the spinal cord.

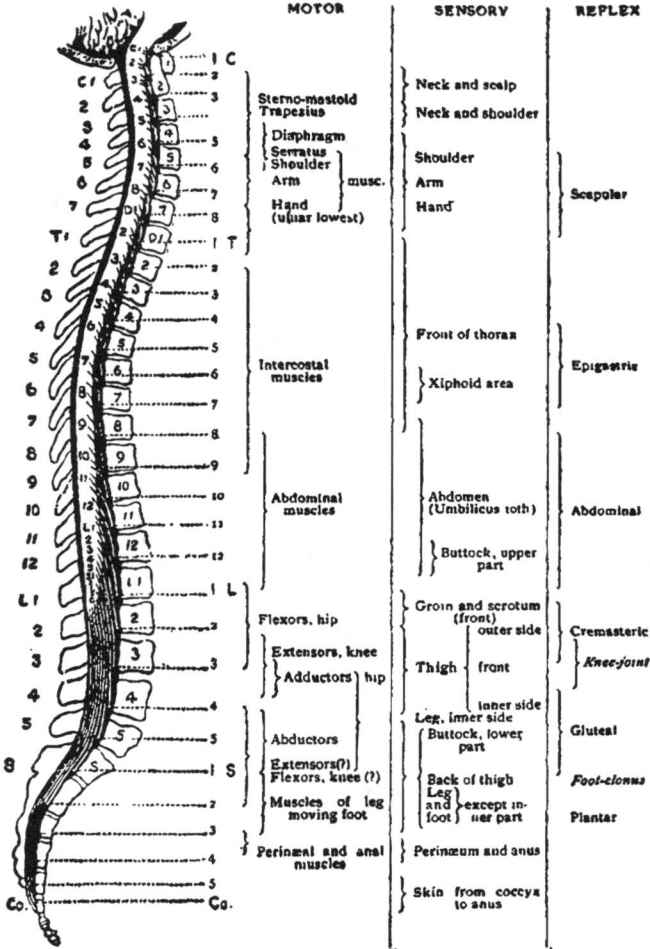

	MOTOR	SENSORY	REFLEX
		Neck and scalp	
	Sterno-mastoid Trapezius	Neck and shoulder	
	Diaphragm		
	Serratus	Shoulder	
	Shoulder		
	Arm musc.	Arm	Scapular
	Hand	Hand	
	(ulnar lowest)		
		Front of thorax	
	Intercostal muscles		Epigastric
		Xiphoid area	
	Abdominal muscles	Abdomen (Umbilicus 10th)	Abdominal
		Buttock, upper part	
		Groin and scrotum (front)	
	Flexors, hip	outer side	Cremasteric
	Extensors, knee		Knee-joint
	Adductors hip	Thigh front	
		inner side	
		Leg, inner side	
	Abductors	Buttock, lower part	Gluteal
	Extensors(?)		
	Flexors, knee (?)	Back of thigh	Foot-clonus
	Muscles of leg moving foot	Leg and except in- foot ner part	Plantar
	Perinæal and anal muscles	Perinæum and anus	
		Skin from coccyx to anus	

Figure 7. Diagram and table showing the approximate relation to the spinal nerves of the various motor, sensory and reflex functions of the spinal cord. (Arranged by Dr. Gowers from anatomical and pathological data.)—Morris' "Anatomy."

Direct cerebellar tract, commencing in the lumbar region, is composed of nerve-fibres from cells in the posterior horn, ascending through the restiform body of the Medulla Oblongata to the Cerebellum.

Antero-lateral Tract lies in front of the direct cerebellar tract, and like it, is an ascending tract. It arises in the posterior

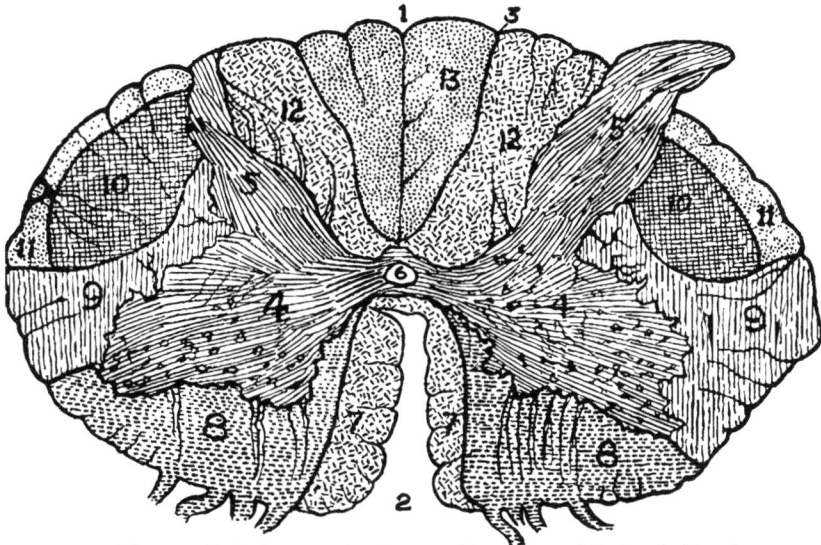

Figure 8. Schematic Cross-Section of Spinal Cord

1, posterior median septum; 2, anterior median fissure; 3, intermediate septum of pia matter between internal and eternal subdivision of posterior column; 4-4,anterior gray horns or cornua (motor); 5-5, posterior gray horns or cornua (sensory); 6, central canal of cord; 7-7, direct pyramidal tracts: 8-8, fundumental part of anterior column; 9-9, antero-lateral tracts; 10-10, crossed pyramidal tract of lateral column; 11 11, direct cerebellar tract; 12-12, column of Burdach; 13-13 column of Goll.

horn and crosses over through the gray commissure (which connects the anterior and posterior horns), and passes up through the Medulla Oblongata, Pons Varolii, to the Cerebellum through its superior peduncles.

Two tracts of Goll and Burdach (posterior columns) consisting of both ascending and descending fibres.

Thirty-one pairs of nerves, termed Spinal Nerves, are given off from the Spinal Cord. These will be described in the next lesson.

1, posterior median septum; 2, anterior median fissure; 3, intermediate septum of pia matter between internal and eternal subdivision of posterior column; 4-4,anterior gray horns or cornua (motor); 5-5, posterior gray horns or cornua (sensory); 6, central caudal of cord; 7-7, direct pyramidal tracts: 8-8, fundumental part of anterior column; 9-9, antero-lateral tracts; 10-10, crossed pyramidal tract of lateral column; 11 11, direct cerebellar tract; 12-12, column of Burdach; 13-13 column of Goll.

FUNCTIONS OF THE CORD
The functions of the Spinal Cord as a whole are as follows: (a) Carries impulses to and from the brain and periphery. (b) Receives Sensory Impulses from the skin and mucus membranes, (c) Originates motor impulses to Skeletal, Visceral and Arterial Muscles, (d) Contains reflex and special nerve centers.

GRAY MATTER (CELLS AND TERMINALS)
The Anterior Horns of the cord (Gray Matter) contain the cells of origin of the anterior roots of the Spinal Nerves and

are therefore concerned with the motor impulses to the voluntary muscles of the body.

The Posterior Horns (Gray Matter) contain the terminations of the Posterior roots of the Spinal Nerves and are therefore relay or way-stations for the Sensory Impulses from the Periphery to the brain.

The Lateral (or middle) portions of the gray matter contain the terminations of the Sensory Nerves from the Viscera and the origin of the motor nerves to the Viscera and the blood vessels. All of the involuntary activities of the organs of the body are carried on through this portion of the Spinal Cord.

WHITE MATTER (FIBRES)

When the sensory impulses reach the Posterior Horns of the cord they are transferred to the motor nerve cells in the Anterior Horns (or lateral masses) of the gray matter and they may or may not be carried to the cortex of the brain. If they reach the cortex of the Cerebrum we are made aware of their presence, (we feel them).

The Nerve Fibres of the White Matter carry sensory impulse to the brain and motor impulses from the brain to the nerve cells in the Cord.

REFLEX ACTION

Most of the involuntary activities in the body are produced by "reflex action" and most diseases are the result of some disturbance of these reflexes. All spinal lesions produce most of their bad effects through "reflex action" and most methods of treatment are effective because they affect the reflex activities.

185

When the sensory impulse reaches the motor cells in the cord a motor impulse is started outward over the motor nerves. When the motor impulses reach muscles, vessels or glands, the activity of these parts is changed in some way. A reflex act, then, is some change in the activity of some tissue or part that is produced by a motor impulse which itself was produced by a sensory impulse passing into the cord or brain.

REFLEX CENTERS

Whenever there is a collection of nerve cells for the purpose of carrying on some special function these groups of cells are called reflex centers. The following reflex centers are located in the Spinal Cord:

(a) Physiological, or Functional, such as, Respiration, Circulation, Vaso-constriction, Perspiration, Digestion, Micturition, Defecation, Parturition.t

(b) Skin, or Tendon, such as, Plantar, Cresmasteric, Gluteal, Abdominal, Epigastric, Scapular, Pupillary, Achilles Patellar, Tricep, Jaw.

NERVES

When a large number of nerve fibres (outside of the brain and cord) are gathered together in one bundle, the collection is called a Nerve. At various places along these nerves there are collections of nerve cells each of which is called a Ganglion. A network of nerves, or nerve fibres and nerve cells, is called a Plexus.

The nerve fibres that carry impulses from the skin, muscles, joints, blood vessels, the serous and mucus membranes to the cord or to the brain are called Sensory Nerves. The nerve fibres

186

that carry impulses from the brain or the cord to the voluntary or visceral muscles, the blood vessels or glands are called Motor Nerves.

Anything that irritates the Sensory Nerve Endings (electricity, chemicals, vibration, 'heat, pressure, light, sound, atmospheric changes, etc.) will start the nerve impulses over the Sensory Nerve Fibres. Motor Nerve impulses are started by sensory impulses or by chemical changes in the nerve cells.

CRANIAL NERVES

There are 12 pairs of nerves given off from the brain. Their point of exit is through some foramen in the cranium, hence they are termed, the Cranial Nerves. These nerves are numbered according to their origin; the nerve with the highest origin being the 1st Cranial Nerve, and the nerve with the lowest origin being the 12th Cranial Nerve. They are also named according to their function and part they supply. Numbers and names are as follows:

The 1st Cranial, or Olfactory Nerve begins in the mucus membrane of the upper portion of the nasal cavity and passes through the ethmoid and above the spenoid bone to the temporal, lobe of the cerebrum. Its function is that of smell.

The 2nd. or Optic, Nerve begins in the retina of the eye and passes backward through the sphenoid bone to the occipital lobe of the cerebrum. Its function is that of sight.

The 3rd, or Motor Oculi, Nerve begins in the Isthmus (between the third and fourth ventricles) and passes forward to supply the ciliary muscle of the eye which is contracted during near vision, and to the internal rectus muscle of the eye.

The 4th, or Trochlear, Nerve begins in the Isthmus and supplies one of the external muscles of the eye.

5th or Trifacial Nerve, arises from the pons by two roots, a sensory and a motor. The sensory nerve expands, at the apex of the petrous portion of the temporal bone, into a ganglia termed the Gasserian Ganglion: from this three large branches arise:

A. Ophthalmic Division, sensory. Above the sphenoid bone it divides into three main branches: to the Lachrymal gland, mucous membrane of eye and nose, also skin of forehead and nose.

B. Superior Maxillary Division, sensory to cheek, temple, nose, lower eyelid, lips, upper teeth, and the palate.

C. Inferior Maxillary Division, motor to the muscles of mastication, sensory to the lower teeth and gums, the skin of temple, external ear, lower face, lower lip, and to the anterior 2/3 of tongue.

The 6th, or Abducens, Nerve begins in the Pons and supplies one of the external muscles of the eye.

The 7th, or Facial, Nerve begins in the Pons and passes outward through the temporal bone to supply the muscles of the face and to the salivary glands. It also carries the sensation of taste from the anterior portion of the tongue.

The 8th, or Auditory. Nerve begins by two divisions. One from the cochlea of the inner ear,and the other from the semi-circular canals of the inner ear. It carries sensations of sound to the anterior portions of the temporal lobe of the cerebrum, and sensations of equilibrium to the Pons and Medulla.

Lesson 13: The Spinal Cord

The 9th, or Glosso-Paryngeal, Nerve originates in the Medulla, and passes downward and forward between the temporal and occipital bones to the muscles of the pharynx and to the parotid gland. The sensation of taste from the posterior portion of the tongue is carried to the brain over this nerve. The 10th, or Vagus, Nerve has the same origin and course as the 9th until it leaves the skull, after which it passes down just inside the Sterno-Cleido-Mastoid Muscle. It supplies the muscles of the throat and all of the organs of the chest and abdomen. It is both motor and sensory in function. (See Figure 9.)

The 11th, or Spinal Accessory, Nerve begins in the Medulla and follows the same path with the 9th to supply the muscles of the throat and neck.

The 12th, or Hypo-Glossal, Nerve also begins in the Medulla and passes through the occipital bone to supply the muscles of the tongue.

Plate 7 of the Charts should be studied with this lesson.

	NAME	SUP. ORIGIN	DEEP ORIGIN	EXIT	DISTRIBUTION	FUNCTION
1	Olfactory	Olfactory Bulb	Temporal lobe	Ethmoid bone	Schneiderian Membrane of Nose	Special Sense (Smell)
2	Optic	Optic Thalmus	Occipital lobe	Sphenoid bone	Retina of Eye	Special Sense (Sight)
3	Motor Oculi	Crus Cerebri	Isthmus	Sphenoid bone	All Muscles of Eye except Oblique and Ext. Rectus	Motor to Eye-Ball
4	Trochlear	Crus Cerebri	Isthmus	Sphenoid bone	Superior Oblique Muscle of Eye	Motor to Eye-Ball
5	Trifacial	Side of Pons	Floor of 4th Ventricle	Sphenoid bone	Head, Face, Teeth, Eyes and Tongue	Motor to Jaw muscles. Sensory to Head, Face, Jaws Eyes and Tongue
6	Abducent	Pons	Floor of 4th Ventricle	Sphenoid bone	External Rectus	Motor to Eye-Ball
7	Facial	Pons	Floor of 4th Ventricle	Temporal Bone	Scalp, Face and Tongue	Motor to Muscles of face and scalp. Special Sense, to Tongue. (Taste)
8	Auditory	Post border of Pons	Floor of 4th Ventricle	Does not leave Cranium	Internal Ear	Special Sense (Hearing)
9	Glossopha-ryngea	Medulla	Floor of 4th Ventricle	Between Temporal and Occipital bones	Tongue, Tonsils, and adja-cent membranes	Sensory and Special Sense (Taste)
10	Pneumogas-tric	Medulla	Floor of 4th Ventricle	Between Temporal and Occipital bones	Larynx, Pharynx, Trachea, all thoracic and abdominal organs	Motor and Sensory
11	Spinal	Medulla and Cord	Floor of 4th Ventricle and gray matter of cord	Between Temporal and Occipital bones	Muscles of tongue and throat	Motor to Muscles
12	Hypo-Glossal	Medulla	Floor of 4th Ventricle	Occipital Bone	Muscles of Tongue and Throat	Motor to throat and tongue

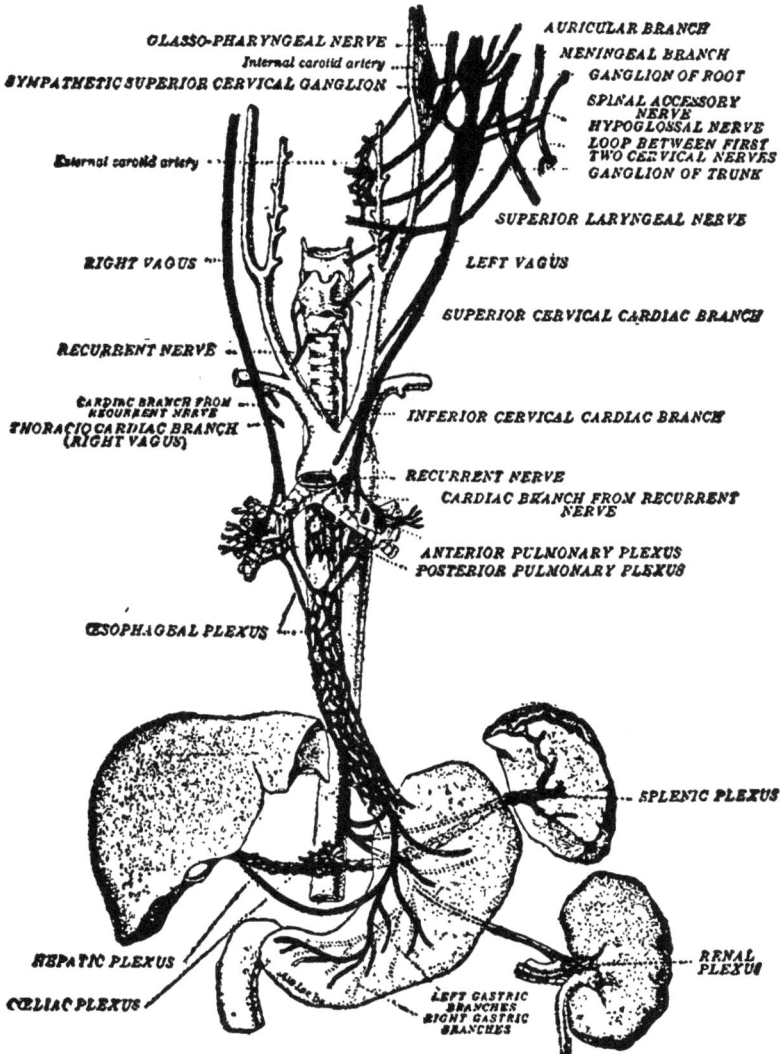

Figure 9. The Vagus Nerves and Their Connections. (Morris)

QUESTIONS—LESSON 13

1. Locate and briefly describe the spinal cord.

2. What is the difference between the gray matter and the white matter of the cord?

3. Name the nerve tracts in the white matter of the spinal cord.

4. If the patient had paralysis of the right leg what part of thecord would you suspect as being diseased?

5. What has the cord to do with involuntary activities, like digestion?

6. Name the Cranial Nerves in their order.

7. Give distribution and functions of the 5th Cranial Nerve.

8. Describe the Vagus, or 10th Cranial Nerve.

9. Which of the Cranial Nerves are Motor nerves?

10. What nerve is affected in toothache.

Lesson 13: The Spinal Cord

EXTENSION COURSE
IN CHIROPRACTIC
AMERICAN UNIVERSITY
CHICAGO, Ill., U.S.A.

LESSON 14

SPINAL NERVES AND PLEXUSES

The Spinal Nerves are arranged in pairs, of which there are thirty-one. They arise from the spinal cord by two roots, an anterior motor root and a posterior sensory one. These roots pierce the Dura Mater in separate places, but join to form the Spinal Nerve before they pass out of the Spinal Canal. The posterior root has a ganglion upon it, while the anterior root has none.

After the two sets of nerve roots join, they are enclosed in a single sheet of Dura Mater and in that form pass through Intervertebral Foramen, emerging from which, the nerve immediately divides into the anterior primary division, and posterior primary division. The former is connected with the sympathetic nerves through gray and white communicantes, making the sympathetic nerves visceral branches of the spinal nerves. These nerves will be described in our next lesson.

The anterior primary divisions divide into many branches which supply the skeletal muscles and the skin over them. The

194

Posterior primary divisions supply the deep muscles of the back and the skin over them and is of extreme importance to the Chiropractor.

The Spinal Nerves are named according to the region of the cord from which they take origin. There are 8 pairs of Cervical Nerves, 12 pairs of Dorsal Nerves, 5 pairs of Lumbar Nerves, 5 pairs of Sacral Nerves, and 1 Coccygeal Nerve. (See Figure 10.)

The anterior primary divisions of the Spinal Nerves (except the second to the eleventh dorsals) are joined together to form four large plexuses, each of which consists of a network of nerve fibres. The anterior primary divisions of the 2nd to the 11th dorsal nerves pass forward between the ribs and are known as the intercostal nerves. They supply the chest and abdominal muscles and the skin of the chest and abdomen. (See Figure 11.)

VISCERAL DIVISIONS

While the spinal nerves have no direct connection to the internal organs of the body, they are very closely connected to all of the organs through the rami-communicantes which connect the anterior divisions of the spinal nerves with the two sympathetic cords that lie in front of the spinal column. (This connection is shown very clearly in the accompanying sketches.) (See Figure 12.) Fibres extending from the ganglia of the sympathetic cords make up the sympathetic plexuses, which control the action of the various organs (See Lesson 15.)

For all practical purposes of diagnosis and treatment each spinal nerve may be considered as having three divisions: Anterior primary division, which supplies the voluntary muscles of the body and the skin overlying them, Posterior primary

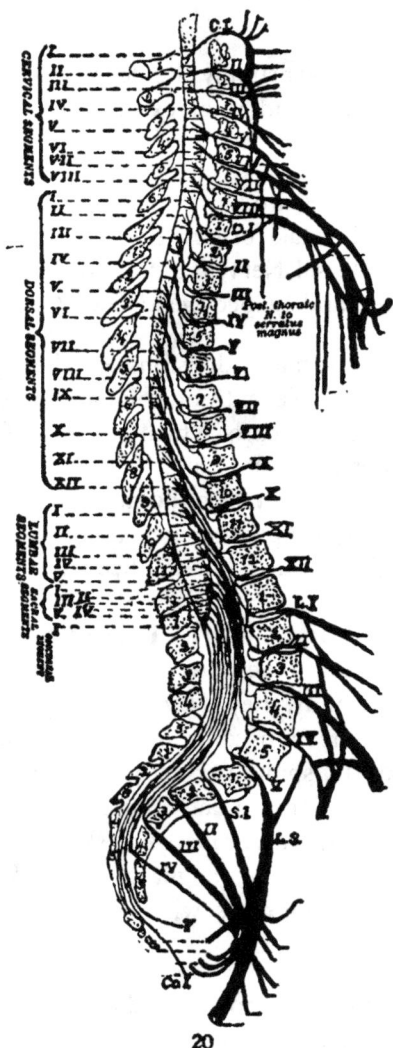

Figure 10. Side View of Spinal Column and Spinal Cord, showing Spinal Nerve and Plexuses

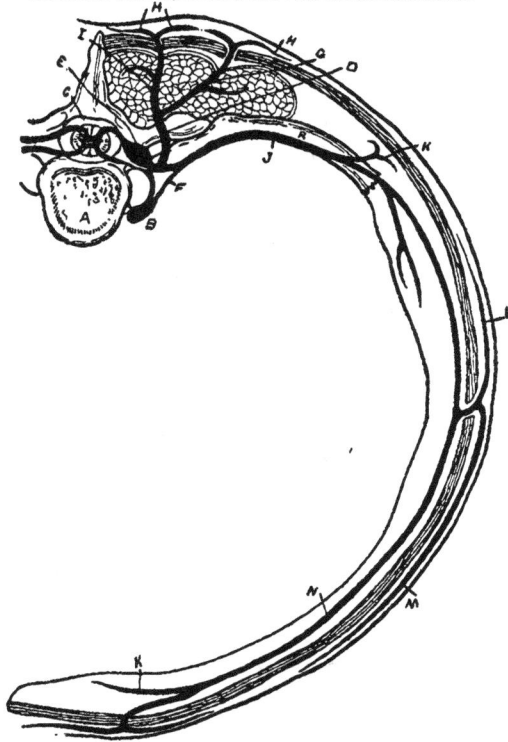

Figure 11.
Diagram of Dorsal Nerve Distribution.
A, body of vertebra; B, sympathetic ganglion; C, spinal cord; D, posterior primary division of dorsal nerve; E, intervertebral or spinal ganglion on the posterior roots; F, rami communicans between the sympathetic and cerebro-spinal nervous systems; G, external branch; H-H, cutaneous branches; I, internal branch: J, anterior primary division; K-K, muscular branches; L, posterior branch of lateral cutaneous nerve; M, anterior branch of lateral cutaneous nerve; N, anterior cutaneous nerve; R, rib, broken off.

division which supplies the deep muscles behind the vertebrae and Visceral division, which supplies some organ or organs of the body (through the rami- communicates and the sympathetic system.) (See Figure 11).

The posterior primary division is very frequently irritated or impinged by spinal lesions. The effects of this irritation, if prolonged or severe, will radiate to all divisions of this same nerve. This will interfere with the functional activity and nutrition of the affected organs and may produce pain, tenderness, or muscular contraction in the parts supplied by the anterior or peripheral divisions of the nerves.

When the visceral division is irritated, through disease in some organ, pain, tenderness and muscular contraction are produced in the parts supplied by the other two divisions of that spinal nerve.

PLEXUSES
There are four Cerebro-Spinal Plexuses named according to their location: Cervical, Brachial, Lumbar and Sacral.

The Cervical Plexus is formed by the four upper cervical nerves. It lies underneath the Sterno-cleido-mastoid muscle. In front of it lies the rectus capitus anticus and behind lies the scalenus merius. It gives off 4 superficial branches and 6 deep. These branches contain both Sensory and Motor fibres and supply the muscles of the neck and shoulders and the skin overlying them.

The Brachial Plexus is located in the neck and axilla, lying between the Anterior and Middle Scaleni muscles, and surrounds the axillary artery. It is formed from the anterior primary divisions of the 5th, 6th, 7th, 8th Cervical and first Dorsal nerves. The divisions unite to form three large trunks. The branches from these trunks supply the muscles of the shoulders, arms, and hands, and the skin overlying these muscles, as well as some of the muscles of the chest. This is the largest of all the Cerebro-Spinal Plexuses. (See Figure 13.)

Schematic Diagram of Brachial Plexus

The Lumbar Plexus is formed by the anterior primary division of the three upper lumbar nerves, a part of the 4th lumbar, and a branch of the 12th dorsal. It is located in the substance of the Psoas Muscle in front of the transverse processes of the lumbar vertebrae. Its branches supply the muscles of the hip, anterior, outer and inner thigh and the skin of the lower abdomen, hips, genitals, thigh, inner and anterior leg.

The Sacral Plexus is placed on the posterior wall of the pelvis and is formed by branches from the anterior primary divisions of the 4th and 5th lumbar and the 1st, 2nd, and 3rd sacral nerves. The branches from this plexus supply the muscles of the leg, foot, and posterior thigh and the skin of the posterior thigh, and the posterior and outer leg.

SPECIAL NERVES

The Phrenic Nerve arises mainly from the 4th cervical, but is reinforced from the roots of the 3rd and 5th cervicals. It passes downward in the neck and enters the thorax between the Subclavian artery and vein, and then traverses the mediastinum to reach the Diaphragm, of which it is the motor nerve.

The Great Sciatic Nerve is the largest nerve in the body, and is formed by two main nerves of the sacral plexus bound

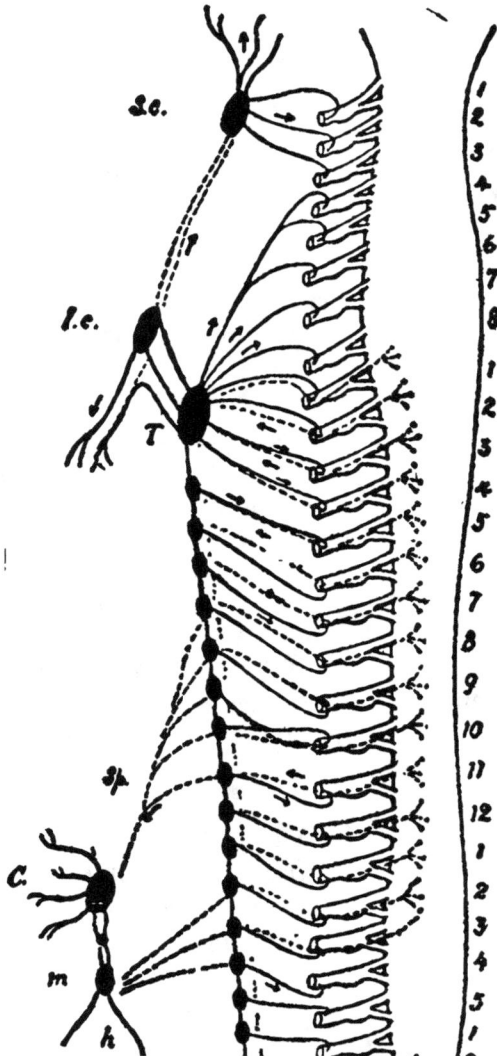

Figure 12. Connections Between Spinal Nerves and Sympathetic Cords. (Abrams.)

together by an investing sheath. After passing through the Great Sacro-sciatic

Foramen, it enters the buttock, passes downward along the back of the thigh to the knee, where it divides into the external

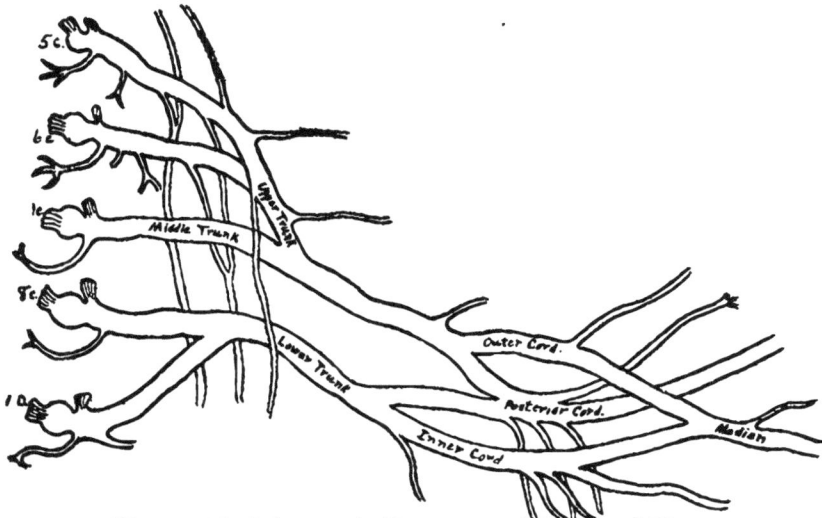

Figure 13. Schematic Diagram of Brachial Plexus.
and internal Popliteal. (See Plate 7 of Charts.)

The Pubic Nerve is formed from the lower portion of the sacral plexus and passes out of the pelvis beneath the pyriformis muscle through the great Sacro-Sciatic Foramen. After crossing the spine of the Ischium it re-enters the pelvis and passes forward to supply the skin and muscles of the perineum and the external genitals.

201

There are also some visceral branches from the 2nd, 3rd and 4th sacral nerves which supply the bladder, rectum and the vagina. Reference will be made to these branches in Lesson 15.

QUESTIONS—LESSON 14

1. Locate all and describe one of the spinal nerve plexuses.

2. Why is the posterior primary division of the spinal nerve so important to a Chiropractor?

3. How can impingement of a spinal nerve affect the stomach when the stomach is supplied by the Sympathetic Nervous System?

4. Describe the Phrenic Nerve.

5. Describe the Great Sciatic Nerve.

6. How do the anterior divisions of the sacral nerves differ from those of the other spinal nerves?

7. What is peculiar about the dorsal spinal nerves?

8. What is the difference in function between the anterior roots and the posterior roots of the spinal nerves?

9. Describe the Intercostal Nerves.

10. Describe the Pubic Nerve.

EXTENSION COURSE
IN CHIROPRACTIC
AMERICAN UNIVERSITY
CHICAGO, Ill., U.S.A.

———

LESSON 15

———

THE SYMPATHETIC NERVOUS SYSTEM

The divisions of the sympathetic nervous system are given in Lesson 12. Each division will be described in detail in this lesson.

The two gangliated cords which make up the central portion of the Sympathetic Nervous System are connected at the top by the ganglion of Ribs which is located near the base of the skull. Their lower extremities are connected by the ganglia of Impar which lies in front of the coccyx. (See Figures 14, 15 and 16.)

The Gangliated cords are connected with a cerebro-spinal system through a set of small fibres termed the Rami Communicantes. The fibres passing from the sympathetic to the cerebro-spinal system are the gray rami communicantes; and the fibres passing from the cerebro-spinal to the sympathetic system are the white rami communicantes.

The cervical portion of the sympathetic cord consists of a superior, a middle and an inferior ganglion, on each side of

Lesson 15: The Sympathetic Nervous System

the neck. This part of the gangliated cord is characterized by the absence of the white rami communcantes. The branches from the cervical part of the sympathetic cord are distributed to various structures of the head, neck and thorax.

The three ganglia on the cervical parts of these cords are much larger than in other regions. These ganglia are located as follows:

The Superior Cervical Ganglion is the largest of all the Sympathetic Ganglions and is about one inch in length. It is located in front of the second and third Cervical Vertebrae.

The Middle Cervical Ganglion is very small and sometimes absent. It is located in front of the fifth Cervical Vertebrae.

The Inferior Cervical Ganglion lies in front of the seventh Cervical Vertebrae.

The Thoracic Ganglia are irregular shaped; each one of them receives a branch from the corresponding dorsal nerve (white rami communicantes). These white rami divide into two main streams; the five upper passing upward to the cervical sympathetic cord and having the same function as it; while the lower rami are distributed to the abdominal and thoracic organs. The gray rami communicantes arise from the ganglia, and following the course of the rami, they connect with the anterior primary divisions of the dorsal nerves.

There are four or five small ganglia in the Lumbar portion of the Gangliated Cords, which lie on either side of the Lumbar Vertebrae. There are also four or five ganglia on the Sacral portion of the cords, which lie in front of the Sacrum.

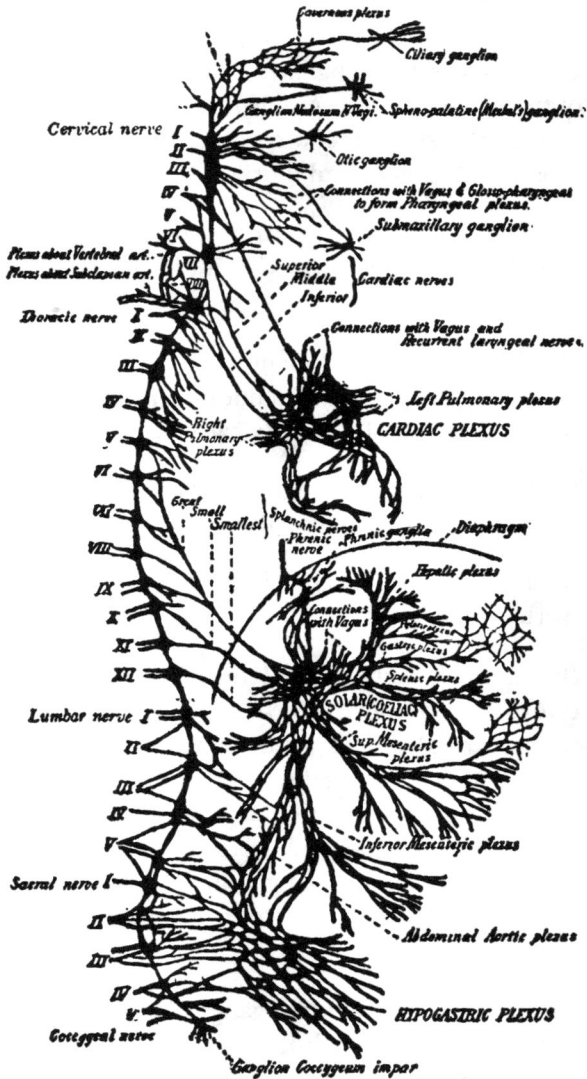

Figure 14. Side View of Sympathetic Nervous System. (Morris.)

Lesson 15: The Sympathetic Nervous System

The Great Plexuses of the sympathetic system are large bundles of nerves located in the thoracic, abdominal, and pelvic cavities, surrounding the visceral branches of the aorta. They are termed Cardiac, Solar, and Hypogastric Plexuses, according to their location. Branches from these plexuses form smaller plexuses which control functions of their individual viscera. (See Figure 14.)

The Cardiac Plexus is located at the origin of the aorta from the heart. It is divided into a deep portion and a superficial portion which are connected very closely with each other. This plexus is made up of branches from the three Cervical Sympathetic ganglia which are interwoven with branches of the Vagus Nerve. (10th Cranial.)

The Solar Plexus, also called the Epigastric Plexus on account of its location above and behind the stomach, is composed of three parts: the Celiac Plexus which surrounds the origin of the Celiac axis from the aorta between the crura of the diaphragm, and the two Semilunar Ganglions which rest upon the crura of the diaphragm and are overlapped by the suprarenal capsules.

The three sets of nerve fibres that connect this plexus with the lower dorsal ganglia are called Splanchnic Nerves. Branches from the Vagus (10th Cranial) Nerve also assist in forming this plexus.

The Hypo-Gastric Plexus is located on the posterior wall of the pelvis and is connected to the Solar Plexus by a large mass of nerve fibres and nerve cells which surround the aorta (called aortic plexus.) Branches from the Lumbar Sympathetic Ganglion combine with branches from the anterior divisions of the 2nd, 3rd, and 4th Sacral Nerves to form this plexus. (These visceral branches of the Sacral Plexus were mentioned in the preceding lesson.)

Surrounding all of the large blood vessels and near, or in, all important organs there are Smaller Individual Plexuses which have the same name as the organ or artery with which they are connected. Branches from these last named plexuses govern the activities of the organs and the size of the arteries (through the vaso-motor system).

THE VASO-MOTOR APPARATUS
This system of nerves governs the distribution of blood to all parts and organs of the body. Its chief center is located in the Medulla Oblongata, but throughout the Dorsal and upper Lumbar region of the Spinal Cord, subsidiary centers are located. The vaso-motor nerves are divided into two sets. Vaso-Constrictors and Vaso-Dilators.

The Vaso-Constrictor Nerves arise from the second dorsal to the second lumbar sympathetic ganglia of the sympathetic and pass through the gray Remi-Communicantes to the Vaso-Constrictor centers in the cord which are located from the second dorsal to the second lumbar region of the cord. From these centers in the cord the vaso-constrictor fibres pass out through the Spinal Nerves to supply the muscles which form the middle coat of the arteries and veins. When the vaso-constrictor nerves are stimulated the vessels contract and decrease the amount of blood in the part supplied by those vessels.

The Vaso Dilator Nerves originate in the Spinal Cord in the same segments that the motor and sensory nerves arise for the part which they supply. In addition to accompanying the Spinal

Nerves the Vaso Dilator fibres are included in the 5th, 7th, 9th, 10th, 11th and 12th Cranial Nerves and in the Visceral branches of the Sacral Plexus.

SPINAL SEGMENTS

For purposes of diagnosis and treatment the spinal cord may be considered as being made up of 31 segments which are placed one above the other. Each segment contains the cells of origin of the motor divisions of the Spinal Nerves and the terminal fibres of the sensory root of the Spinal Nerves as well as the cells which govern the activities of the organs that are supplied by that Spinal Nerve (through the Rami-Communicantes of the Sympathetic).

Each Spinal Segment controls the functional activities of those parts of the body that are supplied by the three branches (Anterior, Posterior, and Visceral) of the two spinal nerves that are connected to that segment. All of the spinal segments are under the control of the brain.

THE AUTONOMIC NERVOUS SYSTEM

The Nervous System is divided anatomically into the Cerebro-Spinal and the Sympathetic System, but this is not a good division from a physiological standpoint, because some of the Cerebro-Spinal Nerves are concerned in the involuntary activities of the body.

The term Autonomic is used to describe those parts of the Nervous System that have to do with the physiological functions of the various organs of the body. Included in this system are the Sympathetic System, the 3rd, 5th, 7th, 9th, 10th, 11th Cranial

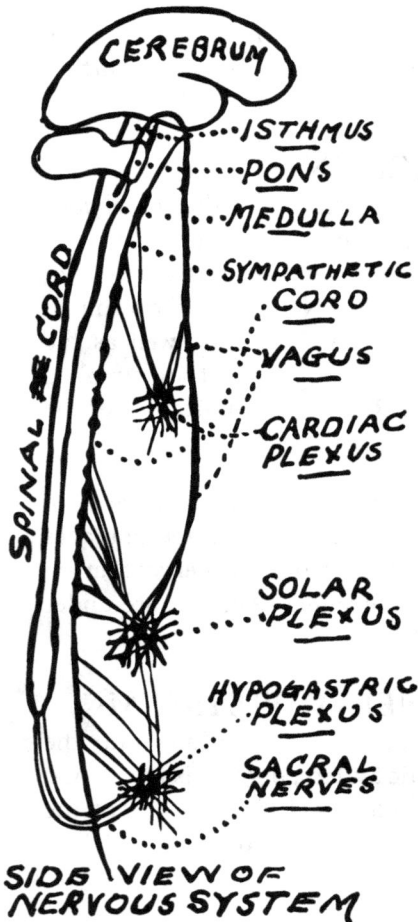

Figure 15.

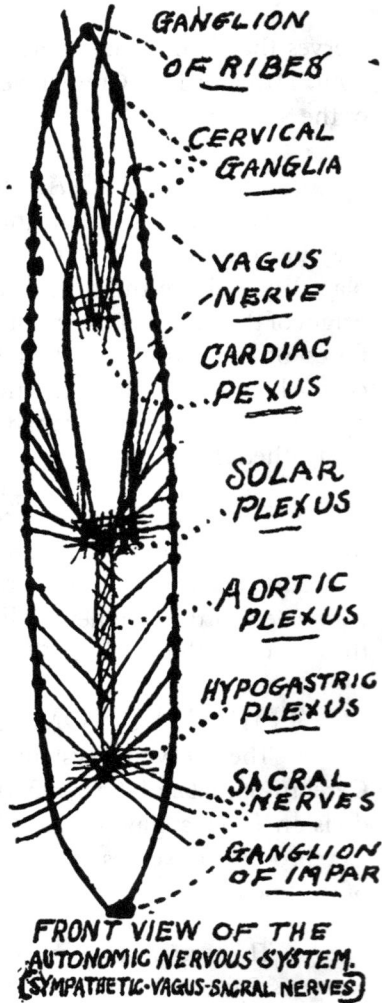

Figure 16.

210

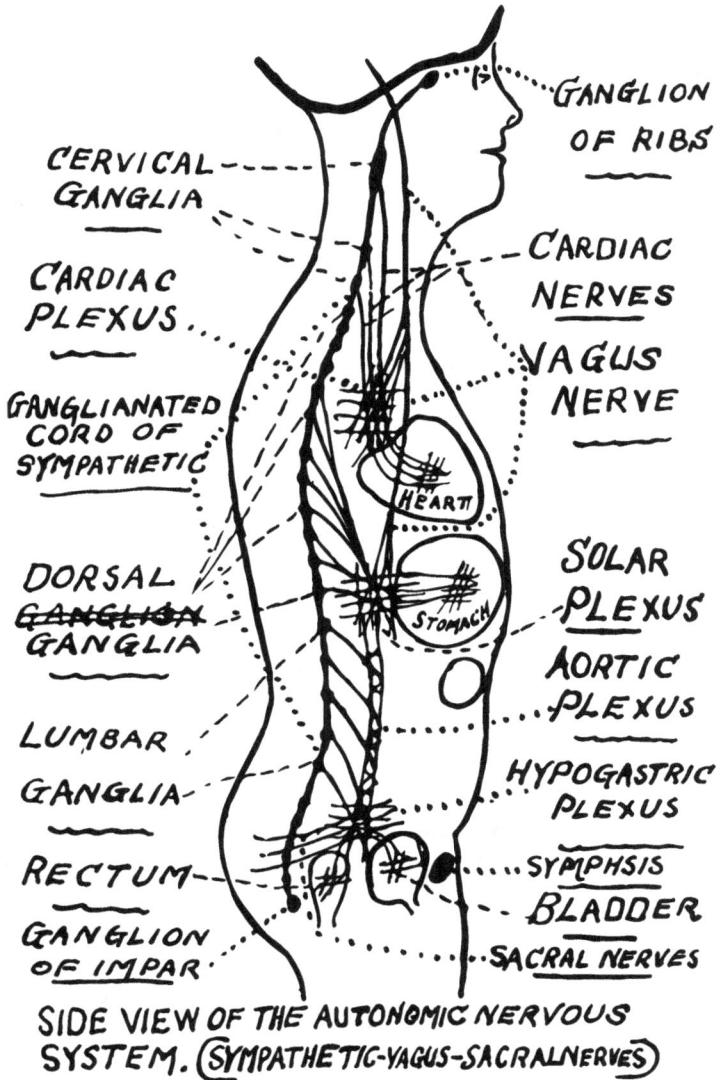

SIDE VIEW OF THE AUTONOMIC NERVOUS SYSTEM. (SYMPATHETIC-VAGUS-SACRAL NERVES)

Figure 17.

211

Nerves and the Visceral Branches of the Sacral plexus as well as the Vaso-motor Nervous System. (See Figures 15, 16 and 17.)

Included in the functions of the autonomic system are digestion, elimination, circulation, respiration, reproduction, mastication, deglutition, accommodation, etc.

Practically every organ in the body is supplied both by fibres from the gangliated cords of the Sympathetic and by fibres from the Cranial (especially vagus) or from the Sacral Nerves.

The effects of impulses through the sympathetic nervous system are just the opposite of those of impulses through the spinal or cranial nerves. The sympathetic increases the rate and force of the muscular contraction of the heart, the bronchial tubes, and maintains the contraction of the muscles of the ileo-cecle valve, the uterine cervix and of the sphincters of the bladder and rectum. It also maintains the normal constriction of the arteries of the chest, abdomen and pelvis as well as all other parts of the body.

The 10th and 11th cranial and the 2nd, 3rd and 4th sacral nerves have an effect exactly the opposite to that of the sympathetic. Impulses over these nerves decrease the frequency and power of the contraction of the muscles of the heart, the bronchial tubes and decreases the contractal power of the ileo-cecle valve, the cervix of the uterus and the sphincters of the bladder and rectum. These nerves increase the tone and contractal power of the muscles of the stomach, intestines, colon, uterus and bladder. Vaso-dilator impulses are also carried over these nerves to the vessels of the chest, abdomen and pelvis. The 5th and 7th cranial nerves are the vaso-dilators of the head.

QUESTIONS–LESSON 15

1. What is the Sympathetic Nervous System?

2. Is the Sympathetic a separate nervous system from the Cerebro-Spinal? Explain your answer.

3. Locate and describe the Solar plexus.

4. Locate and describe the Hypo-gastric plexus.

5. Locate and describe the Cardiac plexus.

6. Describe the Splanchnic nerves.

7. Briefly describe the Vaso-motor Nervous System.

8. What is a spinal segment?

9. What is the Autonomic Nervous System?

10. Give the functions of the Sympathetic Nervous System.

CHIROPRACTIC

The Science of Spinal Adjustment

———

A SERIES OF LESSONS CORRELATING AND
SYSTEMATIZING THE KNOWLEDGE NECESSARY
TO PRACTICE CHIROPRACTIC

Nature's Greatest Ally

IN RESTORING DISEASED CONDITIONS OF THE
BODY TO PERFECT HEALTH, WITHOUT THE AID
OF DRUGS OR SURGERY

———

BOOK 5

GASTRO-INTESTINAL SYSTEM

Lesson 16, 17, 18 19 and 20

———

ORIGINALLY PUBLISHED BY
AMERICAN UNIVERSITY
CHICAGO, ILLINOIS, U.S.A.

Disclaimer

We are proud to republish this series of books on chiropractic medicine.
Originally published as a home-study course in 1913 by American University in Chicago, the 16 volumes give us an historical look at the theory and practice of chiropractic medicine in the early part of the 20th century.

This series is republished for historical interest only. The modern practice of chiropractic has advanced significantly in the century since these books were published. If you want to actually learn modern chiropractic techniques, please consult one of the many fine schools in this country.

The materials in these books are not intended to diagnose or treat disease. If you believe you are ill consult a licensed practitioner for care immediately. The publishers assume no liability for the use, misuse or nonuse of the materials in these books.

Thank you

EXTENSION COURSE
IN CHIROPRACTIC
AMERICAN UNIVERSITY
CHICAGO, Ill., U.S.A.

LESSON 16

DIGESTIVE ORGANS

The Digestive Organs consist of the Alimentary Canal and certain organs that are connected with this canal. The alimentary canal includes the Mouth, Pharynx, Esophagus, Stomach, Small Intestines, Colon and Rectum. (See Figure 1.)

The Appendages are the Teeth, Tongue, Salivary Glands, Liver, Gall Bladder and Pancreas. Each part will be described separately.

The Mouth is an oval-shaped cavity between the upper and lower jaws; it is lined with Mucous Membrane. The part of the mouth between the teeth and the cheeks and lips is called the Vestibule. The Oral Cavity is the part inside of the teeth and in front of the pharynx.

The Palate forms the roof of the mouth. The anterior portion is formed by the maxillary and palate bones and is called the Hard Palate. The posterior portion is formed by muscular and fibrous tissue and is movable. It is the Soft Palate. The Tonsils are two lymphoid glands on either side of the mouth just in front of the pharynx. They lie between two pillars of muscles. (See Figure 2.)

The Salivary Glands are located in the walls and floor of the mouth. The Parotid Glands are in the posterior upper portion of the lateral wall (in front of the ear). The Submaxillary Glands are just inside the angle of the mandible. The Sublingual are in the anterior portion of the floor of the mouth (under tongue). All glands are in pairs, three on each side. (See (a), (b) and (c) of Figure 2 of Plate VI of the Charts.)

The Tongue is one of the digestive organs, but will be described in Lesson 19, as it is also an organ of special sense.

The Teeth are bony appendages of the jaws. They are composed of a special type of bone covered by a hard enamel. Each individual has two sets of teeth. The Temporary Teeth are twenty in number (ten on each jaw); there are eight incisor, four canine and eight milk molar teeth. The Permanent Teeth replace the temporary teeth, beginning at the sixth year and continuing to the twentieth year, at which time there should be thirty-two (eight incisor, four canine, eight bicuspid and twelve molar). (See Figure 5 on Plate VI of Charts.)

The Pharynx is the conical musculo-membranous tube suspended from the base of the skull and behind the mouth and nasal cavity. It is 4 1/2 inches long and has three coats or layers of different kinds of tissue. The outer coat is composed of fibrous tissue; the middle coat of voluntary muscle, and the inner coat is a continuation of the mucous membrane that lines the mouth. (See Figure 1, Plate VIII, of Charts.)

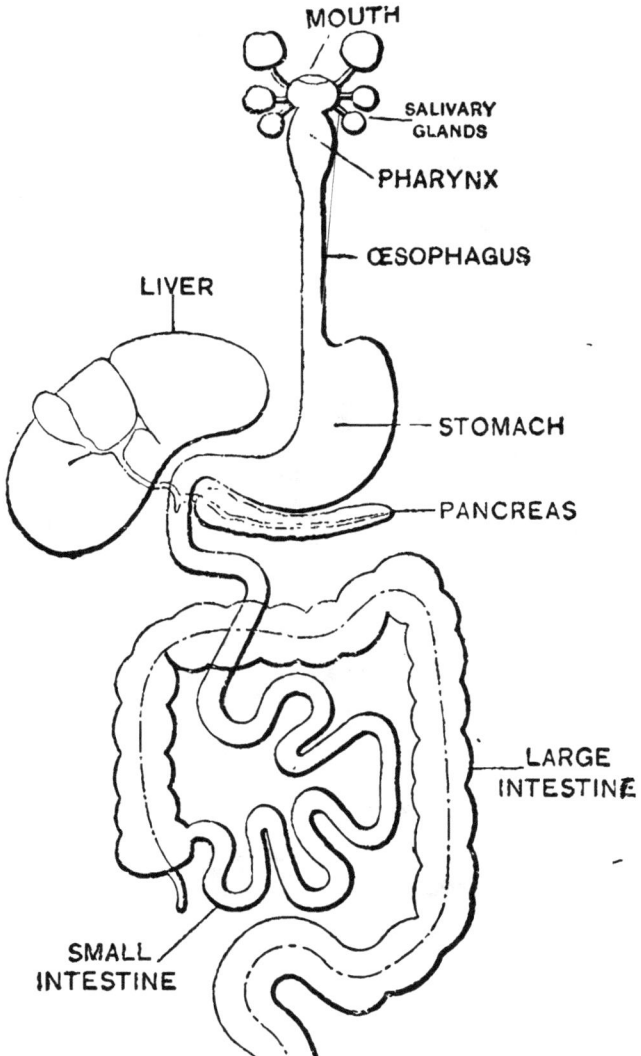

Figure 1

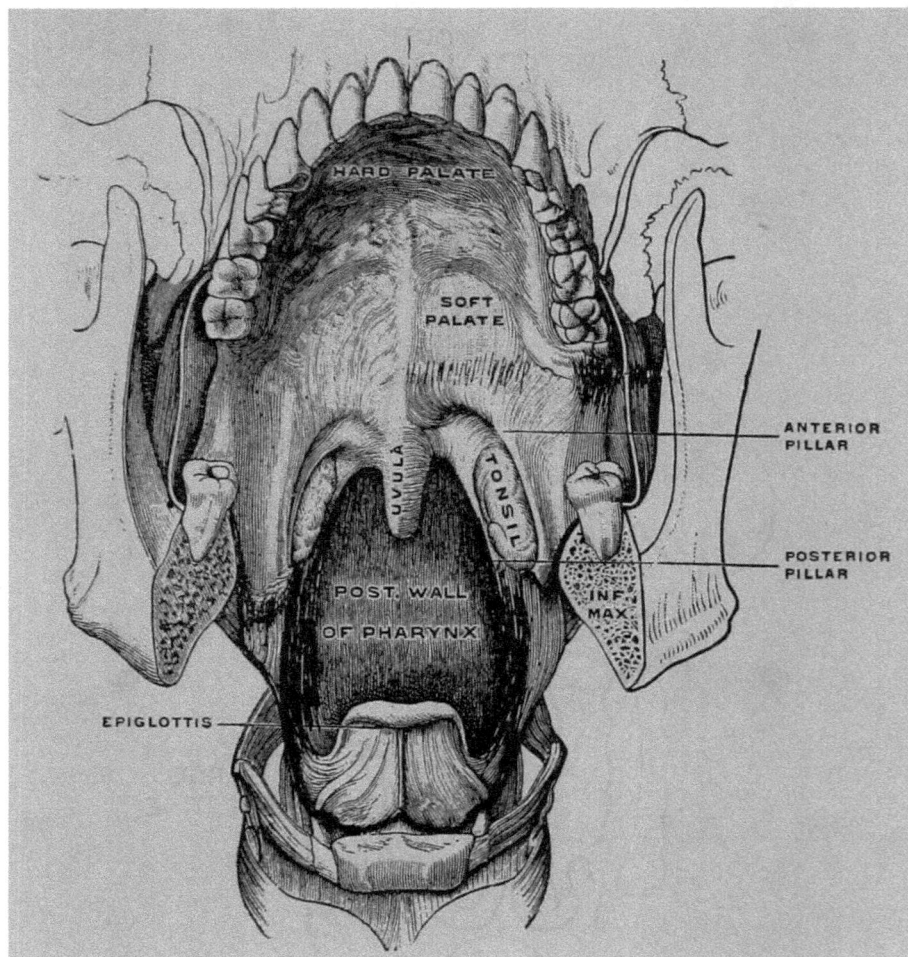

Figure 2

The Esophagus is a musculo-membranous tube connecting the pharynx with the stomach. It lies in front of the vertebral column and is nine inches long. Its outer coat is composed

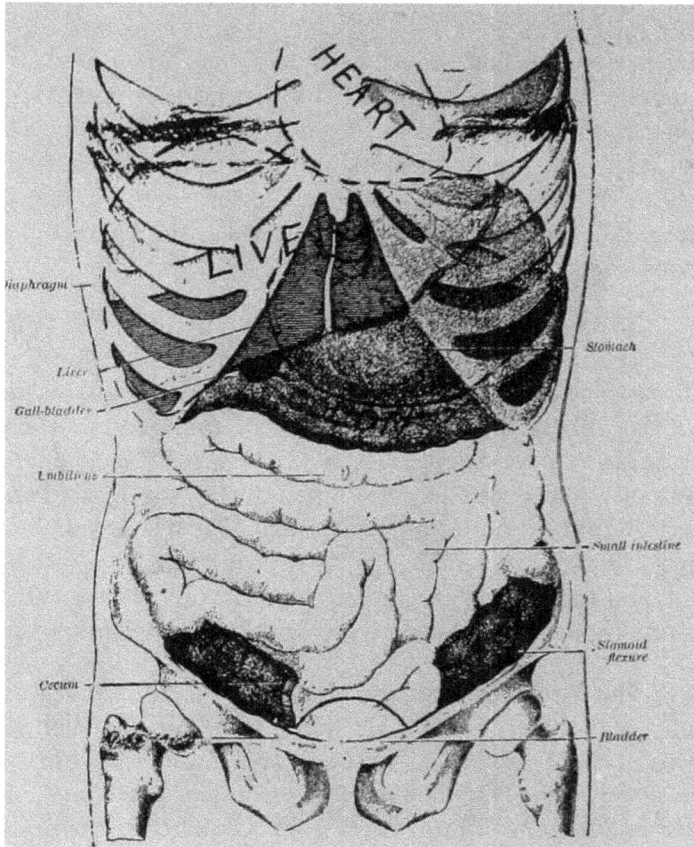

Figure 3

of involuntary muscle which is arranged in both longitudinal and circular layers. The inner coat is mucous membrane and the middle coat is loosely formed connective tissue.

The Stomach is a pear-shaped, hollow, muscular organ situated in the left side of the upper abdomen, just beneath the diaphragm. It is thirteen inches in length (from left to right), four

221

inches in diameter, and holds about five pints. The point where the esophagus joins the stomach (upper surface) is called the Cardiac End. The Pylorus is the constricted right extremity where the stomach joins the duodenum. The muscular coat is very thick at this portion, forming the pyloric sphincter valve. The enlarged portion lying to the left of the cardiac end is the Fundus of the stomach. (See Figures 2 and 3 of Plate VI of Charts.)

The walls of the stomach are made up of three kinds of tissues. The inner coat is mucous membrane (Epithelium). The middle coat is of involuntary muscle which is arranged in three layers, the fibers of the different layers running in different directions. The outer coat of the stomach is a part of the large Serous Membrane that lines the abdominal cavity (the Peritoneum). Imbedded in the inner coat of the stomach are a large number of simple Tubular Glands. Those in the pyloric end having one layer of cells and those in the fundus two layers of cells. The portion of the stomach between these parts has both kinds of glands.

The Small Intestine is a long convoluted tube occupying the middle of the abdomen. It is twenty-one feet long and one and one-half inches in diameter. There are three divisions. The first ten inches is called the Dudodenum. It curls upward and backward to the left and then downward into the right, encircling the head of the pancreas. The Jejunum is the eight feet between the duodenum and the ileum. The last twelve feet is the Ileum. It terminates in the colon. (See Figure 2 of Plate VI of Charts.)

The outer coat of the intestine is a serous membrane (from the peritoneum). The middle coat is composed of involuntary muscle fibres arranged in circular and longitudinal bands. The mucous membrane making up the inner coat is much longer than the other coats so that it contains many transverse ridges. On the surface of this epithelial membrane are a very large number of small projections (Villi) which contain blood vessels. These are most numerous in the duodenum and jejunum and altogether number about four million. (See Figure 10 of Plate VI.) Between these villi are small tubular glands or Crypts. In the duodenum there are also numerous compound tubular glands. In the lower portion of the small intestine (Ileum and Jejunum) are many lymph glands. Some of these are arranged in groups and are called Peyers Patches.

The Colon is the first part of the large intestine. It is a large sacculated tube beginning at the termination of the small intestine and terminating in the rectum. It is five feet long by two and one-half inches in diameter. The Colon has four divisions. (See Figures 1 and 3.)

The Cecum is the large blind tube or pouch forming the beginning of the colon and is situated in the lower right-hand part of the abdomen. The Ileocecal Valve separates the ileum from the cecum. The Vermiform Appendix is a small worm-like blind tube projecting from the lower portion of the cecum.

The Ascending Colon is the vertical portion extending from the cecum to just below the liver on the right side. The horizontal portion extending from the right to the left across the upper abdomen is the Transverse Colon. The Descending Colon is the vertical portion extending downward on the left side from the spleen to the left iliac bone. The terminal portion of the colon forms the loop which extends from the lower extremity of the descending colon to the beginning of the rectum. It is called the Sigmoid Flexure or Pelvic Colon. (See Figure 11.)

The Structure of the large intestine is similar to that of the small intestine except that the mucous membrane has no villi and that the longitudinal muscular fibres are arranged in three bands which are shorter than the other coats of the colon. This produces the bulging or sacculation of the walls of the colon. The large intestine has glands similar to those of the small intestine except that there are no compound tubular glands.

The Rectum is the expanded lower portion of the large intestine situated in the posterior portion of the pelvis. It is about eight inches long and extends from the third sacral vertebrae to just below the tip of the coccyx, where it terminates in the Anal Canal. Its structure is similar to that of the colon. Around the external orifice (Anus) are two circular bands of muscular tissue which are called the Internal and External Sphincters. The inner one is composed of involuntary muscle and the outer one of voluntary muscle. (See Figure 11.)

The Liver is a large glandular organ situated in the right upper portion of the abdomen. It is the largest gland in the body. It is nine inches in length from left to right and five inches in width (from front to back). Its vertical depth is three inches and it weighs four pounds. (See Figures 3 and 4.)

The upper surface of the liver is convex and lies in contact with the under surface of the diaphragm and the inner surfaces of the seven lower ribs. The under surface is concave and covers the stomach, duodenum, the hepatic flexure of the colon and the right kidney. The anterior border is sharp and the posterior border is rounded. The right surface is flattened.

Lesson 16: Digestive Organs

The Liver has five fissures on its under surface which are arranged in the form of the Letter H. These fissures divide the liver into five lobes. The right lobe comprises more than half the liver. The left lobe is the largest of the remaining lobes. (See Figure 9, Plate VI of Charts.) The liver is connected to the under surface of the diaphragm and to the anterior wall of the abdomen by five ligaments. Four of these ligaments are made up of folds of the peritoneum. The ligament extending from the umbilicus is the remains of a fetal vein.

The Liver Substance is composed of a large number of small rounded bodies (lobules) measuring about one-twentieth of an inch in diameter. These lobules are separated by spaces in which are situated blood vessels, nerves, bile ducts and lymphatics. The lobules are composed of many sided cells measuring about one-thousandth of an inch in diameter. (See Figure 6, of Plate VI.)

These cells are grouped around a central vein into which the capillaries of the hepatic artery and the portal vein empty. The capillaries of the hepatic vein drain the central veins of the liver lobules. The liver is very vascular and contains about one-fourth of all of the blood in the body.

The bile is formed in the liver cells and is collected by the bile capillaries in the lobules. These capillaries are fused together to form the bile ducts. The bile ducts coalesce to form the hepatic duct which passes out through the transverse fissure and joins the cystic duct from the gall bladder.

The Gall Bladder is a pear-shaped bag situated in one of the fissures on the under surface of the liver. It is about three inches long by one inch in diameter. Its duct joins the hepatic duct

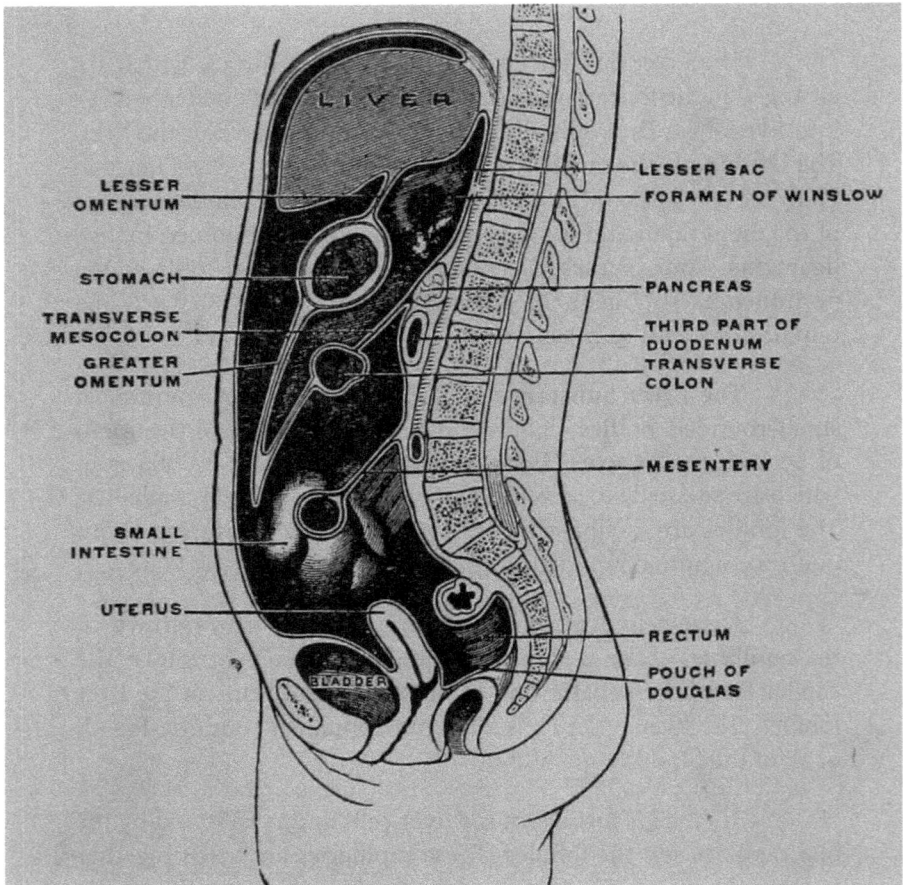

Figure 4

from the liver and forms the common bile duct which empties into the duodenum. (See Figure 2, Plate VI.)

The Pancreas is compound gland situated transversely across the posterior wall of the abdomen (behind the stomach). It is five and one-half inches long and one and one-half inches thick.

226

Lesson 16: Digestive Organs

The right extremity is the largest and is called the Head which is encircled by the duodenum. The left extremity (Tail) lies between the spleen and the left kidney and above the colon. (See Figure 3, Plate VI.)

Extending through the whole length of the pancreas is a duct which empties into the duodenum. This duct divides gradually into many other small ducts that terminate in small sacs which are lined with the epithelial cells, making up the pancreatic substance. Distributed throughout the pancreas are small bodies of connective tissue (Islands of Langerhans) which furnish the internal secretion of the pancreas.

The Peritoneum is a large serous membrane lining the abdominal cavity and covering the abdominal organs. It is composed of endothelial tissue. The outer coat of the stomach, intestines and colon are formed by the peritoneum. It nearly covers the liver and spleen; the kidneys lie behind it. (See Figure 4.)

The peritoneum is divided into two sacs, the greater and the lesser. These are connected by an opening or foramen. In the male these sacs have no opening into the outer air; in the female the Fallopian Tubes open into the greater sac.

The Mesenteries are folds of the peritoneum connecting various parts of the intestinal canal to the posterior abdominal wall; each containing the vessels of the part which it supports.

The Omenta are folds of peritoneum which connect the external surface of the stomach to the liver, spleen and colon. The greater omenta extends from the anterior surface of the stomach downward in front of the colon and small intestines to the lower portion of the abdomen.

Questions—Lesson 16

1. Name the Digestive Organs.

2. Briefly describe the Mouth.

3. Describe the Pharynx and Esophagus.

4. Describe the Stomach.

5. Briefly describe the Small Intestines.

6. In what ways does the Colon differ from the Small Intestine?

7. Locate and briefly describe the Liver.

8. Locate and briefly describe the Pancreas.

9. What is the Peritoneum?

10. Draw a sketch of the Abdomen showing the relative positions of the various organs.

EXTENSION COURSE
IN CHIROPRACTIC
AMERICAN UNIVERSITY
CHICAGO, Ill., U.S.A.

_____

LESSON 17

_____

RESPIRATORY ORGANS

The Lungs are the principal respiratory organs; the Nasal Cavities, Larynx, Trachea, Bronchi and Pleurae are appendages of the lungs. (See Figure 2, Plate V of Charts.)

The Nasal Cavaties will be described in Lesson 19 as the nose is also an organ of special sense.

The Larynx is a cartillaginous box forming the organ of voice and connecting the nose and mouth with the trachea. It is situated in front of the pharynx and extends from the base of the tongue to the beginning of the trachea (in front of the 4th, 5th and 6th Cervical Vertebrae). It is about two inches long. (See Figures 1 and 14 of Plate VIII.)

The Larynx is composed of the following structures:— The Thyroid Cartilage is a wedge shaped box of hyaline cartilage surrounding and supporting the other structures. It is open behind and is covered in front by the skin of the throat. The Cricoid

Cartilage is a ring of hyaline cartilage between the thyroid and the trachea. The Arytenoid Cartilages are two small pyramidal bodies resting on the posterior edge of the cricoid cartilage. They support the posterior ends of the vocal cords. The Epiglottis is a leaf-shaped plate of yellow, elastic cartilage lying between the base of the tongue and the upper edge of the thyroid cartilage. It forms the cover of the larynx. (See Figure 2.)

The Vocal Cords are two pairs of ligamentus bands extending from the arytenoid cartilages to the inner surfaces of the anterior edge of the thyroid cartilage. The lower pair are the True vocal cords; the upper pair are called False vocal cords. The Glottis is the opening between the vocal cords connecting the cavity of the larynx with the trachea. It is one-half inch wide by one inch long. (See Figure 12, Plate VIII.)

The Trachea is the tube connecting the larynx with the bronchial tubes (bronchi). It extends from the sixth cervical to the fourth dorsal vertebrae, lying in front of the esophagus. The trachea is four and one-half inches long and one inch in diameter. It is composed of eighteen rings of cartilage connected to each other by fibrous tissue. The trachea is lined by mucous membrane which is continuous with that of the larynx and that lining the lungs.

The trachea divides at its lower extremity into two tubes (bronchi) each about one inch long. These tubes subdivide many times into successively smaller tubes which finally terminate in the air sacs of the lungs. (See Figure 2, Plate I.)

The Lungs are two conical organs occupying the greater portion of the chest. They are supported by the bronchi. The right

231

lung is the largest, weighing about twenty two ounces; the left lung weighs twenty ounces. The right lung has three lobes; upper, middle and lower; the left lung has an upper and a lower lobe. The lower flat surface is called the Base and the upper pointed portion (in base of neck) is the Apex of the lungs. The point at which the bronchi vessels and nerves enter the lungs is the Root. (See Figure 5.)

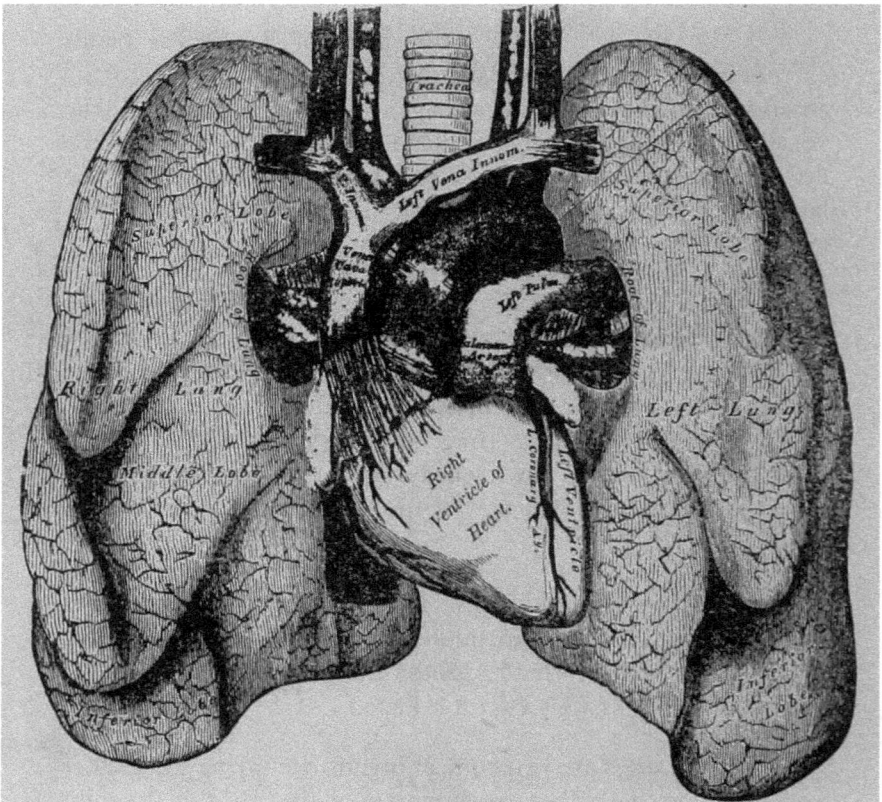

Figure 5

Lesson 17: Respiratory Organs

The Lung Substance is soft, spongy and highly elastic. During life it contains air. The lung may be considered as a mass of air cells (one-hundredth of an inch in diameter) arranged in groups (lobules) around the termination of the smaller bronchial tubes. The walls of these air cells are composed of epithelial tissue. The outer surfaces of these air cells are connected to the others by a very fine network of connective tissue.

The Pulmonary Arteries from the right ventricle of the heart accompany the bronchial tubes to the air cells which are surrounded by a network of capillaries. (See Figure 3, Plate I.) These capillaries are drained by the pulmonary veins which also accompany the bronchial tubes. The pulmonary veins empty into the left auricle of the heart. The bronchial tubes and the lung substance is supplied with nutrition by the bronchial arteries.

The Pleurae are two sacs of serous membrane (endothelium) covering the lungs and lining the chest. Each pleura is a closed sac. The space between the two layers is called the Pleural Cavity. (See Figure 5, Plate I.)

The Mediastinum is the space between the lungs and between the two pleural sacs. It contains all of the thoracic structures except the lungs.

FEMALE GENERATIVE ORGANS
The Female Generative organs consist of the Vulva, Vagina, Uterus, Uterine Appendages and Breasts.

The Vulva is a structure situated in front of and below the pubic symphysis of the female. It is divided for description into the

Labia Majora, Labia Minora, Clitoris, Vestibule, Hymen and the Urinary Meatus. (See Figure 7.)

The Labia Majora are two outer, longitudinal elevations. They are composed of fatty tissue covered by the skin. The Labia Minora are two small longitudinal folds of skin lying inside of the labia majora and surrounding the vaginal orifice and vestibule.

The Clitoris is the small cylindrical body just above the anterior junction of the labia minora. The space between the vaginal orifice and the upper anterior portions of the labia minora is called the Vestibule. The Hymen is a fold of mucous membrane partially enclosing the vaginal orifice.

The Vagina is a curved, cylindrical muscular membranous canal connecting the vulva with the uterus (three inches long). It lies between the bladder and the rectum. Its lower end (orifice) is surrounded by a voluntary sphincter muscle. (See Figure 6.)

The Uterus is a hollow, muscular organ situated in the female pelvis between the sacrum and the pubic symphysis. It lies above the vagina, above and behind the bladder and in front of the rectum. (See Figure 6.)

In shape it resembles a flattened pear with its large end directed upward and forward. Its lower end is contained within the upper extremity of the vagina. The Uterus is three inches long (vertically), two inches wide (laterally) and one inch thick.

The upper rounded portion is called the Fundus; the lower constricted portion the Cervix. The Body is the part between the cervix and fundus. The cavity of the uterus opens into the vagina through the Os. (See Figure 8.) The mass of involuntary muscle

234

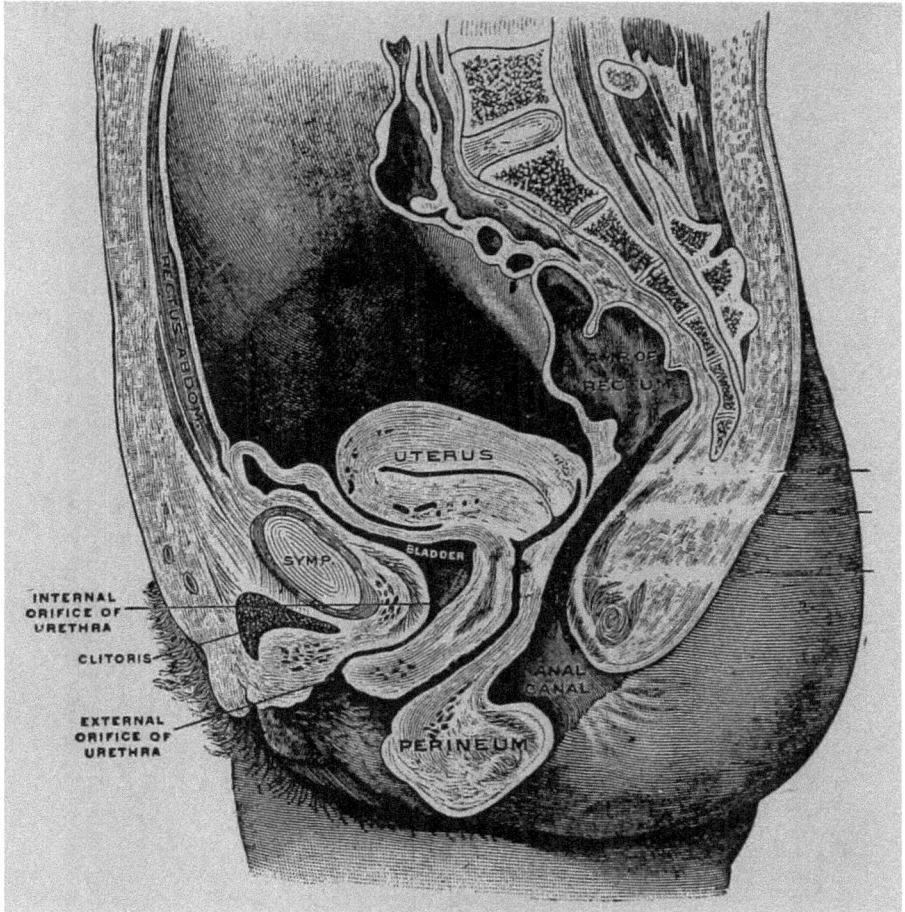

Figure 6

of which the uterus is composed is lined internally by mucous membrane (continuous with that of the vagina) and covered externally by the peritoneum.

235

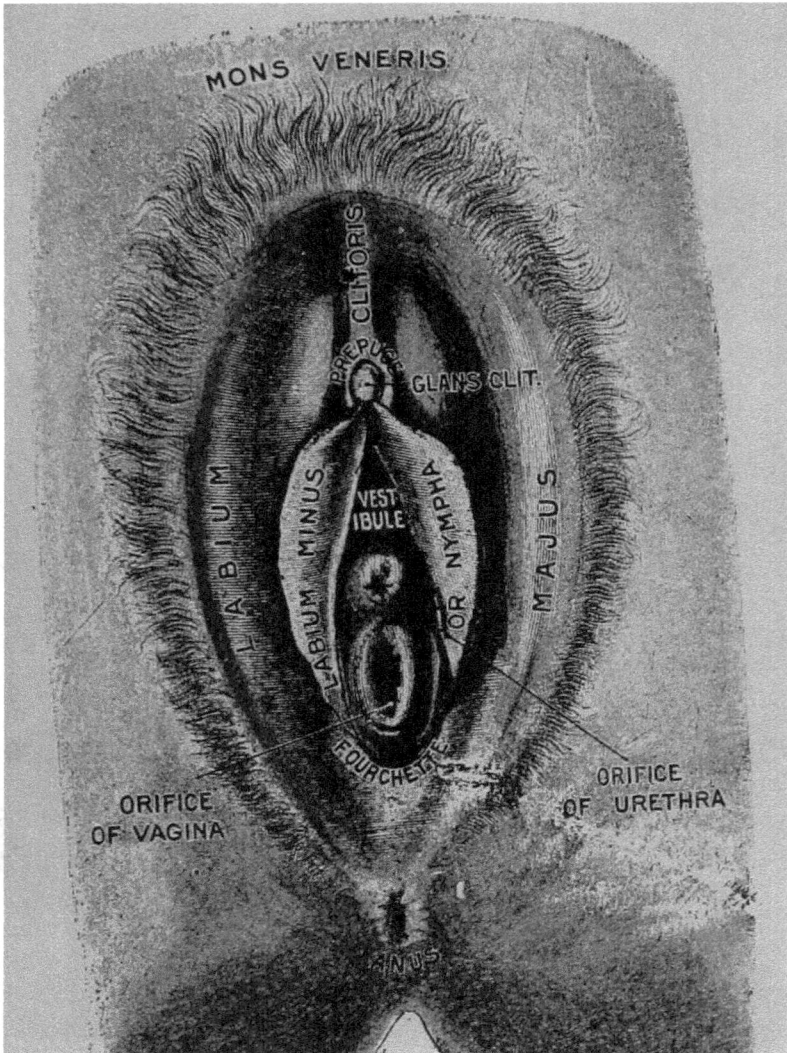

Figure 7

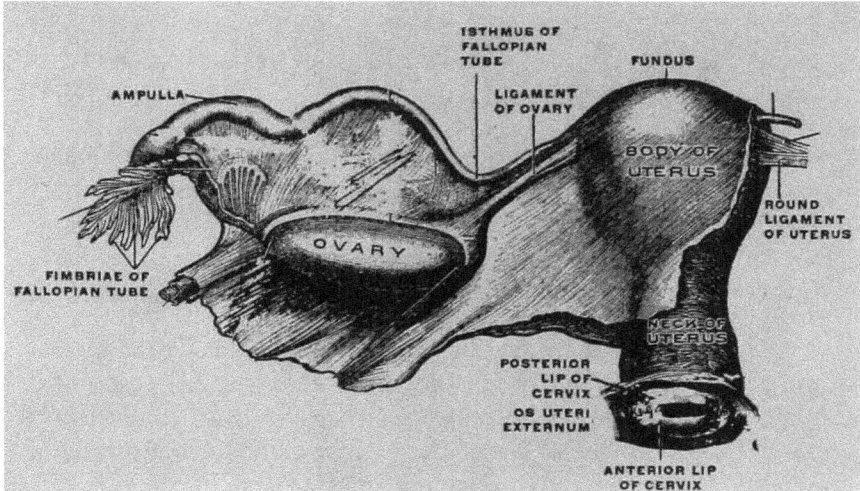

Figure 8

Eight ligaments connect the uterus with the bony pelvis; the most important of these are the Round ligaments and the Broad ligaments. The Broad Ligaments are two folds of peritoneum (one on either side) extending laterally from the sides of the uterus to the lateral walls of the pelvis. The Round Ligaments are two cords of fibrous, muscular tissue extending from the sides of the fundus to the anterior surface of the bodies of the pubic bones. They pass through the Inguinal Canals.

The Uterine Appendages consist of the Ovaries and the Fallopian Tubes. (See Figure 8.) The Ovaries are two oval, glandular bodies situated in the posterior layer of the broad ligaments on either side of the body of the uterus, below and behind the fallopian tubes. Each ovary measures one and one-half by three-fourths by one-third inches. They are composed of connective tissue framework which surrounds and supports the

237

blood vessels and the Graafian Vesicles. The Graafian Vesicles are small sacs containing fluid and the ova.

The Fallopian Tubes are two muscular membranous tubes extending laterally from the lateral surface of the fundus of the uterus to the ovaries. (One on either side.) Each one lies between the two layers of the broad ligament at its superior margin. The tube is four inches long by one-sixteenth to one-half inch in diameter.

The Breasts are two hemispherical, glandular bodies on the anterior-lateral surface of the chest. They are composed of many small lobes of gland cells bound together with connective tissue to form fifteen or twenty larger lobes. The ducts from the lobes unite and pass out through the nipple.

The Ova, or female generative element, is produced in the Graafian Follicles of the ovaries. The ova is liberated by the bursting of the vesicle and is carried by the fallopian tube to the uterus. If it becomes impregnated it becomes imbedded in the wall of the uterus and forms the embryo or fetus. If the ova is not fertilized it passes out through the cervix and the vagina during menstruation.

Questions—Lesson 17

1. Name the Respiratory Organs.

2. Briefly describe the Larynx.

3. Describe the Trachea and the Primary Bronchi.

4. Briefly describe the Lungs.

5. What are the Pleurae?

6. Name the structures included in the Vulva.

7. Describe the Vagina.

8. Briefly describe the Uterus.

9. Name and locate the Uterine Appendages.

10. Describe the Breasts.

EXTENSION COURSE IN CHIROPRACTIC AMERICAN UNIVERSITY CHICAGO, Ill., U.S.A.

LESSON 18

URINARY ORGANS

The Urinary Organs consist of the Kidneys, Ureters, Bladder and Urethra; the Kidneys are the essential organs and the others are the appendages of the kidneys.

The Kidneys are two bean-shaped glandular organs situated in the posterior upper part of the abdominal cavity. There is one on either side of the spinal column (Twelfth Dorsal to Third Lumbar Vertebrae.) (See Figure 10.) Both kidneys lie behind the peritoneum and the other abdominal organs except the liver which is above the right kidney. The kidney lies between two sheets of fibrous tissue which are connected to the diaphragm and the posterior abdominal wall. This fibrous tissue together with the mass of fat surrounding each kidney holds it in its proper position. The right one is about one-half inch lower than the left.

Each kidney is four inches long (vertically) two inches wide (left to right) and one inch thick (front to back). Each one weighs about five ounces. The edge nearest the spinal column is

240

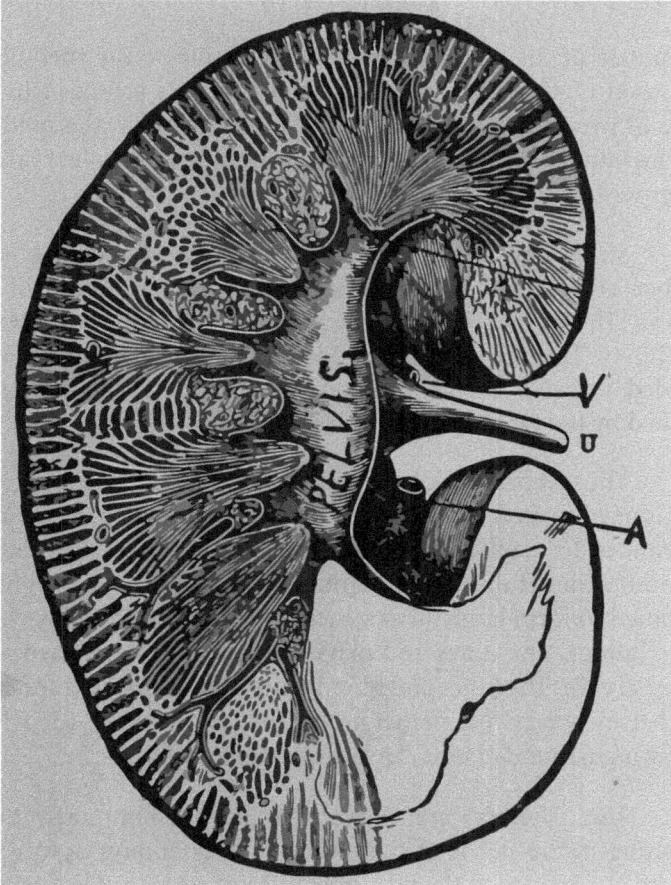

Figure 9

slightly concave and is called the Hilum. The vessels, nerves and ureters pass in and out the kidney at this point.

For description the kidney is divided from within outward into the Pelvis, the Medulla and the Cortex. The Cortex is made up of a large mass of coiled tubules, capillaries and the rounded

241

extremities of the tubules (Bowman's Capsules). The medulla is composed of straight tubules and blood vessels arranged in the shape of pyramids. The Pelvis is the cavity between the medulla and the hilum. The structure of the kidneys is shown very clearly in Figure 9.

Structurally, each kidney may be considered as a large number of very fine tubes which empty into the hilum of the kidneys. These tubes begin in the outer portion or the cortex of the kidney. They begin in a rounded capsule which surrounds a rounded mass of capillary blood vessels. These capillaries are supplied by the renal artery and are drained by the renal vein.

Those portions of the tubules that lie in the cortex of the kidney are very much coiled upon themselves and are also surrounded by capillaries. In the central or medullary portion of the kidney these tubes are straight. Many of these smaller tubules are joined to form large tubes which empty into the hollow pelvis of the kidney. The tubes and pelvis of the kidney are lined with epithelial cells. The tubes and blood vessels are connected and held together by a very fine network of connective tissues. The whole kidney is surrounded by a capsule of connective tissue.

The Ureters are two muscular-membranous tubes beginning in the pelvis of the kidney and extending downward, forward and inward to the posterior-inferior surface of the urinary bladder. Each ureter is sixteen inches long and one-sixteenth of an inch in diameter.

The Bladder is an ovoid, hollow, muscular organ situated in the anterior portion of the pelvis just behind the pubic symphysis. (See Figures 3, 6 and 11.) It is about four inches in diameter and

242

Lesson 18: Urinary Organs

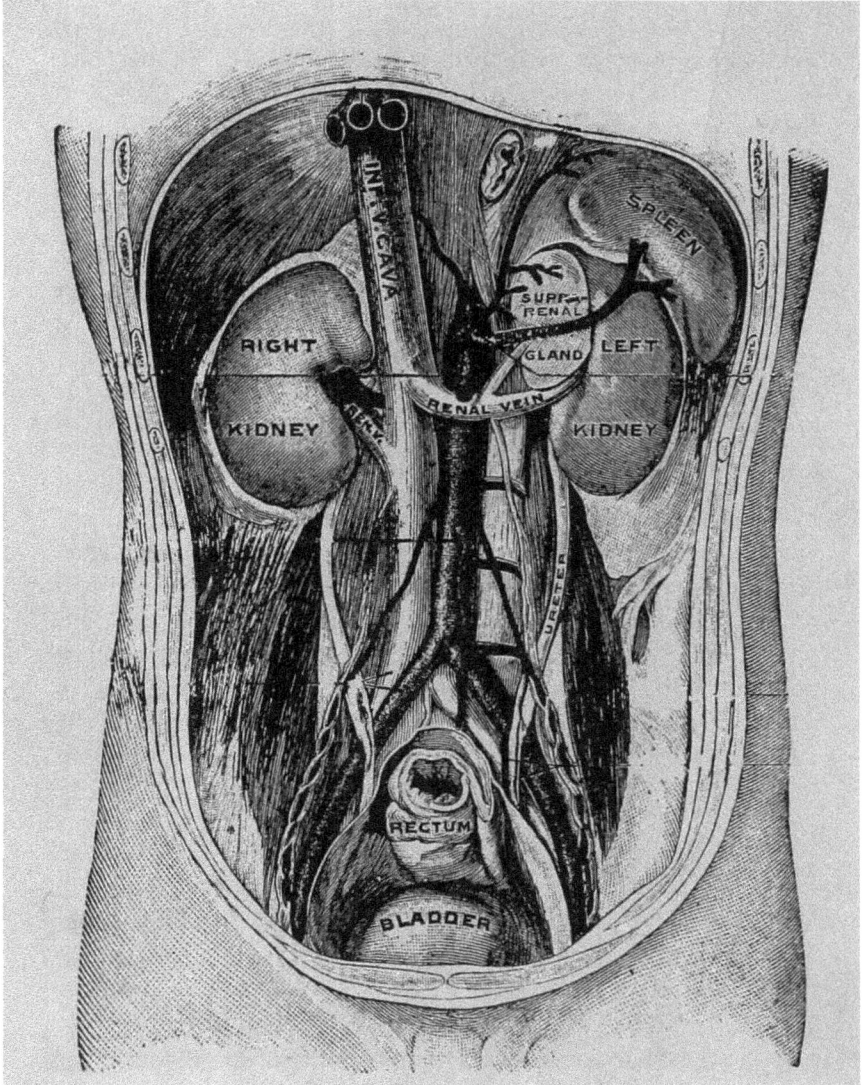

Figure 10

243

holds about one pint. Its anterior-superior pole is called the Apex; its posterior-inferior pole is the Base. The Neck of the Bladder is the constricted anterior portion where the urethra begins.

The middle coat of the bladder is much the thickest and is composed of three layers of involuntary muscle, the fibres of which run in different directions. The inner coat is epithelial tissue (mucous membrane) which is continuous with that of the ureter and the kidney. The upper surface of the bladder is covered by the peritoneum (serous membrane). Around the neck of the bladder the muscular tissue is arranged in circular bands forming the Sphincter.

The Male Urethra is an epithelial tube extending from the neck of the bladder to the end of the penis. (Figure 11.) It is about eight inches long and from one-half to one-third inch in diameter. The Prostatic portion (one and one-fourth inch long by one-half inch in diameter) lies within the prostate gland. The Membranous portion lies within the structures that form the perineum, just below the pubic symphysis. It is one-half inch long by one-third of an inch in diameter and is surrounded by a voluntary muscle. The Penile portion is contained within the spongy posterior portion of the penis. The external opening of the urethra is called the Meatus.

The Female Urethra resembles the male urethra in structure and location, but is only one and one-half inches in length and one-fourth of an inch in diameter. The meatus lies between the clitoris and the vaginal opening. (See Figures 6 and 7.)

MALE GENERATIVE ORGANS

The Male Generative Organs consist of the Prostate, the Seminal Vesicles, the Testes and the Penis. (See Figure 11.)

Lesson 18: Urinary Organs

The Prostate is a gland behind and partially surrounding the first part of the Urethra. It lies between the neck of the bladder and the rectum. In shape it resembles a large chestnut about one and one- quarter inch in its greatest diameter. The prostate is composed of muscle tissue which surrounds and supports the gland cells. The whole is covered by a fibrous tissue capsule. The ducts from the gland cells empty into the urethra.

The Testes are two glandular organs situated in the scrotum. They are suspended below the arch of the pubis by the spermatic cords. The glandular structure of the testes consists of a large number of small lobules which are separated and held together by fibrous tissue which also forms the capsule. The ducts from these lobules converge to form the spermatic duct. Immediately after leaving the testicle this duct is coiled upon itself to form the epididymis which lies behind and above the testicle.

The Scrotum is a fibrous sac surrounding both testes, the two being separated by a fibrous partition or septum. It is covered externally by the skin.

The Spermatic Duct together with the nerves and vessels of the testes form the Spermatic Cords (one on either side) which pass upward through the inguinal canals to the seminal vesicles.

The Seminal Vesicles are the dilated portions of the spermatic ducts. They lie between the bladder and above and on either side of the prostate. Each one empties into the urethra through a small duct which passes through the prostate gland.

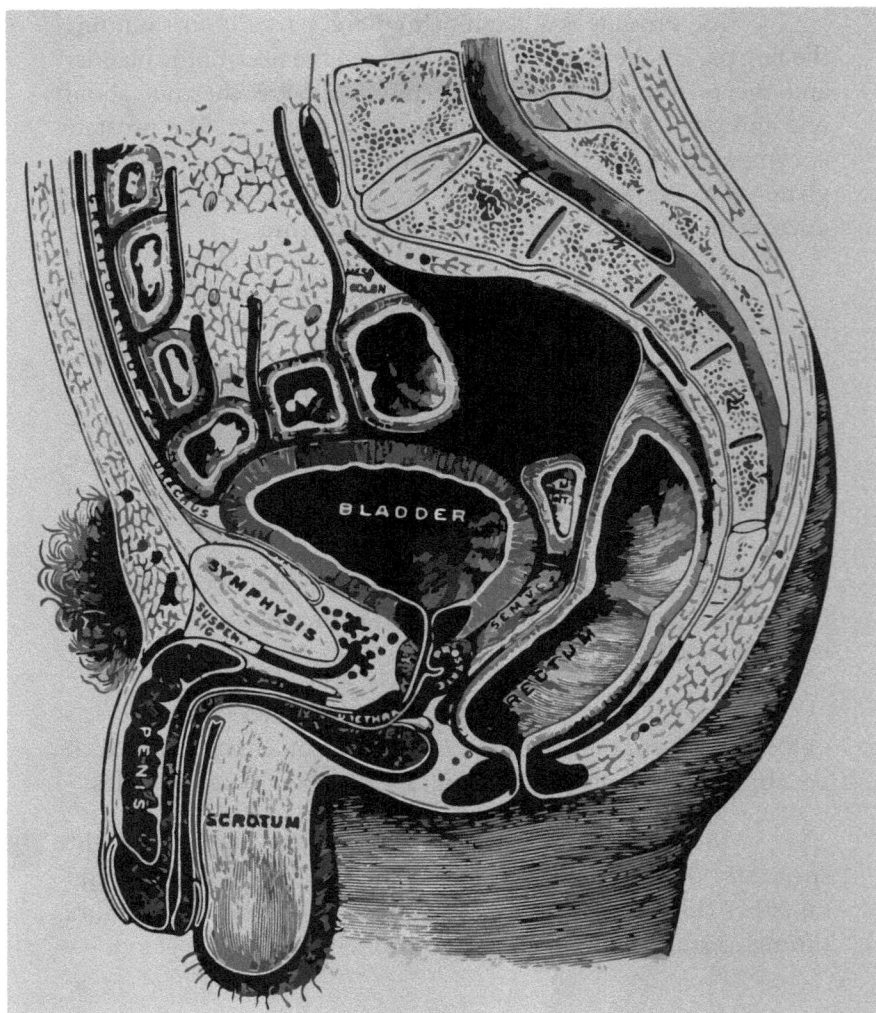

Figure 11

The Penis is a long mass of erectile tissue composed of three compartments, each surrounded by a fibrous sheet. It consists of a Root, a Body and a Glans. (Figure 11.)

The Body is cylindrical and is covered by the skin which is loosely attached. The distal portion of the skin hangs loosely about the glans forming the Prepuce. The Glans, or extremity, is a flattened cone.

The Spermatazoa or male generative elements are produced in the lobules of the testes from whence they are carried in the seminal fluid through the spermatic ducts to the seminal vesicles. The seminal vesicles serve as reservoirs for the seminal fluid. The seminal fluid is thrown out through the urethra by the contraction of the seminal vesicles, the prostate, and the voluntary muscle which surrounds the urethra.

Questions—Lesson 18

1. Name and locate the Urinary Organs.

2. Briefly describe the Kidneys.

3. Describe the Ureters.

4. Briefly describe the Bladder.

5. Briefly describe the Male Urethra.

6. Name and locate the Male Generative Organs.

7. Briefly describe the Prostate.

8. Briefly describe the Scrotum and its contents.

9. Describe the Seminal Vesicles.

10. Describe the Penis.

EXTENSION COURSE IN CHIROPRACTIC AMERICAN UNIVERSITY CHICAGO, Ill., U.S.A.

LESSON 19

ORGANS OF SPECIAL SENSE

EYE

The Eye is the organ of vision. It is situated in the anterior part of the orbital cavity surrounded by fat and connective tissue. It is held in position by its muscles which extend backwards to the posterior portion of the orbit. The front of the eyeball is protected by the eyelids and the eyebrow. The body of the eyeball is spherical with the exception of the anterior portion which projects forward. (See Figures 4 and 6 of Plate VIII of the Charts.)

The **Outer Coat** of the eye is formed by the Sclerotic and the Cornea. The sclerotic coat covers the posterior five-sixths of the eyeball; the cornea forming the anterior one-sixth. The Sclerotic is a tough white membrane (white of eye). The Cornea is a hard colorless disk resembling a watch crystal.

The **Middle Coat** is formed by the Choroid, Ciliary Body, and the Iris. The Choroid is a thin, brownish, vascular membrane lying beneath the sclerotic. The Ciliary Body connects the anterior

249

edge of the choroid with the outer edge of the iris. It is composed principally of a circular muscle (ciliary muscle). The anterior edge of the choroid is gathered into sixty or eighty folds which are called ciliary processes.

The Iris is a circular curtain lying just behind the cornea. The color of the iris varies with the individual; usually it is some shade of blue or brown. The opening in the iris is called the Pupil. The size of the pupil controls the amount of light entering the eye. There are two sets of muscle fibres in the iris. These extending from the center outward enlarge the pupil by their contraction and the circular fibres diminish the size of the pupil when they contract.

The Inner Coat of the eye is formed by the retina, which is the expanded anterior extremity of the optic nerve. It is a delicate, grayish, transparent membrane lining the posterior two-thirds of the eyeball.

Rays of light are focused on the retina by the Aqueous Humor, the Vitreous Body and the Crystalline Lens. These are called the Refracting Media.

The Aqueous Humor is a clear, colorless fluid composed of water, albumin and salts. It fills the space behind the cornea and in front of the ciliary body and crystalline lens. The Vitreous Body is a transparent, jelly-like substance filling the space behind the ciliary body and crystalline lens. It makes up four-fifths of the globe of the eye. The Crystalline Lens is a bi-convex elastic, transparent body enclosed in a capsule. It is surrounded by the ciliary body and is held in place by a suspensory ligament which encloses it and connects it to the anterior margin of the ciliary body.

250

Lesson 19: Organs of Special Sense

The Optic Nerves (second cranial) originate in the retina and pass out on the inner side of the posterior pole of the eyeball. After leaving the orbit the two nerves join and form the Optic Commissure or Chiasm which lies on the body of the sphenoid bone. From here the Optic Tracts carry the fibres of the optic nerves back through the optic thalmi to the posterior portion of the occipital lobe of the cerebrum.

The Appendages of the Eye are the Conjunctiva, the Lachrymal Apparatus, the Eyebrows, the Eyelids and the External Eye Muscles. (See Figures 6 and 7 of Plate VIII.)

The Lids are composed of muscle tissue and plates of fibrous cartilage. They are covered in front by the skin. Their free margin contains a large number of long stiff hairs. The conjunctiva is a thin, transparent, epithelial membrane lining the posterior portion of the eyelids and covering the anterior part of the eyeball.

The Lachrymal Gland is an oval body situated above the outer angle of the orbit. (See Figure 7 of Plate VIII.) It has twelve ducts which open on the inner surface of the upper lid (outer portion). After passing over the eyeball the tears are carried to the Lachrymal Sac in the inner angle of the orbit by two small canals. The Nasal Duct connects the lachrymal sac with the nasal cavity.

The external muscles of the eye have been described in Lesson 9. (See Figure 6 of Plate VIII.)

Light Rays coming directly from luminous objects or reflecting from non-luminous objects pass through the refracting media of the eye to the retina. These light rays produce some chemical changes in the retina which are carried over the optic nerve to the brain where they form the visual impressions which constitute the Sense of Light.

When viewing objects at a distance greater than twenty feet no muscular effort is required. If the object viewed is less than twenty feet from the eye, the light rays must be focused on the retina by a process known as Accommodation. The ciliary muscle contracts allowing relaxation of the suspensory ligaments of the crystalline lens. The lens, being elastic, expands and increases its anterior-posterior diameter. This increases its focusing power.

The eyes must be turned inward when they are used for close work. This Convergence is produced by the contraction of the Internal Recti Muscles. The internal rectus muscle and the ciliary muscle of the same eye are supplied by the same cranial nerve (third), so that in the normal eye convergence and accommodation are always properly coordinated.

EAR

The Ear is the organ of hearing and is divided for description into three parts, External, Middle and Internal Ear. (See Figure 3, Plate VIII.) .

The External Ear (Auricle) is an irregular leaf-like appendage on the outer surface of the malar and temporal bones. It consists of a thin plate of yellow, elastic cartilage covered by the skin. The Auditory Canal is a cylindrical tube one and one-quarter inches long connecting the external ear with the middle ear. It is lined with skin which contains numerous glands and hairs.

The Tympanic Membrane (or drumhead) is an oval, elastic, semi-transparent membrane across the inner part of the auditory canal. It is composed of fibrous tissue covered on the outer side by the skin and on the inner side by mucous membrane (epithelial tissue). (Figure 3, Plate VIII.)

The Middle Ear is an irregular cavity lying within the body of the temporal bone. It is about one-half inch in diameter and contains the three bones of the ear (osicles) and air. The Eustachian Tube connects the cavity with the upper part of the pharynx (naso-pharynx). The osicles are shown in Figure 15 of Plate VIII.

The Inner Ear is the essential part of the organ of hearing. It lies internal to the middle ear within the body of the temporal bone and consists of a series of chambers lined by membranous tissue in which the fibres of the auditory nerve begin. The cavities are divided for description into the Vestibule, the Cochlea and the Semi-circular Canals. (See Figures 3, 13 and 16, Plate VIII.)

The Vestibule is the central cavity connecting the other two with each other and with the middle ear. It contains lymph. The Cochlea is a spiral canal lying internal to and in front of the vestibule. It is about one and one-half inches long by one-tenth to one-twentieth of an inch in diameter. It is coiled around a central axis like a small shell. (Figures 13 and 16.)

The Semi-circular Canals are three C-shaped bony tubes each about one-twentieth of an inch in diameter. (See Figures 3 and 16.) They are situated above and behind the vestibule into which they open. Each canal lies at a right angle with the other two. These canals contain a special form of lymph and aid in maintaining the equilibrium or balance of the body.

The Auditory Nerve (8th Cranial) originates by two branches, one from the semi-circular canals and one from the cochlea. It passes inward through the body of the temporal bone and into the medulla. From the medulla the fibres extend to the auditory areas in the cortex of the temporal lobe of the cerebrum.

Sound Waves are collected by the external ear and are carried to the tympanic membrane by the auditory canal. The vibrations produced upon the tympanic membrane are transmitted by the osicles of the ear to the fluid which fills the vestibule and cochlea. These vibrations are taken up by small hair-like processes on the membranous lining of the cochlea and are transmitted to the brain over the auditory nerve, the fibres of which originate in these processes. The brain translates these impressions into the Sense of Sound.

When the Position or Posture of the Body is Changed, it produces a movement of the fluid in the semi-circular canals. The movement of this fluid produces impressions upon the fibres of the branch of the auditory nerve that supplies these canals. This enables the individual to know the position of his body and to contract the proper muscles to maintain his balance.

NOSE

The Nose is the organ of smell. It consists of the outer nose and the nasal cavities. The Outer Nose projects from the center of the face and is composed of a framework of bone and cartilage covered by the skin. At its base are two oval openings called the Nostrils or Nares.

The Nasal Cavities are two irregular cavities in the middle of the face. (Figures 1 and 2, Plate VIII.) These have been partially described in Lesson 6's section on the face. The bony walls of the eavity are covered by a special form of epithelial tissue (Schneiderian Membrane).

The Olfactory Nerves (1st Cranial) arise in spindle-shaped cells in the mucous membrane of the upper portion of the nasal cavities. These fibres pass through the horizontal plate of the ethmoid bone and form the two olfactory bulbs which lie above the ethmoid. From the bulbs the fibres extend backward to the temporal lobes of the cerebrum.

Odorous Substances in the air produce chemical changes in the olfactory nerve fibres of the Schneiderian Membrane. These changes produce impressions which are carried to the brain and constitute the Sense of Smell.

TONGUE

The Tongue is an organ of Taste in addition to being used in speech and mastication. It is composed of voluntary muscle and is attached to the Hyoid Bone and the posterior portion of the Floor of the Mouth. Its anterior extremity is freely movable. The tongue is covered by mucous membrane in which the nerves of taste originate. On the upper surface of the tongue are numerous small elevations (Papillae). The largest of these lie near the root of the tongue and are arranged in the form of a V. (See Figure 10, Plate VIII.)

Soluble Matter produces chemical changes in the papillae covering the tongue. These impressions are carried over the 7th and 9th cranial nerves to the brain making known to us the taste of various substances.

SKIN

The Organs of Touch are sensory nerve endings contained in the skin and in the mucous membranes lining the orifices of the body. They are composed of connective tissue masses which surround the nerve endings. Their size and shape vary with their location.

Sensations of Weight, Pressure, Heat, Cold and Pain affect the organs of touch and stimulate nerve impulses which are carried over the sensory nerves to the brain and the cord. Impressions are also carried from the joints, ligaments and muscles which give us a sense of the position and the movements of the limbs and of the amount of muscular effort required to perform certain acts.

The structure of the skin will be given in Lesson 20.

Questions—Lesson 19

1. Name and locate the Organs of Special Sense.

2. Briefly describe the Three Coats of the Eye.

3. Briefly describe the Refracting Media of the Eye.

4. Name and locate the Appendages of the Eye.

5. Describe the Middle Ear.

6. Name and locate the Principal Parts of the Inner Ear.

7. Briefly describe the Nasal Cavities.

8. Briefly describe the Tongue.

9. Explain how Sound Waves reach the Brain.

10. Explain the process of Accommodation.

EXTENSION COURSE
IN CHIROPRACTIC
AMERICAN UNIVERSITY
CHICAGO, Ill., U.S.A.

———————

LESSON 20

———————

HISTOLOGY

In previous lessons you have studied the form and structure of various organs and tissues as seen by the naked eye. In this lesson will be given the structure of the tissues viewed through the microscope.

STRUCTURE OF SKIN, NAILS AND HAIR

The Skin is divided into the Epidermis or Cuticle, and the Derma or True Skin. (See Figure 9 of Plate VI.)

The Epidermis is composed of superficial epithelial layers, and pigmentary layers called the Rete Mucosum. It has no nerves or blood vessels. The lowest layers contain the pigment cells which give color to the skin.

The Dermis is tough, protective, elastic tissue composed of a papillary layer and the Corium or deepest layer. Within the papillary layer is contained the sensory nerve ends and the Tactile Corpuscles. The deep layer consists of white fibrous tissue, yellow elastic fibres intermixed with muscular fibres, blood vessels, nerves and the sebaceous glands.

Within the sub-cutaneous cellular tissue are located the sweat glands, also the hair follicles, which perforate both the epidermis and the dermis. The Sweat Glands are long coiled tubes lying just below the true skin. Their ducts pass through the dermis and empty upon the outer surface of the epidermis.

Nails are a modification of epidermis formed on the outer ends of the fingers and toes, the Root being imbedded into a fold of the skin. The Matrix, or part of the dermis directly beneath the nail, is covered with highly vascular papillae. The Lunula is the crescent near the root; its whiteness is due to the small number of papillae underneath.

Hairs are tube-like processes of modified epidermis. Each hair consists of a Root lodged in a hair-follicle which supplies it with nourishment, and a Shaft or projecting portion consisting of a medulla surrounded by a fibrous and a scaly covering.

STRUCTURE OF BONE

Long Bones are composed of an outer compact layer, and an inner cellular or spongy substance. It is surrounded, except at the articular cartilages, by a vescular fibrous membrane, called the Periosteum, which receives the insertions of ligaments and tendons.

The transverse section of a bone examined microscopically shows: Haversian canals, 1/500 of inch in diameter, for the passage of vessels; Canaliculi, 1/16000 inch in diameter, radiating from the canals and connecting these with the lacunae; Lacunae, arranged

259

circularly around the canals, and containing bone cells which appear as dark spots.

A Haversian System consists of a Haversian canal with its lacunae and canaliculi as is shown in Figure 2 of Plate I of the Charts. The bone salts fill in the spaces between the canals, canaliculi and lacunae.

Flat bones do not have Haversian Systems. The outer layers are composed of dense, compact bone. Between the outer layers are spike-shaped fragments of bone salts surrounded by bone marrow.

STRUCTURE OF THE NERVES

The Nervous System is made up of a large number of Neurones. Each Neurone consists of a cell body from which projects the fibres or processes. (See Figures 6 and 7 of Plate VII of the Charts.) One process branches like a tree and is called the Dendrite. The other process does not branch like the dendrite. It is called the Axone. The nerve impulses pass through the dendrite to the nerve cell and from the nerve cell outward over the axone. When examined under a microscope the axone appears as is shown in Figure 12.

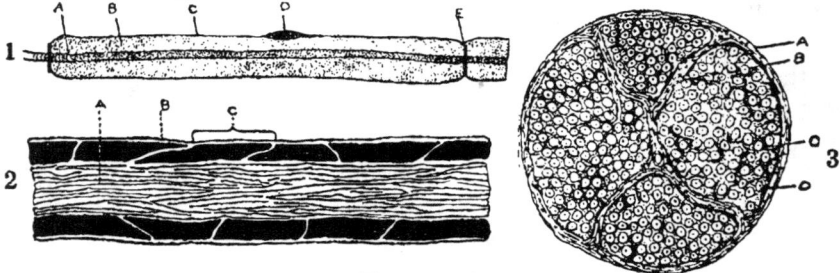

Figure 12

Lesson 20: Histology

Spinal nerves and similar nerve trunks when examined under the microscope are found to consist of large numbers of nerve fibres bound together by connective tissue as is shown in Figure 12.

Nerve fibres are principally of two types, those consisting of the medullated or white fibres, and those consisting of non-medullated or gray fibres.

A medullated fibre consists of a very delicate thread-like axis-cylinder. Surrounding the axis-cylinder is a fatty material (myelin) called the medullary sheath. Surrounding the medullary sheath is a delicate sheath called the neurilemma. About every 1/25 of an inch the neurilemma dips down to the axis-cylinder, forming periodic constrictions called the Nodes of Ranvier.

Ganglia are fusiform enlargments occasionally occurring in the course of some of the nerve trunks. These are composed of nerve fibres, connecting with large spherical cells.

STRUCTURE OF MUSCLES
The Muscular Tissues form a group of specialized cells possessing contractility in a marked degree. Three distinct types of muscle are recognized: Voluntary, Smooth, and Heart Muscle.

Voluntary, Striated or Skeletal Muscle is the most abundant. It forms all the skeletal muscles and is under the control of the will. When examined microscopically, it is seen to be composed of parallel cylindrical fibres, about 1/500 of an inch wide and 3/4 to 1 1/2 inches long. Each fibre is covered by a very delicate structureless membrane, corresponding to a cell wall, called a Sarcolemma. Under this and at the outer edge

261

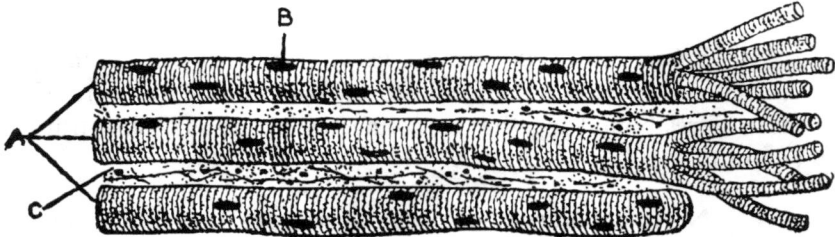

Figure 13

of the fibre are numerous oval nuclei; each fibre exhibits cross striations consisting of dark and light bands. The individual fibres of voluntary muscle are bound together by very delicate fibres of white fibrous tissue called the endomysium, and form bundles (the fasciculi). (See Figure 13.) These bundles are bound together by white fibrous tissue, (the perimysium), to form the large muscles.

Smooth Muscle is composed of spindle-shaped cells, covered by a fine sheath; they average in size about 1/250 of an inch in length and 1/5000 in width. (See Figure 14.) In the center of each is an elongated rod shaped nucleus. Very fine longitudinal striations may be seen in each fibre. They are held together by cement substance and by the interlacing of their ends.

Heart or Cardiac Muscle is found only in the heart; it is composed of rectangular branching cells, placed end to end and joined by cement substance. They possess fine longitudinal

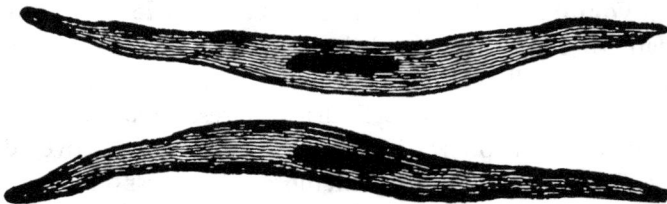

Figure 14

262

striations. A single oval nucleus is formed in the center of each cell. (See Figure 15.)

Generally speaking, the heart muscles begin at the top of the heart, pass downward on one side of the auricles, cross over between the auricles and the ventricles, thence downward on the side of the ventricles to the apex where they whorl like a figure 8 then pass upward on the opposite side of the ventricles cross over as before, and up on the other side of the auricles to the place of beginning.

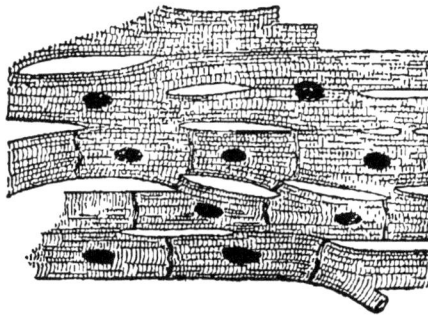

Figure 15

STRUCTURE OF BLOOD VESSELS

The Blood Vessels compose a system of tubes, divided into Arteries, Veins and Capillaries.

An Artery has three coats, an Outer, Middle and Inner. The Inner Coat consists of a single layer of thin, flat, elongated endothelial cells, united by a delicate cement substance. The Middle Coat consists principally of smooth muscle. The Outer Coat consists of fibrous tissue in dense bundles.

The Veins differ from the arteries only in the relatively small size of their muscular coat and the large amount of fibrous tissue; their walls are thinner in proportion to the lumen, and when they cut they tend to collapse.

Capillaries. The arteries branch repeatedly until the finest arterioles are reached, when they lose their outer two coats and continue as the capillaries, which are thin tubes consisting of only a single layer of endothelial cells.

Lesson 20: Histology

Questions—Lesson 20

1. Briefly describe the Skin.

2. Briefly describe the Nails.

3. Briefly describe the structure of the Long Bones.

4. What is a Neurone?

5. In what way does a Medullated Nerve Fibre differ from one that is not Medullated?

6. What are Ganglia?

7. Briefly describe the structure of Voluntary Muscle.

8. Give the structure of Heart Muscle.

9. Draw a sketch of a Smooth Muscle Cell.

10. Briefly describe an Artery.

CHIROPRACTIC

The Science of Spinal Adjustment

————

A SERIES OF LESSONS CORRELATING AND
SYSTEMATIZING THE KNOWLEDGE NECESSARY
TO PRACTICE CHIROPRACTIC

Nature's Greatest Ally

IN RESTORING DISEASED CONDITIONS OF THE
BODY TO PERFECT HEALTH, WITHOUT THE AID
OF DRUGS OR SURGERY

————

BOOK 6

PATHOLOGY

Lessons 21, 22, 23A and 23B

————

ORIGINALLY PUBLISHED BY
AMERICAN UNIVERSITY
CHICAGO, ILLINOIS, U.S.A.

Disclaimer

We are proud to republish this series of books on chiropractic medicine.
Originally published as a home-study course in 1913 by American University in Chicago, the 16 volumes give us an historical look at the theory and practice of chiropractic medicine in the early part of the 20th century.

This series is republished for historical interest only. The modern practice of chiropractic has advanced significantly in the century since these books were published. If you want to actually learn modern chiropractic techniques, please consult one of the many fine schools in this country.

The materials in these books are not intended to diagnose or treat disease. If you believe you are ill consult a licensed practitioner for care immediately. The publishers assume no liability for the use, misuse or nonuse of the materials in these books.

Thank you

EXTENSION COURSE IN CHIROPRACTIC AMERICAN UNIVERSITY CHICAGO, Ill., U.S.A.

LESSON 21

PATHOLOGY

Pathology is the science that deals with the structural, chemical and functional changes that take place or are present in disease. In previous lessons you have studied the normal anatomy and physiology. In this lesson you will study the abnormal or morbid anatomy and physiology.

Before any treatment can be intelligently applied, it is absolutely necessary that you know what conditions are present in the body to produce the symptoms about which the patient complains. All rational treatment must be founded upon the pathology of the disorder as well as being directed towards the removal of its cause. (The causes of disease will be considered in Lesson 22.)

Pathology is divided for study into General Pathology and Special Pathology; the first division includes the changes that occur in many diseases and the second the conditions that are present in individual diseases. This lesson will deal with General

Pathology. Special Pathology will be studied in the lessons on Symptomatology.

BLOOD CHANGES

In all constitutional and practically all of the local disorders there is some change in the quantity or quality of the blood.

Anemia is a term applied to a condition in which there is a deficiency in the total quantity of the blood or some of its separate elements. Usually there is too little coloring matter (Hemoglobin) or a decrease in the number of red blood cells in addition to changes in the blood plasma.

Leukocytosis means that there is an increased number of white blood cells, usually poly-nuclear. (This condition is normal after exercise, after meals and during pregnancy.)

Leukemia is a form of Anemia in which the number of white cells is greatly increased and there is some disorder of the blood-forming organs.

Toxemia denotes the presence of poisonous materials in the blood. (See below.)

An Embolus is a particle of foreign matter floating in the blood stream. When the blood clots in a blood vessel during life, the condition is known as Thrombosis.

TOXEMIA

This term is applied to a condition in which there is poisoning of the body cells and tissues by harmful materials in the blood stream. They may be formed within the body or taken in from without.

The **External Toxins** that may produce disease include gases, minerals, drugs, animal poisons, improper diet and parasites. Examples of each class are: Minerals—lead, mercury; Drugs—arsenic, strychnine, opium, acids; Animal Poisons—bites of insects and reptiles; Parasites—worms, bacteria; Dietary—decomposed food, excessive food.

Internal Toxins may include those produced by excessive, diminished or perverted activity of glands and glandular organs, toxins from the malignant tumors and abscesses, the waste products of metabolism, retained carbon-dioxide or bile, and poisonous material absorbed from the decomposition of fecal matter in the colon.

CIRCULATORY CHANGES
Ischemia (or Local Anemia) denotes an abnormal decrease in the amount of blood in an organ or part.

Hyperemia (or **Congestion**) means that there is an abnormal increase in the amount of blood remaining within the vessels.)

If an excessive amount of blood plasma or lymph passes through the vessel walls into the surrounding tissues, the condition is known as **Edema**.

When there is an escape of blood (plasma and cells) from the blood vessels, due to the rupture or injury of the vessel walls a **Hemorrhage** is said to have taken place.

When an Embolus or Thrombus (see above) lodges in a small artery, it may produce degeneration of the tissues that are supplied by this vessel. This condition is known as **Infarction.**

INFLAMMATION

Whenever living tissue is irritated or slightly injured, an effort is made to remove the irritation and to repair the damage done. This phenomenon is known as Inflammation.

Formerly inflammation was considered a destructive process—a condition to be combated. Now it is known that it is really a constructive process and no effort should be made to interfere with it unless the reaction is too great.

The irritation produces first a dilatation of the blood vessel supplying the part. This is followed by a slowing of the local circulation producing Stasis. Next the blood cells and the blood plasma pass through the vessel wall into the surrounding tissues.

The tissue cells increase in size and multiply and if the irritation has been severe enough, they undergo degeneration.

Inflammation may terminate in several ways. If the reaction has not been too great, the tissue returns to nearly its normal state. There may be an increase in the amount of connective tissue. The affected area may undergo suppuration or necrosis. (See below). If the inflammation has been improperly treated it may become chronic.

Special types of inflammation are given special names. If the working structure of an organ is affected, it is called Parenchymatous Inflammation. When the connective tissue supporting the structure of the part is affected, it is called Interstitial. Catarrhal Inflammation refers to mucous membranes; Serous Inflammation to endothelial membranes. If accompanied by an increase in the amount of connective or fibrous tissue in or upon the surface of a part, it is Fibrinous Inflammation. Purulent Inflammation is present when pus is formed in a tissue or part.

If the irritation is severe and of short duration Acute Inflammation is produced. In this condition the blood vessels and the working cells of the part are principally affected and the tissues become infiltrated with leukocytes.

When the irritation is mild and extends over a long period a Chronic Inflammation is produced. There is an increased amount of connective tissue in the affected part and an infiltration of blood plasma or lymph.

DESTRUCTIVE PROCESSES

All disorders of marked intensity or prolonged duration produce degenerative or destructive changes in the cells and tissues. The most important of these changes are given below.

Atrophy is a term applied to a condition in which there is a decrease in the size or amount of a certain tissue due to a decrease in the number or size of its cells.

Sometimes these cells or tissues are changed into another type of cells or tissues that is of a lower order and incapable of performing the required functions. These changes are included under the term **Metaplasia**.

Some disorders are accompanied by a deposit of connective tissue, fat or calcium salts in or around the other tissue cells, producing a condition known as **Infiltration.**

The destructive changes in the cells that are produced by deficient nutrition, defective elimination or poisonous materials are grouped under the general head of **Degeneration.** The most common varieties are given below.

In Granular Degeneration the cell becomes swollen, cloudy and is filled with a granular material. The nucleous and capsule are destroyed and the cell disintegrates.

In Fatty Degeneration the normal protoplasm of the cells is changed into fat.

Mucoid, Hyaline, Colloid or Amyloid Degeneration are terms used when the normal cell material changes to a colorless albuminous substance. The various types can be differentiated only by chemical tests.

There may be an increased amount of connective or fibrous tissue in a part following some other condition, producing **Fibrosis.** It may follow wounds or injury to the tissues or be secondary to inflammation. Prolonged mild irritation may cause it. When there is a destruction of the working tissues or cells, they may be replaced by fibrous tissue.

When masses of tissue die, Necrosis is said to have taken place. This term is usually applied to the death of hard tissue (bone.)

Lesson 21: Pathology

Gangrene occurs when the soft tissues undergo death and decomposition. If the blood supply is diminished, dry gangrene is present. The part is dry, brittle and black. When the blood supply is good but there is some interference with the venous drainage, the part becomes swollen, soft and putrid, producing moist gangrene.

If the cells on a free surface die a few at a time and are thrown off by the underlying cells the process is called **Ulceration**.

Suppuration is a process in which the tissue cells, leukocytes and bacteria undergo decomposition and form, with the blood cells, a fluid or semi-fluid mass known as pus.

If the pus is enclosed in a newly formed cavity the collection is called an **Abscess**.

Suppurating or ulcerating canals connecting cavities with each other or with the outer surface are called Sinuses or **Fistulae**.

CONSTRUCTIVE PROCESSES

The body, in its effort to counteract or reduce the injury of the tissue or part, may bring about certain constructive or regenerative changes which include repair, renewal or replacement of cells or tissues.

Hypertrophy means that there has been an increase in the size of the tissue cells usually because there is an increased amount of work for them to do.

If the increase in the size of a part is due to an increase in the number of cells the condition is known as **Hyperplasia**.

275

Regeneration is the term applied to the repair or replacement of cells or tissues that have been injured or that have undergone physiological degeneration.

Wounds that sever tissues and allow separation of the cut surfaces are healed by the formation of granulation tissue and scar tissue. The blood vessels surrounding the cavity produce new capillaries which line the cavity. This is called Granulation tissue. The opening soon becomes filled with newly formed connective tissue interwoven with blood vessels (Scar tissue). The connective tissue contracts and draws the surfaces of the wound together, usually with a mass of fibrous tissue between them.

Foreign substances within the tissues may be surrounded, absorbed or replaced by scar tissue. This process is called **Organization**.

TUMORS

A tumor is a new formation without a physiological function or reason for its existence. They are classified as benign (or innocent) and malignant; the difference between the two types is given below.

Benign Tumors resemble the tissue in which they grow, do not spread to other tissues or parts, do not recur after removal and do not directly affect the general health. They are harmful because they produce pressure upon nerves, blood vessels, and organs.

Lesson 21: Pathology

Malignant Tumors do not resemble tissues in which they grow, they spread to other tissues and parts, they recur after removal, and directly affect the general health.

A Cancer is a malignant tumor composed of abnormal epithelial cells. A Sarcoma is a malignant tumor composed of undeveloped connective tissue cells.

The name of a benign tumor is determined by the type of predominating tissue it contains. If composed of fibrous tissue, it is a Fibroma; if of muscle tissue, Myoma; if of fat tissue, Lipoma; if of bone, Osteoma, and Neuroma if it is made up of nerve tissue.

CYSTS
A Cyst is a closed sac of fibrous or epithelial tissue that contains fluid which is secreted by its lining membrane.

Cysts are divided according to the manner in which they are formed into four classes. A Retention Cyst is formed by the obstruction of the duct or gland. A Distention Cyst is formed by the accumulation of fluid in a preexisting sac or cavity. The internal structure of a tumor may undergo degeneration and form a Degenerative Cyst. Some animal parasites surround themselves with a capsule, producing what is known as a Parasitic Cyst.

GRANULOMA
This term is applied to accumulations of connective tissue, blood vessels, leukocytes, or special abnormal cells around a collection of bacteria. In Tuberculosis it is called a Tubercle. In Syphilis, it is given the name of Gumma. Similar masses are found in Leprosy, Glanders, and Actinomycosis.

FEVER

When the body temperature is above 98 6-10 the condition is known as Fever. It is due to perverted metabolism, toxemia, or some nervous disturbance of the heat-regulating mechanism.

Except in the latter case, it may be considered as an effort of the body to destroy the poisonous material. Prolonged or severe fever is accompanied by granular degeneration of the heart, liver, kidney, spleen and muscles.

QUESTIONS—LESSON 21

1.   What is Pathology and why is it necessary to study it?

2.   Name the Pathological Blood Changes and describe one of them.

3.   Name the Circulatory Changes and define one of them.

4.   Write a brief description of the changes that take place during Inflammation.

5.   What is the difference between a Destructive and a Constructive Process?

6.   Describe Granular Degeneration.

7.   Explain how Wounds are healed.

8.   What is a Tumor and what is the difference between a Benign and a Malignant Tumor?

9.   What is a Cyst?

10. What is Fever?

EXTENSION COURSE IN CHIROPRACTIC AMERICAN UNIVERSITY CHICAGO, Ill., U.S.A.

LESSON 22

ETIOLOGY

Etiology is that branch of science that treats of the cause or causes of disease.

Causes may be divided into Indirect, or Predisposing, and Direct, or Exciting. Predisposing causes act by lowering the resistance of certain tissues, or of the body as a whole, making them more susceptible to the effects of the exciting causes. The factors that have an immediate effect in the production of disease are called Active or Exciting causes.

For example: improper diet, lack of exercise, too little fresh air and sunshine may lower the resistance of the individual so that a short exposure to extreme cold may produce Pneumonia, while the same exposure would have no effect upon an individual whose resistance was up to normal. A subluxation of the 6th Dorsal vertebrae will lower the resisting power of the tissues of the stomach so that slight errors in diet will produce digestive disturbances when they would not do so in an individual who had no such subluxation.

The cause that is predisposing in one case may, in another case, be an exciting cause. The effect of each agent can be determined in each individual case only by taking a careful history and making a thorough examination of the patient.

A more practical classification of etiological factors in disease is that of External Causes and Internal Causes; the former referring to those factors that exist outside of the body and the latter to conditions present in the body that produce the disorders that we know as diseases.

EXTERNAL CAUSES

Atmospheric. Climate is unquestionably a factor in lowering the bodily resistance. A climate in which the temperature varies with the seasons from zero to 100 degrees, with the average temperature about 60 is the best for maintenance of vitality, vigor and mental and physical energy.

A climate in which the temperature remains practically the same for long periods is not conducive to good health; temperatures above 60 are more injurious than those below this point.

In addition to the proper temperature, it is necessary that the air contain the proper percentage of moisture; a humidity of from 60 to 80 being the best, It is also desirable that the air be in motion.

Those spending a large portion of their time indoors should see that the atmospheric conditions approach those outside as near as possible. In addition to having a plentiful supply of pure, fresh air, the room temperature should not be much above 60 when physical work is being done and not above 65 when the work is mental. All artificial means of heating houses decrease the amount of moisture in the air; this must be overcome by the evaporation of water in the room. Fresh, pure air of correct temperature and humidity is not sufficient in itself. The air in the room must be kept in circulation.

Occupation. Certain occupations have an injurious effect because they require the individual to stand or sit in an incorrect position or because of poor ventilation or sanitation.

Prolonged standing or sitting in the same position or constant use of certain muscles without the use of other muscles are also factors in lowering the resistance.

Work requiring long hours with insufficient rest uses more nervous energy than can be replaced during sleep and makes the individual more susceptible to disease.

Gaseous, mineral or animal poisons are elements of danger in some trades.

Home Life. In addition to the factors mentioned above under occupation, it is essential that the home life be congenial, free from irritation and monotony. Constant quarreling and emotional disturbances use up an immense amount of nervous energy that should be utilized by the body functions in addition to disturbing the activity of the entire nervous system.

Lesson 22: Etiology

Clothing. The influence of clothing in the production of disease is too often overlooked. Most individuals wear more clothing than is really necessary. Excessive clothing decreases the activity and lowers the resistance of the skin, making the individual more susceptible to slight changes in temperature.

A few persons wear too little clothing in cool weather; this wastes nervous energy that is required to maintain the proper body temperature.

Clothing should produce no pressure or restriction upon any part of the body. Free movement of the chest and abdomen during respiration is absolutely essential to normal health. Respiration is one of the fundamental functions of the body and interference with it may produce practically any disorder. The tight belts worn by men, as well as the corsets worn by the women restrict the abdominal respiratory movements. Both are very important factors in the production of abdominal and pelvic disorders.

The rubbing of some articles of clothing upon the body produces a constant irritation that may disturb the activity of the entire nervous system. Incorrect shoes deform the feet, and produce incorrect posture. Undergarments hung from the shoulders may produce dorsal kyphosis and round shoulders, especially in children.

Exercise. No individual can long maintain a normal degree of health unless he has the proper amount and kind of exercise. The form of exercise necessary depends somewhat upon the individual, but in every case he should move every vertebrae of his spine through its full normal range of movement and the exercise should be sufficiently strenuous to increase the rate and force of the heart beat and depth of Respiration.

At least fifteen minutes should be spent daily in special forms of exercise. If the occupation requires that the individual remain for long periods in one position, he should take light active exercises for the arms, legs, neck and waist several times a day.

Too much exercise is nearly as bad as too little. Exercise should never be so prolonged or severe that it requires more than one hour to become fully rested.

Rest and relaxation are fully as important as exercise. Some persons are never relaxed; their muscles are in a constant state of tension, misusing nervous energy that could be profitably used for other purposes.

Sleep. Just what vital force or nervous energy is and where it comes from is still a matter of dispute, but it is certain that it is replenished during sleep. If a sufficient amount of good sound sleep is not secured, your therapeutic measures will have a limited effect in restoring the patient to health. The amount of sleep required varies considerably with different individuals; generally speaking, about eight hours each night is necessary.

The sleeping room must be cool, dark, quiet and well ventilated. It is not sufficient to have a window open a few inches at the top or bottom. Whenever possible, arrangements should be made to have an opening on two sides of the room and place the bed between the two of them so that it is reasonably certain that the individual will be sleeping in air that is in motion. If necessary,

284

a screen may be used to prevent the draft falling directly upon the patient's body.

The posture during sleep is very important, especially if the patient has any spinal lesions. Soft beds that settle down in the middle and the use of too thick or too thin pillows may produce spinal lesions. The lateral or prone positions are the best during sleep; no person should sleep on his back unless it is impossible for him to sleep in any other position.

Bathing. Generally speaking, one warm bath with soap each week is sufficient unless the person perspires very freely or is engaged in some dirty occupation. Most individuals will be benefited by a short cold bath each morning, but it should never be taken unless there is good reaction following it and the individual feels better in every way after the bath than before. Excessive use of prolonged hot baths lowers the body tone and makes the skin more susceptible to external influences.

Diet. Of all things that relate to health, diet is the most important and the least understood. If the diet does not supply the element the body needs in the form that can be digested and assimilated, the cells and tissues will degenerate no matter how correct his other habits of living may be.

The most common as well as the most injurious dietary error is the use of foods that are deficient in organic salts. Other common dietary errors are the excessive use of sugars and starches, condiments and, less often, proteids. Most of the foods in common use are so changed in their preparation for the table that the greater portion of their organic salts is removed or changed so much that they cannot be utilized by the body.

(Dietetics will be more fully discussed in Lesson 57.)

Poisons. In addition to the poisons that may be taken in with the air breathed or absorbed through the skin (gases and minerals), injurious substances may be taken through the mouth. Among these may be mentioned alcohol, tobacco and drugs. Animal parasites (worms) and bacteria may find entrance to the body through the mouth, nose or skin. The effect of bacteria in the causation of disease is still a matter of dispute, but it is certain that they have no bad effect upon the body unless the resistance of the tissues or the body as a whole has been lowered by other causes. Vaccination and serum treatment for the prevention of disease unquestionably have a bad effect upon the body, even though they do prevent certain diseases, which is very doubtful.

Habits. Alcohol, tobacco and drugs have been mentioned above. Many individuals eat an excessive amount of candy. Excessive venery and other forms of dissipation are factors in the production of some disorders, especially those due to low vitality. The influence of worry and uncontrolled fits of temper must not be overlooked.

Trauma. Blows, falls, strains and similar accidents may directly produce injuries to the tissues, may lower the vitality of the parts so that other agents are more effective in producing disease, or they may reflexly produce diseases in other parts through their effect upon the nerve supply or circulation to organs or tissues in other regions of the body. Faulty posture is a common cause of spinal lesions and may also interfere with the respiratory movement of the chest and abdomen.

INTERNAL CAUSES

The conditions within the body which may produce a disease of the affected part, of some remote part, or of the body as a whole may be classified as spinal, constitutional, reflex, local and mental.

Spinal Causes. Subluxations are the most important spinal lesions when their effect upon remote parts is considered. Curvatures may produce all of the effects of subluxations in addition to more general effects through their influence on posture and respiration. A rigid spine may cause considerable trouble even though the vertebrae are in their normal positions.

Contraction or infiltration of the spinal muscles and shortening of the spinal ligaments may also interfere with the blood or nerve supply to other parts. Abnormal constriction or dilation of the spinal vessels or irritation of the spinal nerves are usually produced by other spinal lesions, although they may exist independently.

(Spinal Lesions will be more fully discussed in Books 10 and 11.)

Constitutional Causes. Toxemia or Anemia may produce diseases of any part of the body; the former because of the poisonous effects of the material in the blood and the latter because the blood does not supply the cells and tissues with the required elements. If the amount of Nervous Energy or bodily force is insufficient for the needs of the body, some organ or tissue is bound to suffer.

Reflex Causes. Many symptoms, as well as local and general pathological changes, are brought about by other conditions in other parts of the body because there is a direct or indirect nervous connection between them. Spinal lesions may be included in the reflex causes. Likewise, the reflexes may be from the colon, rectum, pelvic organs, nasal cavities or eyes. Lesions of these parts directly affect the sympathetic nervous system and may affect the activity of the brain or cord.

Local Causes. Displacement of an organ may interfere with the blood or nerve supply of that organ or one in close relation to it. It may also, through the effects of pressure, disturb the function of some adjacent organ. Injury to or irritation of any tissue will affect the circulation through it and in this way may produce practically any local disorder.

Mental Causes. No real physician can afford to overlook the effect of the patient's mind upon the bodily activities. Emotional disturbances, fits of temper, worry, and mental shock have a profound effect upon the functions of the autonomic nervous system. This division of the nervous system which controls all involuntary activity is under the control of the subconscious or instinctive mind which in turn can be influenced by the conscious mind. It is possible to bring on certain symptoms and disorders by merely thinking you have them. Many individuals are chronic invalids because they believe that their condition is incurable.

(The influence of mind in producing disease will be more fully discussed in Lesson 61.)

QUESTIONS—LESSON 22

1. What is Etiology and why should it be studied?

2. What Atmospheric Conditions are unhealthy?

3. In what ways can the Occupation affect the health?

4. Explain how improper Clothing may produce disease.

5. What kind and how much Exercise should be taken daily?

6. What conditions should be present in a healthful Sleeping Room?

7. What are the most common Dietary Errors?

8. Name the Habits that are injurious to health.

9. In what way does the Spine influence other parts of the body?

10. Name some Reflex Causes of Disease.

EXTENSION COURSE
IN CHIROPRACTIC
AMERICAN UNIVERSITY
CHICAGO, Ill., U.S.A.

LESSON 23 A

DIAGNOSIS

The process of deciding which of several diseases the patient may have is called Diagnosis. A Diagnosis may be made in either of two ways; you may learn the patient's symptoms and compare them with those of the different diseases, or you may make a systematic examination of his body and base your conclusion upon the results of your examination. The symptoms that are present in each of the common diseases will be given in lessons 24 to 38; the methods of examining the patient and the meaning of the abnormal signs found will be taught in this lesson.

No treatment should ever be given without learning beforehand the location, nature and extent of the patient's trouble as well as the internal or external causes that may be producing it.

Generally speaking, no great amount of skill is needed to learn enough about the patient's disorder to satisfactorily apply any drugless method of treatment that may be necessary. If you know the normal anatomy and physiology, how to detect variations from the normal and then make a thorough examination, you will in practically all cases be able to make a satisfactory diagnosis.

PHYSICAL DIAGNOSIS

Physical Diagnosis is the method of discriminating diseases by the direct aid of the special senses, namely, the eye,

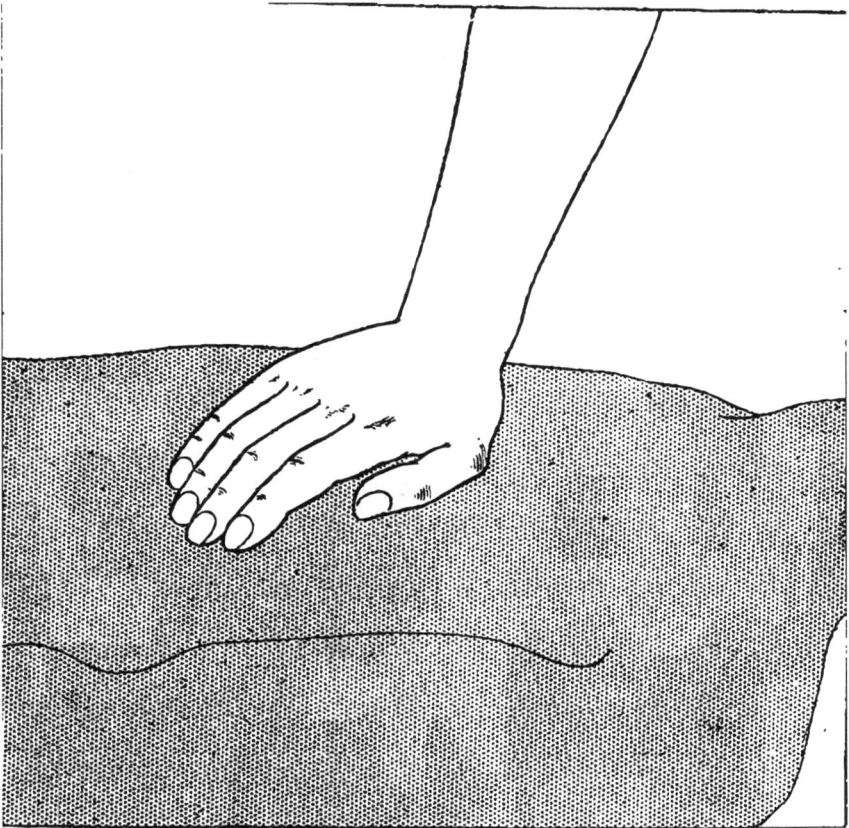

Figure 1

the ear and the touch. The diagnostic evidences thus obtained are known as Physical Signs.

They depend upon the physical nature and structure of the organs or parts examined, and vary with the changes caused by disease. Hence they are divided into two groups: Normal, or Healthy, and Abnormal, or Morbid, Physical Signs.

Physical diagnosis is constantly employed in the study of general maladies and in local diseases of all parts of the body but it is of special service in the investigation of the diseases of the respiratory or circulatory organs. This is the most important of all methods of diagnosis and forms the basis for many other diagnostic methods. It should be used in the examination of every case.

Methods of physical diagnosis are Inspection (seeing), Palpation (feeling), Percussion (striking) and Auscultation (listening). Mensuration (measurement) is sometimes used.

In the examination of the patient these methods are used systematically and in the order given, the signs discovered by one serve to confirm or control the knowledge obtained by the other. Physical examination must under all circumstances be conducted carefully and according to a definite plan. More errors are made from want of system than from want of knowledge. It is best, whenever practical, that the part examined be bare.

METHODS

A good light is necessary for Inspection; the part should be uncovered. You should note any variations from the normal size, shape, color, surface, or movement of the part examined.

When **Palpation** is used, the muscles of the region examined must be relaxed as much as possible. Use the Flat of Hands or Palmar Surfaces of the Fingers, keeping them relaxed as much as possible. Use no more pressure than is absolutely necessary. Make the movements slow and apply the pressure gradually. Palpate tender areas last. You should determine the size,

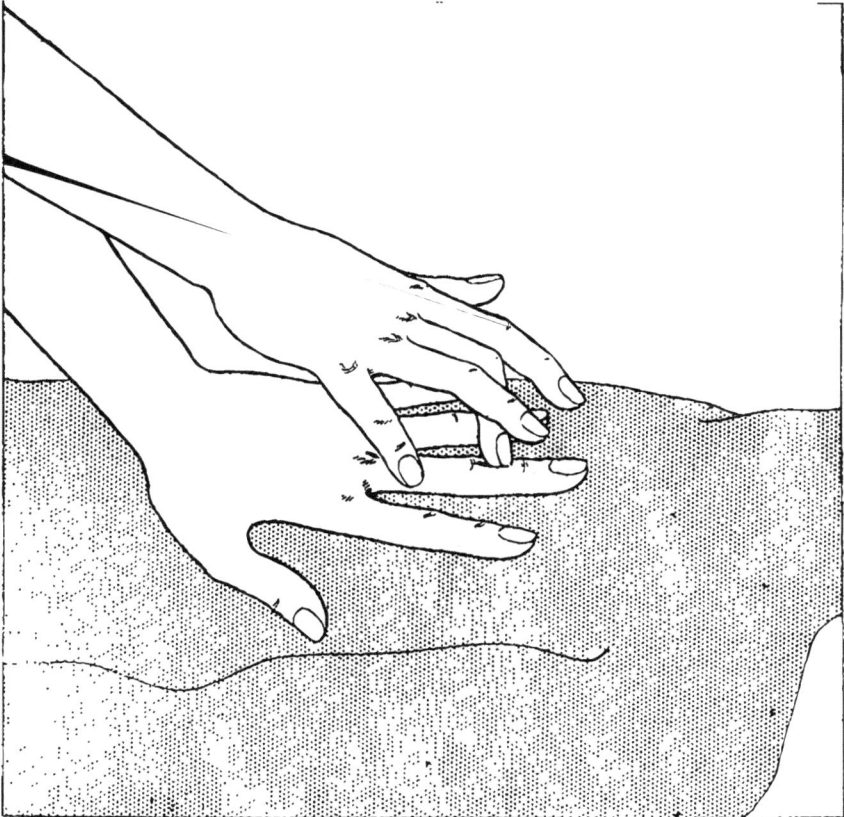

Figure No. 2. Percussion

293

shape, consistency, surface and mobility of the parts as well as their relation to other parts and the presence or absence of tenderness.

The surface outlines of the viscera as determined by Percussion

In **Percussion**, the second finger of the left hand is placed in contact with the skin. The back of the middle phalanx of the finger is struck with the tip of the second finger of the right hand. The left finger should be kept in firm contact with the body. All blows must strike this finger on the same place with the same force. Do not strike any harder than is absolutely necessary to bring out the sound you want to hear. You should listen to the quality, pitch, intensity and length of the sound produced by your blows. Different tissues produce notes of different character, making it possible to determine the kind of tissue or its condition.

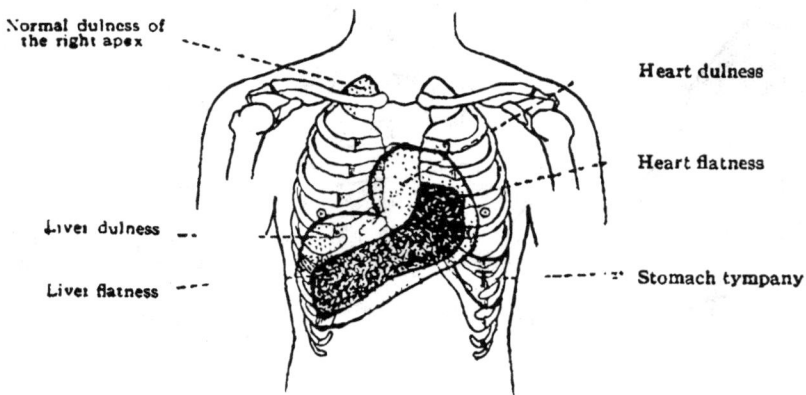

Figure No. 3.
The surface outlines of the viscera as determined by Percussion

For convenience of description four terms are used in describing the notes produced by percussion.

Over the stomach the note is drum-like, low in pitch, loud and long. This is called **Tympany**. Over the lungs the note is more vibrating in character and is medium in pitch, intensity and length. This is **Pulmonary Resonance**.

When the liver is percussed the note is soft, short and high pitched and has a dead sound. The term **Flatness** is applied to this note. When a solid body is not in direct contact with the surface percussed, as is the case with those parts of the heart and liver that

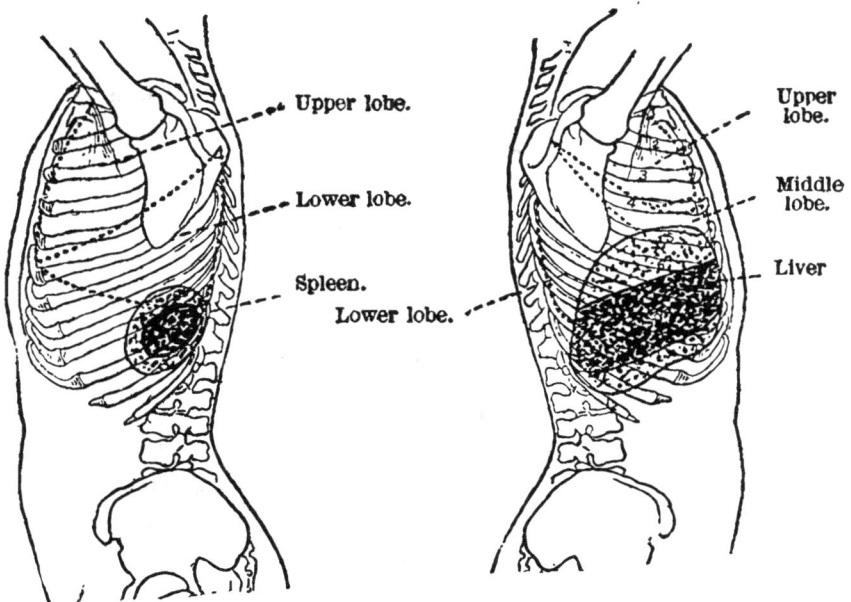

Figures No. 4 and 5.

are covered by the lungs, the note has a quality between that of resonance and flatness. This is known as **Dullness**.

By the use of percussion it is possible to determine the size, shape and position of the different solid and hollow organs, whether there has been any consolidation the softer tissues, and the presence or absence of fluid in hollow organs.

The positions of the Liver and Spleen as outlined by Percussion. The heavily shaded areas indicate Flatness. The lightly shaded areas are Dull on Percussion.

To be able to determine whether an organ is in an abnormal position or of abnormal size or shape, you must know the normal position, size and shape of the organ. The borders of an organ, as determined by percussion or palpation, do not always correspond with the real size and shape of the organ. The illustrations (See figures 3 to 7) show the surface relations of the normal thoracic and abdominal organs.

The Stethoscope is generally used for **Auscultation**. The bell of the instrument must be pressed firmly against the skin and held still. Movement of the bell on the body or of the fingers on the stethoscope will produce the sounds that will confuse you. This method is most valuable in the examination of the heart and lungs.

When examining the lungs the patient should breathe deeply but easily and noiselessly. If the stethoscope is placed over the trachea or large bronchi, the respiratory sounds will be very loud; during expiration it is louder, longer and higher in pitch than during inspiration. This is called **Bronchial Breathing**.

Over the body of the lungs (except right apex) the sounds are very faint. The inspiratory sound is louder, longer and higher in pitch than that during expiration. (Many times the expiratory sound cannot be heard). This is called **Vesicular Breathing**.

Broncho-vesicular Breathing is heard in the middle of the chest between the large bronchi and the body of the lungs. It is also heard over the right apex. When the patient speaks, the vibration of his voice can be heard through the stethoscope; its intensity decreases as the distance from the trachea increases. It is not possible to recognize the words he speaks.

GENERAL PHYSICAL EXAMINATION

Observe the General Appearance of the patient, paying special attention to his Posture, Gait, Rate of Movement, General Behavior and Mental Condition.

Study His Face, paying particular attention to Expression, Color, State of Nutrition, Movement and Condition of the Eyes.

Learn the Present Weight as well as the weight for some time previous to the examination, also the weight that the patient considers normal for himself.

Use the Thermometer and determine the patient's temperature. You should also know the duration of the change of temperature and what variations of temperature have taken place.

Palpate the Radial Artery (with three fingers). Make a note of Rate, Volume, the Regularity of Time and Force, and the Compressibility of the Artery.

Examine the Skin, paying attention to the Color, Moisture, Temperature, Consistency and Condition of its surface.

Watch the Respiratory Movements of the chest and abdominal walls, noting the Rate, Depth and Freedom of the Movement and whether the movement is the same on both sides of the chest and abdomen.

Palpate, or Inspect the Movement of the Apex of the heart. Note the Position, Strength, and Regularity of Time and Force of the apex beat.

Inspect and Palpate the Abdomen. Nothing can be seen or felt in the normal abdomen except the bodies of the Lumbar Vertebrae, the Psoas Muscles and the Abdominal Aorta in thin individuals. If anything is seen or felt, determine its size, shape, surface, consistency and sensitiveness as well as its relationship to the abdominal organs and abdominal wall.

Examine the Spine, noting Shape, Contour, Movement and Sensitiveness. (The detailed examination for detection of subluxations and other spinal lesions will be given in lessons 44 to 48.)

PHYSICAL SIGNS

GENERAL

The Weight is increased or above normal in Obesity, Dropsy and during Convalescence. Loss of weight may be due to Malnutrition, Infectious Fevers, Toxemia, Tuberculosis, Loss of Sleep, Emotional Disturbances or Worry.

Lesson 23 A: Diagnosis

Fever may be present in Infection, Severe Inflammation, Toxemia, or Nervous Disturbances. The temperature may be below normal in Prostration, Wasting Diseases, or Nervous Disturbances. Chills may accompany the onset of Fever, Severe Infections, or Nervous States. Sweats occur at the termination of a period of fever and may be present in Low Vitality or Neurasthenia.

The Pulse is more rapid than normal in Fevers, Heart Diseases, Hemorrhage, Collapse, Exophthalmic Goitre, Menopause, Emotional Disturbances and after Exercise. The pulse rate may be decreased in Exhaustion, Toxemia, Pressure on the Brain, and in some Nervous Disorders. The rate or force of the pulse beat may become irregular in Exhaustion, Toxemia, Heart Disease or Excitement.

The Pulse Wave is small in Exhaustion, Peritonitis, and some Heart Lesions. The pulse wave is large in Fever, after Exercise, and in some Heart Lesions. Generally speaking, the wave is small when the beat is rapid and large when the beat is slow.

The Tension of the Artery is increased in Arteriosclerosis, Chronic Nephritis, Hypertrophied Heart, and when the patient is under a nervous tension. The tension of the artery is low in Wasting Diseases, Low Vitality and Exhaustion. The artery feels hard and incompressible in Arteriosclerosis.

The Skin is bluish (Cyanosis) in Lung and Heart diseases; pale in Anemia, Tuberculosis and in Vaso-motor Disturbances and yellow (Jaundice) whenever there is an Obstruction to the outflow of the Bile or when the Liver Cells are Rapidly Destroyed as well as in severe Toxemia. A peculiar color (Cachexia) is present in Syphilis, Malaria, Cancer and Adrenal Diseases.

Skin Eruptions may be due to Skin Diseases, Toxemias, Drugs, or accompany some of the Acute Infectious Fevers. The skin is dry in Fevers, Severe Diarrhea, Polyuria and Cachexia. It is hot in Fever, Inflammation and wherever there is Hyperemia. Cold skin may be due to an Obstructed or Failing Circulation or to Constriction of the Blood Vessels.

Excessive Moisture is present at the Breaking of a Fever, in Debility, Rheumatism, Prostration and in Vaso-motor Disturbances.

The Skin Pits on Pressure (Edema) in Heart Disease, Nephritis, Anemia, Obstructed Veins and when there is an Abscess beneath the surface.

LUNGS

The Size and Shape of the Chest is not of much diagnostic importance except where there is a deformity covering a small area. Local flattening may be due to Chronic Tuberculosis, Chronic Pleurisy or Fibrosis of the Lungs; local bulging may be caused by Pleurisy with effusion or Thoracic Tumors.

The Movement of the Chest in respiration should be free, painless, and of the same amount on both sides of the chest. The normal respiration is one-fourth the pulse rate.

Rapid Breathing may be due to Heart or Lung Diseases, Anemia, Weakness from any cause or Emotional Disturbances. Slow Breathing may be due to Exhaustion, Toxemia or Pressure on the Brain. Breathing is Difficult in Heart, Lung, or Kidney Diseases, Intercostal Neuralgia, Obstruction to the Trachea or Glottis or in any painful chest condition.

Lesson 23 A: Diagnosis

The Movement of the Chest may be increased in Painful Disorders of the Abdominal Organs. In Painful Chest Conditions, Asthma or Emphysema, the abdominal respiratory movements are increased. The Respiratory Movement of one side of the chest may be decreased with that region distended or retracted; when the restricted side bulges, it may be due to Pleurisy with effusion, or to a Thoracic Tumor, when the restricted side is flattened, Tuberculosis, Pleurisy with adhesions, Obstruction of a Bronchus, Fibrosis of the Lungs, Atelectasis, Thoracic pain or Paralysis of the Respiratory Muscles may be present.

The Resonance of the Chest on percussion is increased when there is a Cavity present and when the Lung is Distended. Decreased Pulmonary Resonance may be caused by Consolidation, Tumor or any condition that interferes with the expansion of that region of the lungs.

Dullness may be present (in the regions where there should be resonance) in Pulmonary Edema or when there is Fluid in the pleural sac. The lung may be diminished in size in Fibrosis or Destruction of the lung tissue, Atrophy or when there is any interference with the expansion of the lung. The lung may be increased in size in Hypertrophy or Distention.

The Breath Sounds are Increased in intensity in Consolidation, Hypertrophy or Compression of the lung. The Breath Sounds are Diminished in intensity when there is Fluid, Air or Solid Matter in the pleural cavity, Obstruction to the Bronchi, Atrophy, or Diminished Activity of the lung.

When Bronchial Respiration is heard over an area in which it should not be present, it indicates that a Cavity is present or that portion of the lung has undergone Consolidation.

Rales are abnormal sounds heard during auscultation. Dry Rales are whistling or blowing sounds caused by Diminished Calibre of the Bronchial Tubes as in Bronchial Asthma. Small, Bubbling Rales are produced by Loose Fluid in the Bronchial Tubes which may be caused by inflammation of these tubes or of the lung tissue as well as congestion of the lungs. Crackling Rales are produced by thick mucous in the lung cells or in any condition in which the cells are collapsed. (Coughing may bring out, intensify or clear away rales.)

The Voice Sounds may be Increased in intensity in Cavity, Consolidation, or when the chest wall is very thin. The Voice Sounds may be Diminished in intensity, or absent, when there is Air or Fluid in the Pleural Cavity, Obstruction to the Bronchi, Thickened Pleura or when the chest wall is fat. Rubbing Sounds are heard close to the chest walls in dry pleurisy.

HEART
If the Apex Beat of the Heart is in its Normal position, and Regular in Time and Force, the heart may, for all practical purposes, be considered Normal.

The Apex may be Displaced when the Heart is Enlarged, in Lung Diseases and when there is an accumulation of Gas in the Stomach or Intestines. The Impulse may be Absent in Pleurisy, Pericarditis, Heart Weakness, or when the apex is behind a rib or the chest is fat. The Impulse may be Irregular in time or force in

Toxemia, Brain Disease, Exhaustion, or Heart Failure from any cause.

The Size, Shape and Position of the Heart may be determined by percussion. It is Enlarged in Valvular Heart Diseases and in any condition that increases the work of the heart. The Heart may be Displaced in any disease of the thoracic contents that causes pressure on one side or diminishes the volume of the tissues on one side of the heart.

Mitral Valve Sounds are heard by placing the stethoscope over the apex of the heart; the Tricuspid over the lower end of the sternum. Both valves sound nearly alike. The First Sound is a long, loud and dull sound, the Second Sound is short and snappy.

The Pulmonary Valve Sounds are heard near the sternum in the second left inter-space; the Aortic in the second right interspace near the sternum. Both sounds of these two valves are of nearly the same length. Before 35 years of age, the Second Pulmonic is louder than the first; after 35 the Second Aortic is louder than the first aortic sound.

The Intensity of the First Mitral sound is Increased whenever the heart is enlarged or whenever the heart beats more forcibly. It is Decreased in intensity in Myocardial Degeneration, some Valve Lesions, Pericarditis, and in Heart Failure from any cause.

The Second Pulmonic sound is Increased whenever there is an increase in the resistance to the flow of the blood through the lungs. Weakening of this sound indicates a serious condition; it may be caused by Degeneration of the Heart Muscle or by Valvular Lesions.

The Second Aortic sound is Intensified when the Heart is Hypertrophied or whenever there is an increase in the resistance to the flow of the blood through the peripheral vessels as in Arteriosclerosis.

Normally, the two valve sounds are heard close together and then there is a period of rest before the sounds are repeated. When this Silent Period becomes Shortened, it is an indication of heart failure, due usually to a degeneration of the heart substance. If the first heart sound (at apex) should be split into two sounds (Gallop Rythm), it is an indication of grave cardiac weakness.

Heart Murmurs are not usually difficult to detect, but they rarely give any information of value in treatment that cannot be obtained from interpretation of the signs given above.

CONDITION OF HEART
The most important thing to determine in regard to the heart is how well it can perform the work required of it. The function of the heart is to aid in the circulation of the blood and it should be capable of responding to any reasonable demand upon it. If the heart functions normally, any anatomical lesions or conditions present in it may be safely disregarded. The best test for the functional capacity of the heart is to have the patient exercise until it markedly increases the rate and depth of his respiration.

Normally, the heart beats more rapidly and more forcibly after exercise. There should be no difficulty in breathing, no faintness, no cyanosis, no signs of venous stasis, nor should the pulse be weak or irregular. If any of the foregoing symptoms are present after a reasonable amount of exercise, the heart should be considered incompetent.

If the heart action is seriously weakened, there will be some interference with the circulation even when the individual is at rest.

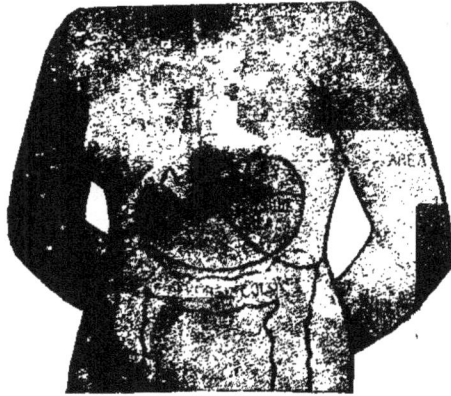

Figure No. 6.

If the circulation through the lungs is retarded, there will be Cough, Dyspnea, Hemoptysis, Rales, or Cyanosis. If the venous blood accumulates in the liver, it will be enlarged and tender and the heart beat may be felt when the hand is placed over it. Dyspepsia will also be present. Venous stasis in the head may produce Vertigo, Syncope, Insomnia, or Pulsation of the jugular veins. Edema may be caused by an incompetent heart. It is usually present in the feet and ankles,

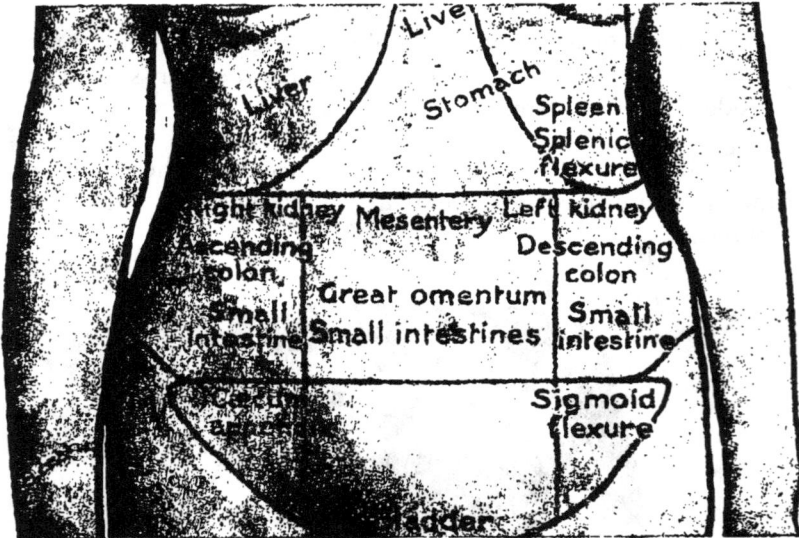

Figure No. 7. Showing the positions and relations of the Abdominal Viscera.

The size, shape and position of the normal Stomach and its relation to the adjacent organs. The portion marked by circles is covered by the lung; the shaded area is overlapped by the liver

Showing the positions and relations of the Abdominal Viscera.

ABDOMEN

The Abdomen may be Enlarged in Ascites, Flatulency, Abdominal or Pelvic Tumors, Pregnancy or in Obesity. The Abdomen is Retracted in Wasting Diseases and in Malnutrition. Local Regions of the Abdomen may Bulge when an Organ is Displaced or Enlarged, or when an Abscess, Tumor or Aneurysm is present. Local Bulging may also be due to a Distended Bladder or to Contraction of the Abdominal Muscles.

If any Mass is Felt in the abdomen (except the vertebrae, aorta, or psoas muscles) you should suspect an Enlarged or Displaced Organ, Tumor, Abscess, Aneurysm, Intestinal Obstruction, or Constipation.

The Abdominal Muscles are Contracted whenever there is Abdominal Inflammation or when there is Irritation of any of the Abdominal Organs or of the Nerves that supply the abdominal muscles. Extreme Muscle Rigidity is caused by Peritonitis (local or general.)

THE SPINE

The Spine may be Deformed in Curvature, Spinal Diseases, or because the patient sits or stands in an incorrect position. Bulging may be due to Subluxated Vertebrae, Contracted Spinal Muscles, Tumors of the spinal tissues or to Curvatures.

The Spine is Rigid in some Spinal Diseases, in most Spinal Lesions and in Spinal Pain or Tenderness. Tenderness of the spinal tissues may be caused by Spinal Lesions, Spinal Diseases or it may be a reflex from some Viscera.

QUESTIONS—LESSON 23 A

1. What is Diagnosis and why should it be studied?

2. What is Physical Diagnosis?

3. Briefly describe the technic of Palpation.

4. What sounds are produced by Percussion?

5. What is Auscultation and what organs are usually examined by this method?

6. Give a brief outline of the General Physical Examination. (Need not give the conditions examined for).

7. What conditions may interfere with the Normal Movement of the Chest?

8. What conditions may produce Abnormal Breath Sounds, or Rales?

9. What is the most important thing to learn about the Heart?

10. If you felt a Mass in the Abdomen what would you suspect?

EXTENSION COURSE
IN CHIROPRACTIC
AMERICAN UNIVERSITY
CHICAGO, Ill., U.S.A.

LESSON 23 B

EXAMINATION OF THE PATIENT

Symptoms are divided into Subjective and Objective symptoms; the former term is applied to those symptoms of which the patient himself is conscious, the latter to those which are discovered by the physician when he examines the patient.

Objective symptoms are also known as Signs. The objective symptoms and the conditions that produce them are discussed in the sections on Diagnosis. The subjective symptoms are learned by carefully questioning the patient. It is often necessary to know the patient's previous condition of health, habits, etc. These facts are included under the term of History.

It is essential that you learn every important condition, change, or symptom that may have any influence upon the diagnosis or treatment of the patient's condition. This makes it necessary to follow some definite plan when questioning the patient if you are to get all of the desired information within a reasonable length of time. Below is given a schedule that will answer every purpose.

TAKING PATIENT'S HISTORY

Learn and record the patient's Age, Sex, Civil State and Occupation, also street address and phone number.

PREVIOUS DISEASES

Some diseases makes the patient more susceptible to other diseases and some acute disorders may later develop into chronic diseases. In certain chronic conditions the symptoms are manifested at regular or irregular intervals. It will do no harm to have the complete record of the patient's previous condition of health.

FAMILY HISTORY

While it has not been definitely proven that any disease is hereditary, there is no doubt that the resisting power of the various tissues and organs is considerably influenced by heredity. It is also true that certain types of individuals are more susceptible to certain disorders than other types. The physical and mental characteristics are very largely determined by heredity. If the patient's ancestors are stout or thin and he is of the same type, it will be difficult to increase or decrease his weight. If the parents are of a neurotic disposition the child too will be more susceptible to functional nervous disorders.

PRESENT COMPLAINT

Allow the patient to tell you in his own way just what symptoms induced him to come to you. These are the ones that most concern him and that he is most anxious to have relieved. You may relieve all other symptoms, but he will not be satisfied until you overcome the symptoms that brought him to you.

TREATMENT

Learn what treatment the patient has used and what effect these measures have had upon his condition.

COMMON SYMPTOMS

A symptom that seems very important to the patient may be of very little value to you in diagnosis and he may entirely overlook some symptom that is absolutely essential to diagnosis. This makes it necessary for you to carefully question him about the presence or absence of the following common symptoms:

Pain (head, neck, back, chest, abdomen, pelvis and extremities), Headache, Dizziness, Sore Mouth, Sore Throat, Catarrh, Eye Trouble, Palpitation, Dyspnea, Cough, Expectoration, Flatulency, Constipation, Diarrhea, Foul Stool, Piles, Urinary Difficulties, Abnormal Urine, Leukorrhea, Dysmenorrhea, Convulsions, Paralysis, Muscular Rigidity, Ataxia, Weakness, Emaciation, Jaundice, Skin Eruptions, Edema, Fever, Chills, Cold Extremities, Cramps and Nervousness.

If he has none of the above symptoms there is nothing serious the matter with him; the presence of any of them will guide you in further questioning and in examination.

SPECIAL SYMPTOMS

Each physiological system of the body produces symptoms that are peculiar to it when it becomes diseased. Listed below are the signs and symptoms that indicate disorders of the different systems.

Nervous System. Convulsions, Localized Spasms, Paralysis, Anesthesia, Numbness, Tremor, Vertigo, Coma, Difficulty in

Walking or Standing, Mental or Speech Disturbances, Rectal or Bladder Disturbances, Frequent or Continuous Headache, Frequent Vomiting.

Blood. Pallor, Dyspnea, Palpitation, Headache, Vertigo, Hemorrhages, Debility, Emaciation, Cachexia, Edema of Feet, Dyspepsia.

Heart and Vessels. Dyspnea, Cyanosis, Palpitation, Cough, Edema, Precordial distress, Sudden Vertigo, Restless Sleep, Bronchitis, Piles, Pulsating Liver, Dyspepsia, Obesity.

Lungs. Cough, Hemoptysis, Dyspnea, Chest Pain, Cyanosis, Loss of Weight and Strength, Night Sweats, Fever.

Stomach and Intestines. Abdominal Pain, Pyrosis, Eructations, Flatulency, Nausea, Vomiting, Headache, Foul Breath, Stomatitis, Coated Tongue, Rapid Wasting, Hematamesis, Costiveness, Diarrhea, Foul Stools, Mental Depression.

Liver and Gall Bladder. Right Hypochrondial Pain, Jaundice, Dark Urine, Grey Stools, Pruritis, Dyspepsia, Hematamesis, Nausea, Melancholia, Irregular Chills and Fever.

Kidneys and Bladder. Lumbar Pain, Painful or Frequent Micturition, Smoky or Turbid Urine, Polyuria, Oliguria, Dyspnea, Facial Edema, Anasarca, Headache, Drowsiness, Nausea, Vomiting, Asthma, Amblyopia, Dyspepsia, Convulsions.

Pelvic Organs. Pelvic, Abdominal or Spinal Pain, Vaginal Discharge, Backache, Menstrual Disturbances, Costiveness, Bladder Disturbances, Nervousness.

The "Pain Area" Charts will also aid you in deciding which organs are most probably diseased.

PHYSICAL EXAMINATION

First make a thorough physical examination of the organs that you suspect as being the seat of the patient's disorder. Next make a brief general examination. (See Lesson 23.)

SPINAL EXAMINATION

Make a thorough spinal examination. (See Lesson 44 to 48.)

OTHER EXAMINATIONS

Examine the Urine, and use any Special Method of examination that may be necessary.

ETIOLOGICAL HISTORY

No treatment can have much permanent effect unless the cause of the patient's disorder is found and removed or counteracted. The causes of disease are given in Lesson 22. Below is given a schedule that may be followed to enable you to secure the most information in the least time.

Diet. Breakfast, Lunch, Supper, Between Meals, Amount, Meat and Eggs, Bread and Cereals, Vegetables, Fruits, Raw Food, Condiments, Coffee, Tea, Milk, Water, Sugar, Appetite, Mastication, Digestion, Satisfaction.

Habits. Bowel, Bladder, Sleep, Baths, Exercise, Work, Rest, Recreation, Sexual, Acquired, Candy.

Occupation. Posture, Fatigue, Sanitation, Ventilation, Poisons, Temperature, Associates, Surroundings.

Clothing. Amount, Pressure, Friction, Constriction, Shoes, Hanging from Waist.

Home. Family, Associates, Surroundings, Ventilation, Temperature, Heating, Humidity.

Mentality. Disposition, Emotions, Worry, Shock, Contentment, Idea of Present Illness, Temperament, Fits of Temper.

Trauma. Falls, Blows, Strains, Temperature Extremes, Operations, Shocks.

Infection. Parasites, Chemicals, Vegetables, Gasses, Drugs.

URINALYSIS
Much information relative to the patient's condition can be obtained by examination of the urine. The amount, appearance and composition of the urine varies with the weight of the individual, the temperature of the surrounding atmosphere, the amount of physical work he does, the amount of water taken each day and upon his diet. These factors must always be taken into consideration when the urine is examined, otherwise the findings will be unreliable and misleading.

NORMAL URINE
The urine of a normal, healthy man, weighing 150 pounds, doing a moderate amount of physical labor in a moderate temperature, living on a normal diet and drinking five pints of water each day will have the following characteristics and composition:

Physical Characteristics:

Amount: 1500 cc	Solids: 50 grams
Color: Amber	Transparency: Clear
Odor: Urinous	Specific Gravity: 1.015 to 1.025
Reaction: Acid (15 degrees - 22,500 acid units per day.)	

Chemical Composition:

Water: 1450 cc	
Organic Solids -	Inorganic Solids -
Urea: 23 grams	Chlorides: 12 grams
Uric Acid: 1/2 gram	Phosphates: 3 grams
Proteids: 1 1/2 grams	Sulphates: 3 grams
Pigments, etc.: 5 grams	Other Salts: 2 grams

ABNORMAL URINE
PHYSICAL CHANGES

The Amount may be Increased in Diabetes, Interstitial Nephritis, High Blood Pressure, Hysteria and when the skin is cold. Also when more than five pints of water are drunk each day.

The Amount may be Decreased in Parenchymatous Nephritis, Acute Rheumatic Fever, Acute Infectious Fevers, Renal Congestion, Vomiting, Diarrhea, Excessive Perspiration or when too little water is taken.

The Color is Pale in Interstitial Nephritis, Diabetes, Epilepsy, Hysteria, and when there is a decreased amount of solids in it. The Color is Dark in Acute Nephritis and when there is an increased amount of solids or when the amount of urine is less than normal. The urine is Smoky when it contains Decomposed Blood; Pink when Fresh Blood is present, and Dark Yellow or Brown when it contains Bile.

An Odor resembling Ammonia indicates Decomposition of the urine either in the bladder or after it has been passed. A Putrid odor is caused by the presence of decomposed Blood, Pus or Albumin. In Diabetes Mellitis it may have a Sweetish Odor.

The Urine is Cloudy whenever it contains an Excess of Solids of any kind. This solid matter may be Blood, Pus, Phosphates or Mucus, or it may be due to a diminished quantity of urine.

The Specific Gravity is Increased when there is Sugar or Albumin present and when there is an increased amount of solids or a decreased amount of urine. The Specific Gravity is Decreased in Interstitial Nephritis, Diabetes, Hysteria, Neurasthenia, and when the quantity of solids is decreased or the amount of urine is increased.

The Amount of the Solids in the urine is Increased when there is an Excessive Waste of the Body Tissues, when an Excessive Amount of Food is eaten (especially proteids) and when it contains Sugar or Albumin. The Solids may be Diminished in any Kidney Disease and in Constitutional Disorders accompanied by Diminished Metabolism.

316

Alkaline Reaction indicates Fermentation of the urine either in the bladder or after it has been voided. Increased Acidity may be due to an Excessive Amount of Acid-forming Food, to a Decreased Alkalinity of the Body Fluids and Tissues (Acidosis) or to Excessive Muscular Activity.

Sediment at the bottom of the glass may be due to Scanty or Concentrated urine, changes in the acidity or because the urine has Decomposed from standing.

MICROSCOPIC CHANGES

Red and white blood cells indicate a hemorrhage from some part of the genito-urinary tract; degenerated polynuclear leukocytes indicate suppuration. Bacteria are present if there is an infection.

Granular or Hyalin Casts are present in Chronic Interstital Nephritis, Renal Stasis and after prolonged physical exertion. Blood or Epithelial Casts indicate an Active Inflammation of the Kidneys. Pus Casts indicate Suppuration in the Kidneys. Fatty Casts are present in Fatty Degeneration of the Kidneys.

Urate, Uric Acid, Phosphate and Oxalate Crystals may be found in the urine.

CHEMICAL CHANGES

Albumen is present in Nephritis, Renal Stasis, Poisoning, Anemia, when there is an Excessive Waste of Tissue or an Excessive amount of Proteid in the diet. (Blood or pus in the urine will also give the reaction for albumin.)

317

Sugar (Glucose) may indicate Diabetes, Mellitus or an Excessive amount of Carbohydrates in the diet. Indican is present when there is putrifaction of proteid food material in the Colon.

Bile is an indication of Jaundice. Pus is present in Renal, Vesical or Urethral Infection. Blood is present in Renal, Vesical or Urethral Inflammation, Stone or Tumor in the Kidney or Bladder, Acute Infectious Fevers and in poisoning.

Acetone or Diacetic Acid in the urine may be the result of too much Fat or too little Carbohydrates in the diet. It is commonly present in Diabetes and of serious consequence.

The Amount of Urea may be Increased (over 35 grams) in Acute Infectious Fevers, Excessive Tissue Waste, Fasting, or may be due to an Excess or Proteid in the diet or to Increased Acidity of the urine. The Amount of Urea may be Diminished (under 10 grams) in Kidney Diseases, Liver Diseases, Diminished Tissue Waste or when there is a Deficiency of Proteid in the diet.

The Amount of Uric Acid may be Increased (over one gram) in Acute Infectious Fevers, Excessive Tissue Waste, Fasting, Acute Rheumatic Fever, Renal or Vesical Stones, or it may be due to the Diet (excess of purine bodies). The Amount of Uric Acid may be Diminished (less than 1/4 gram) in Kidney Diseases, Diminished Tissue Waste, Deficiency of Proteid in the diet (vegetarian or purine free diet.)

CHEMICAL TESTS

Whenever possible you should take a sample of the whole amount of urine passed during twenty-four hours; otherwise, take the urine first voided in the morning. Urine will decompose in

318

a few hours unless kept cold. (A few drops of chloroform in the container will prevent decomposition.)

Albumin. If urine is turbid filter it before testing. Place urine in the test tube and heat it over an alcohol lamp. If albumin is present, a white cloud will be formed and this white cloud will remain after you have added two drops of acetic acid. If the white material, after settling to the bottom of the tube, equals 1/4 of the urine, there is 1/4 of one per cent of albumin present; if it equals 1/2 of the urine, there is one per cent, and if the whole tube is filled, there is two to three per cent of albumin in the urine.

Sugar. You should test the urine for albumin first and filter out any albumin that may be present before testing for sugar. Take 4 cc of Fehling's Solutions (2 cc of each solution) and add 12 cc of water. Heat in a test tube until it boils. While it is hot, add the suspected urine drop by drop. If sugar is present a red or yellow deposit will be formed. If 15 drops of urine are required to produce this deposit, there is two per cent of sugar in the urine. If 60 drops are used there is one-half per cent of sugar in the urine.

Bile. Filter the urine through filter paper and then drop one drop of Nitric Acid on the wet filter paper. If bile is present there will be a play of colors (green predominating.)

Blood. Add enough Potassium Hydroxide (caustic potash) to make the urine strongly alkaline. Boil the urine. If blood is present there will be a red or brown deposit.

Pus. Take equal parts of urine and solution of Sodium Hydroxide and shake together. White ropy strings or white jelly-like deposit indicate pus.

Indican. Mix the following chemicals in the order given: 4 cc filtered Urine, 1 drop of one per cent Solution of Potassium Chlorate, 2 cc Chloroform and 4 cc pure Hydrochloric Acid. Mix thoroughly and allow it to stand for ten minutes, shaking it several times during this period. The presence of indican is indicated by a blue color. The amount can be estimated by the shade of the blue; the greater the amount of indican the darker the color.

Urea. Use a Doremus Ureometer. Fill it with a Sodium Hypobromite Solution (water 250 cc, sodium hydroxide 25 grams and bromine 5 cc) Add exactly 1 cc of urine which will form a gas. When no more gas is formed note the figure at the top of the tube at which the urine stands. The figure will give you the number of grams of urea in one cubic centimeter of urine. To determine the total amount of urea passed in a day it will be necessary to multiply this figure by the number of cc of urine passed that day.

Uric Acid. Take 5 cc of Carbon Bisulphite and add 2 cc of Ruheman's Solution. Pour the urine slowly into the tube (shaking often) until the lower portion of the mixture becomes white. Then note the amount of urine that has been used to produce this change. If 3 cc of urine has been used there is two grams of uric acid in each 1,000 cc of urine; if 5 cc of urine has been used there is gram in each 1,000 cc of urine; if 19 cc are required there is 1-10 gram in each 1,000 cc

Acidity. If the urine is acid it will turn Blue Litmus paper Red; if alkaline, Red Litmus paper Blue. The simplest and most reliable method for determining the degree of acidity and the number of acid units is with Harrower's Acidimeter. Full directions accompany this instrument.

Sediment. Place urine in a conical glass and allow it to stand for twenty-four hours (keep cool). Urates are indicated by Yellow Grains which will disappear when the urine is Heated. Phosphates are indicated by a White Cloud which will disappear when a few drops of Acetic Acid has been added. If the sediment does not disappear after the urine has been heated or acetic acid has been added it, may be due to Calcium Oxalate or Uric Acid. Calcium Oxalate is Colorless and will disappear when Hydrochloric Acid has been added. Uric Acid appears as Reddish Specks which do not disappear with Heat, Acetic or Hydrochloric Acid. The addition of Sodium Hydroxide will cause their disappearance.

Specific Gravity. This can be determined with a Urinometer. Partly fill tube with urine and carefully place the urinometer in it. The figure at the top of the urine will indicate the Specific Gravity.

The Amount of Solids in any specimen of urine may be determined by taking the specific gravity and then multiplying the last two figures of the specific gravity by two and one-third. This will give the number of grams of solids in one thousand cubic centimeters of urine.

QUESTIONS—LESSON 23 B

1.   What is the difference between Subjective and Objective Symptoms, and how are Subjective Symptoms found?

2.   What influence has Heredity on Disease?

3.   What special symptoms may be present when the Nervous System is diseased?

4.   What special symptoms may be present when the Heart and Blood Vessels are diseased?

5.   What special symptoms would make you suspect disease of the Genito-urinary Organs?

6.   What conditions may influence the Amount, Appearance and Composition of the Urine?

7.   Give the physical characteristics of Normal Urine.

8.   What disorders may produce changes in the Color of the Urine?

9.   Does the presence of Casts in the urine always indicate disease of the Kidneys?

10. What disorders may produce Albumin in the Urine?

CHIROPRACTIC

The Science of Spinal Adjustment

———

A SERIES OF LESSONS CORRELATING AND
SYSTEMATIZING THE KNOWLEDGE NECESSARY
TO PRACTICE CHIROPRACTIC

Nature's Greatest Ally

IN RESTORING DISEASED CONDITIONS OF THE
BODY TO PERFECT HEALTH, WITHOUT THE AID
OF DRUGS OR SURGERY

———

BOOK 7
DISEASE AND TREATMENT
SYMPTOMATOLOGY
CONSTITUTIONAL DISEASES

Lessons 24, 25, 26, 27 and 28

———

ORIGINALLY PUBLISHED BY
AMERICAN UNIVERSITY
CHICAGO, ILLINOIS, U.S.A.

Organic MD Media
PO Box 50399
Palo Alto, CA 94303

First Published 1913, 1916
American University
Chicago, Ill, USA

Second Edition 2017
Published by OrganicMD Media
eBook Edition copyright © Organic MD Media 2017

Printed in the United States of America

Organic MD Media   2012 -

Chiropractic - The Science of Spinal Adjustment - Book 7

ISBN: 978-1-946036-06-3

Disclaimer

We are proud to republish this series of books on chiropractic medicine.
Originally published as a home-study course in 1913 by American University in Chicago, the 16 volumes give us an historical look at the theory and practice of chiropractic medicine in the early part of the 20th century.

This series is republished for historical interest only. The modern practice of chiropractic has advanced significantly in the century since these books were published. If you want to actually learn modern chiropractic techniques, please consult one of the many fine schools in this country.

The materials in these books are not intended to diagnose or treat disease. If you believe you are ill consult a licensed practitioner for care immediately. The publishers assume no liability for the use, misuse or nonuse of the materials in these books.

Thank you

EXTENSION COURSE
IN CHIROPRACTIC
AMERICAN UNIVERSITY
CHICAGO, Ill., U.S.A.

LESSON 24

PHILOSOPHY OF DISEASE AND
TREATMENT

Spinal Lesions are the sole, or contributing, causes of the great majority of the acute and chronic diseases and Spinal Adjustment will cure a larger proportion of them than any other plan of treatment.

It has been found necessary in a great many cases to use some other measures with Chiropractic if results are to be secured in a reasonable length of time. To use these adjuncts intelligently, it is essential that you know just what disease is and what should be done to eradicate it. If this is understood, you will be able to successfully use any measure with which you are familiar.

Disease may be defined as any alteration in the body or any of its organs interrupting or disturbing the performance of vital functions. Disease is not something that attacks the body from without, but is an abnormal condition originating within the body. It may consist of chemical or functional processes or it may be accompanied by structural changes in the tissues or organs.

The conditions before and at the time of his birth, his previous surroundings, diet, mental and physical activity, and his present physical and mental condition determine for each individual what shall be his best diet, surroundings, mental and physical activity for the present and future. So long as his diet, surroundings, mental and physical activity are approximately correct for him, the individual will remain in a state of health.

When the conditions under which he lives are not approximately correct for him, his body becomes unable to adapt itself to its environment, to eliminate the harmful factors, or to compensate for the disturbed function of certain organs or tissues and the body is said to be diseased.

Disease may be either a protective process, a constructive process, or evidence of the body's inability to successfully combat the harmful agencies.

The diarrhea following the eating of spoiled food is an effort on the part of the body to protect itself from the poisons the food contains. The changes occurring in the tissues during the acute inflammation following a severe irritation may be considered a constructive effort on the part of the body to repair the damage done by the irritant. The prostration accompanying severe general toxemias is evidence of the body's inability to successfully deal with the poisons being produced.

327

CLASSIFICATION OF DISEASES

The classification of diseases commonly used is not a good one from the standpoint of treatment. It is best to consider diseases from the standpoint of the primary pathological conditions present in the body.

The external causes given in the lesson on Etiology (Number 22) may produce one or more of the following conditions within the body: Abnormal Composition of the Blood, Lowered Vitality, Morbid Accumulations, Perverted Nerve Activity, Circulatory Disturbances, Functional Mental Disorders, or Deformities. These primary pathological conditions may produce the constitutional or local conditions and symptoms that are commonly known as disease. The symptomatology of these diseases will be given in Lessons 25 to 38.

Abnormal Composition of the Blood may be due to an excess or a lack of normal ingredients or to the presence of abnormal elements.

Lowered Vitality may be the result of a diminished supply or an excessive expenditure of nervous energy.

Morbid Accumulations may represent an excess of normal tissue or the presence of abnormal tissues.

Perverted Nerve Activity may be in the nature of an increase or decrease in the number or strength of the normal impulses or the presence of abnormal impulses.

Circulatory Disturbances may produce an excessive or diminished amount of blood in the affected part or a decrease in its rate of flow through the part.

328

Functional Mental Disorders may be conditions in which there is a functional disorder of the brain itself, or a condition in which the individual's state of mind produces or maintains disorders in other parts of the body.

Deformity may be said to be present when an organ or part is of an abnormal size or shape or is displaced from its normal position.

If the symptoms of the disorder are severe and of short duration the disease is said to be Acute; if the symptoms are mild and persist over a longer period, the disease is called Chronic. If the etiological factors are relatively severe and of short duration, acute diseases are produced. When the harmful agencies or conditions are relatively mild and are present for a long period, chronic diseases are produced. If the reactive power of the body is good, the influences that usually produce chronic diseases may produce acute diseases. If the reactive power of the body is relatively poor, chronic diseases may be produced by any of the etiological factors.

RATIONAL TREATMENT OF CHRONIC DISEASES

No method or plan of treatment can cure any disease unless it overcomes the primary pathology of the disorder. If the cure is to be permanent, the cause of the disorder must receive attention. It is also desirable in many cases to treat the secondary pathology (symptoms). As many different conditions within or without the body may produce the primary pathology and one or more of several primary pathological conditions may be present in the body, it is evident that no one plan of treatment will be effective in all cases. It is usually desirable, and many times

329

absolutely necessary, to use several different methods of treatment at the same time.

The first step in treatment is to **Find the Cause of the primary pathology** (see Sections on Etiology, Diagnosis and Examination). When found, the cause should be removed, if possible. If not possible to remove it, you should attempt to lessen its activity or to counteract its effects.

The Primary Pathology should be corrected if possible. To do this, you should purify the blood, increase the vital resistance, eliminate morbid accumulations, restore normal nerve activity, control the blood distribution, correct deformities, or rectify the mental condition, as may be necessary.

Compensation and Adaptation may be brought about by increasing the activity of some normal organ so that it will be able to do part of the work of some abnormal organ. Changing the patient's environment will also aid compensation and adaptation.

Mental suggestion is a powerful factor in the treatment of practically all disorders and should be used whenever it is possible to use it. It is usually best to mask suggestion with some other form of treatment. The object of the mental treatment should be to stimulate faith, hope, courage and optimism.

Sometimes the body becomes accustomed to and tolerates a chronic disorder and makes no attempt to rid itself of the condition. In these cases it is desirable to use some measure to arouse the body's activity and produce reaction against the disease or the factors that are producing it. This can be done by quickening the metabolic processes, raising the vitality, or stimulating nerve and circulatory activity. The patient's own blood or discharges from his body may also be used for this purpose.

Treatment should be directed to the symptoms when the symptoms tend to aggravate the primary pathology or to interfere with its treatment. Symptoms should never be suppressed, but it is possible, in many cases, to alleviate them without interfering with your other treatment.

RATIONAL TREATMENT OF ACUTE DISEASE

The patient should be put at rest in bed in a quiet, well ventilated room, and should be disturbed no more than is absolutely necessary. The physician and attendants should allay fear and anxiety and should stimulate courage and optimism. If fever or digestive disturbances are present no food should be given except water and fruit juices, which should be given freely. It is usually best to give no food for twenty-four hours after the temperature is normal and the digestive symptoms have been relieved.

The patient should have a hot sponge bath and a warm enema each morning and each evening. The spine and neck should be thoroughly but carefully relaxed by use of manipulation or prolonged hot applications.

AVOID OVER-TREATMENT

You should always be very careful not to treat your patient too severely, too long or too often. The body cannot react to the treatment if too great a demand is made upon its healing forces. It is understood, of course, that only a few of the many measures suggested should be used on any one patient.

You should carefully search for and remove any condition within or without his body that may be causing or aggravating the trouble. In addition to this you may increase, decrease, or control visceral or bodily activities as may be necessary. Symptoms that aggravate the patient's condition may be treated if this can be done without suppressing them or interfering with the body's efforts to overcome the disorder.

In practically all acute disorders you will find spinal lesions that are producing or aggravating his condition or the symptoms. In a few cases nothing but spinal treatment will be needed. Usually, however, it is necessary, or at least desirable, to follow the plan given above.

TREATMENT OF ACCIDENTS AND EMERGENCIES

First find and remove or counteract the activity of whatever may be responsible for the condition. The patient should be put at rest in a recumbent position where he will have plenty of fresh air. If necessary, he should be prevented from injuring himself.

Open wounds should be protected and hemorrhages should be controlled. The patient should be kept warm and an effort should be made to overcome the effect of the shock or collapse. Cardiac, respiratory or nervous activity should be stimulated if necessary.

CORRECTION OF PRIMARY PATHOLOGY

Blood may be purified by removing the abnormal material through fasting or eliminative treatment or by supplying the deficient normal elements through correct diet, fresh air, sunshine or ozone.

Vital Resistance may be raised by increasing the supply of nervous energy through sleep, food, exercise, sunshine, ozone and ultra violet light or by decreasing the expenditure of nervous energy through rest, correction of faulty habits, correction of refractive errors, removal of orificial or spinal lesions and by preventing excessive functional demands upon the supply of energy.

Morbid Matter may be eliminated through the Skin by the use of prolonged hot or short cold baths, hot sponge baths, wet sheet packs, electric light, vapor, or hot air baths, sinusoidal or faradic baths, sun, air, or friction baths, endurance or strength-building exercises, slow sinusoidal current to large groups of muscles, high frequency auto-condensation, static charging, and adjustment of the 10th dorsal vertebrae; through the Bowels by the use of enemas, laxative diet, abdominal massage, exercises for the waist, abdomen or lumbar spine, slow sinusoidal, rapid sinusoidal, or faradic current to abdomen or lumbar spine, vibration, alternate hot and cold sitz baths, abdominal douches, abdominal breathing and spinal stimulation; through the Kidneys by the use of hot enemas, water drinking, fruit juices, spinal stimulation or prolonged hot applications to the lower dorsal spine; through the Liver by use of waist exercise, vibration, alternate hot and cold applications to liver or middle dorsal spine, prolonged hot applications to middle dorsal spine or by fasting, and through the Lungs by the use of breathing or endurance exercises.

Nerve Activity may be normalized by removing the causes of the abnormal activity through spinal treatment, orificial treatment, correction of eyestrain, manipulation, or suggestion.

In addition to removing the causes of the abnormal activity, nerve activity may be decreased through the use of manipulation, hydrotherapy, electrotherapy, phototherapy, chromo therapy, vibration, zone therapy, hyperemia, traction, massage, abdominal breathing, rest, suggestion, or by the use of strong plus lenses and it may be increased by the use of manipulation, hydrotherapy, electrotherapy, chromo therapy, vibration, exercise, sunshine, ozone or ultra violet light.

Blood Distribution may be controlled through spinal treatment, orificial treatment, manipulation, massage, Swedish movements, lymphatic treatment, hydrotherapy, phototherapy, vibration, hyperemia, electrotherapy, exercise, posture, abdominal breathing, rest, or bandaging.

Functional Mental Disorders may be corrected by the use of suggestion, masked suggestion, conversational psychology, or education of the patient.

Deformities may be corrected by the use of manipulation, exercise, apparatus, or surgery.

TREATMENT FOR GENERAL EFFECTS

In addition to the removal of the causes and the correction of the primary pathology of a disorder, it is often desirable to produce certain functional changes in the body for the purpose of counteracting the effects of the disease.

The Metabolic Processes may be quickened by the use of prolonged hot or short cold baths, wet sheet packs, hot sponge baths, electric light, hot air, or vapor baths, exercise, massage, lymphatic treatment, faradic and sinusoidal baths, slow sinusoidal to large muscles, auto condensation, positive charging, faradic massage, vibratory kneading, sun, air, and ultra violet baths, ozone, and rectal dilatation.

The Activity of the Nervous System may be Stimulated by short cold baths, short very hot baths, alternate hot and cold application to the spine, stimulation of the 7th cervical vertebra, slow sinusoidal, faradic, high frequency sparking, or rapid sinusoidal to the spine, spinal vibration, short heavy traction, adjustment of the atlas, short hot enemas, faradic massage, faradic baths, general massage, spinal massage, exercise, Swedish movements, red or yellow light, ultra violet light, sunshine and ozone. It should be remembered that overstimulation always produces the opposite effect. All stimulative treatment should be short and relatively severe.

The Activity of the Nervous System may be Decreased by the use of neutral prolonged cool or hot baths, prolonged moderate heat or moderate cold to the spine, spinal and neck relaxation, prolonged pressure behind the 1st and 2nd cervical vertebra, electric light, hot air, or vapor baths, deep breathing, mild traction, rest, suggestion, auto-condensation, negative breeze, high frequency effleurage or rapid sinusoidal to the spine, sinusoidal bath, spinal vibration, massage, zone therapy, blue or green light.

Circulatory Activity may be Increased by stimulation of the 7th cervical and 5th to 8th dorsal vertebrae, alternate hot and cold baths, alternate hot and cold spinal applications, rectal dilatation, faradic current to dorsal spine or chest, strength building or endurance exercises, massage, lymphatic treatment, stimulation of heart activity through the spine, faradic massage, slow sinusoidal current, vibration, Swedish movements, and milk diet.

Respiratory Activity may be Stimulated by rectal dilatation, concussion of the chest or abdomen, stimulation of the 4th and 5th cervical and 5th to 8th dorsal vertebrae, short cold or alternate hot and cold applications and passive chest movements.

QUESTIONS—LESSON 24

1. Why is it necessary to study the philosophy of disease and treatment?

2. What is disease?

3. Explain how disease is produced.

4. Name the seven primary pathological conditions that may be present in disease.

5. What is the principal object of treatment in chronic diseases?

6. How can the primary pathology be corrected?

7. When and how should symptoms be treated?

8. Briefly outline the plan of treatment to be used in chronic diseases.

9. Briefly outline the treatment of accidents and emergencies.

10. What measures may be used in the treatment of abnormal nerve activity?

EXTENSION COURSE
IN CHIROPRACTIC
AMERICAN UNIVERSITY
CHICAGO, Ill., U.S.A.

LESSON 25

SYMPTOMATOLOGY

The presence of symptoms is an indication of abnormal functional, chemical or structural changes (Pathology) somewhere in the body. Certain changes in certain parts produce certain groups of symptoms and signs. When a patient has this group of symptoms and signs, he is said to have a certain disease. It is immaterial whether we name this disease or not, but we must recognize and group the symptoms and signs before we can know what Pathology is present.

Diseases may be recognized and distinguished from each other in two ways. You may learn the characteristic symptoms of each disease (Symptomatology) and then compare the patient's symptoms with those of the diseases it most closely resembles, or you may examine the body in various ways and by the discovery of certain abnormal conditions or signs (Diagnosis) thus learn the seat and nature of the patient's trouble. Each plan has its place; both should be used together whenever possible.

338

NECESSITY OF DIAGNOSIS

The determination of the seat, nature, progress and probable course of the patient's disease is an absolute necessity if your treatment is to be anything but experimental. More failures result from inability to discover what is the trouble with the patient than inability to treat the disease after it is correctly diagnosed. Nine-tenths of all consultations between physicians are for the purpose of diagnosing the patient's disorder.

In this course you will be taught how to recognize and differentiate all but the very rare diseases by the symptoms that are manifested when the diseases are present. Many diseases of the same organ very closely resemble each other, that is, they have many symptoms in common. One can be told from the other only by the presence or absence of one or more characteristic symptoms.

The examination to ascertain the necessary facts should be conducted in an orderly and systematic manner. Time is thus saved, a general survey of the clinical phenomena made, and those of chief importance brought into contrast and proper relation with those of subordinate value. Data not otherwise obvious are brought to light and the chances of oversight minimized. Vague and pointless inquiries are omitted. The interrogation is precise and explicit. Above all leading questions are to be avoided. Tact and patience are necessary. An examination thus conducted has a favorable influence upon the patient, especially in chronic and difficult cases, and always inspires confidence. The investigation should not be unduly extended or minute. On the other hand, the inquiry may be too concise and brief. The middle course is the best. There are two principal modes of case-taking the Synthetic and the Analytic.

In the synthetic, sometimes spoken of as the historical method, the inquiry begins with the history of the patient, rather than with his present condition. His place of birth, age, social state, occupation, previous diseases, hereditary and constitutional tendencies are first ascertained, then follows an investigation into the beginning and progress of the present illness. All this constitutes the history.

The present symptoms are then considered. The condition of the several physiological systems, the digestive, the circulatory, the respiratory, the genitourinary, the nervous, and so on, being carefully inquired into in regular order. Finally, the symptoms and signs referable to the organs or structures especially affected are carefully studied. The next step in the process is the diagnosis, upon which the prognosis, treatment and general management of the case depend. Case-taking by this method follows the natural order. It is scientific and useful in obscure cases. The chief objections to it are the time it consumes and the fact that in the progress of the inquiry unnecessary attention must be given to facts which are found later to have little or no bearing upon the patient's present conditions.

In the analytical method the order of procedure is reversed. The principal symptoms are taken as the point of departure for the investigation. The organ or region to which these symptoms are referred is examined by the proper diagnostic measures. The general condition of the patient, his facies, the state of nutrition of his body, his posture, his movements, are carefully observed; meanwhile he is questioned as to the duration and progress of his present illness and an inquiry is made into such facts in his previous history and antecedents as may bear upon the case. The clinical study is then extended the condition of the other organs

Lesson 25: Symptomatology

investigated, the history of the case more systematically reviewed, an opinion formed as to whether the malady is general or local and a diagnosis reached. This is the plan commonly pursued in ordinary professional work where the data is sufficient for a diagnosis by the direct method, and is available in all cases except those where the symptoms are obscure and ill defined.

The section "Examination of the Patient" in Lesson 23 B should be studied with these lessons on Symptomatology. The schedule for the examination will be found on those pages.

The presence or absence of any of the common symptoms (Lesson 23 B) will give you a clue to the line of questions to follow or the examination to make to find the seat and cause of the patient's trouble in the shortest possible time. If he has any of the common symptoms you should compare them with the groups of special symptoms (in Lesson 23 B) which will aid you in determining which organ or systems are most probably effected. Next question him very carefully about the other symptoms that may be present in diseases of the part that is suspected. You should lean the order, time and character of onset of each symptom together with the treatment that had been used and that results of the treatment of the condition.

If you will carefully follow the plan outlined you will have eliminated from your consideration all but a very small number of diseases. The diagnosis will rest upon your knowledge of these few diseases.

DIAGNOSIS

The diagnosis may be made in several ways. Very rarely it can be made by the presence of some one peculiar symptom, as the opaque lens in cataract of the eye. Usually diagnosis depends upon certain combinations of symptoms, e.g., the enlarged thyroid, rapid heart, protrusion of the eyeball, tremors and vasomotor disturbances in exophthalmic goiter. The patient may have all of the cardinal symptoms of a certain disease and no other symptoms. In this case a Direct Diagnosis may be made. Many times, however, he does not have all of the important symptoms or he has some additional symptoms. Differential Diagnosis must be used in this case, i.e., you must compare his group of symptoms with those of all of the diseases that closely resemble his to determine which one presents the most symptoms in common with those he has.

Occasionally, a Provisional Diagnosis must be made until more information can be obtained by further study of the case. It should be remembered that a patient may have two diseases at the same time (e.g., Bronchial Asthma and Gastric Ulcer), and that he may have some acute disease while suffering from a chronic disorder of the same or another organ. Rare diseases require much more conclusive evidence of their presence than the common disorders, but they should always be considered as a possibility.

DIAGNOSIS OF THE PRIMARY PATHOLOGY
Abnormal Composition of the Blood is present when there is anemia, emaciation, toxemia, skin eruptions, fever, abnormal or excessive discharges, atrophy, or degeneration of any part.

Lowered Vitality is present when there is debility, prostration, lack of energy, diminished endurance, brain fag, poor circulation, diminished tissue tone, degeneration, gangrene, and many functional disorders.

Morbid Accumulations are represented by tumors, abscesses, stones, hypertrophies, infiltrations, obesity and many structural changes.

Perverted Nerve Activity may produce pain, anesthesia, paresthesia, muscular spasms, paralysis, contractures, tremors, and increased, decreased, or perverted activity of the affected part.

Circulatory Disturbances are revealed by the presence of ischemia, congestion, stasis, atrophy, hypertrophy, degeneration, infiltration, and increased, decreased, or perverted activity of the part supplied.

Functional Mental Disorders are accompanied by disturbances of perception, reason, will or emotion or changes in the disposition, temperament or manner of thinking.

Deformities can be diagnosed by the malformation or displacement of an organ or part.

ETIOLOGY

Lessons 24 to 37 will be devoted to Symptomatology. The Etiology of disease has been given in Lesson 22 and no mention of it will be made in these lessons except when certain factors are commonly concerned in the causation of the disease. It is understood that any or all of the etiological factors given in Lesson 22 may be present in any disorder.

PROGNOSIS

The Prognosis, or possibility of cure, depends upon how far the disease has progressed and whether or not the etiological factors can be found and removed. It is also influenced very much by the treatment used. There are no incurable diseases, but there are incurable cases. All disorders can be cured if the proper treatment is instituted early enough in the disease. All diseases are incurable if the cause is not found and removed, if improper treatment is used, or if the disorder has progressed so far that there has been too much destruction of vital tissue or the vitality is too much lowered to react to treatment. Some conditions are much more stubborn than others and require much longer treatment, while some respond very quickly to treatment.

TREATMENT

The treatment of any disorder will depend almost entirely upon the cause of that disorder and the pathological conditions present in the patient's body. Unless the cause is found and removed, no treatment can be anything but palliative. In addition to finding and removing the cause, it is usually necessary to use some measure to overcome the pathology of the disease. It is understood that in every case a thorough spinal examination must be made and any spinal lesions present must be corrected.

The principles and technic of spinal examination and adjustment will be given in Lessons 39 to 55. The general principles that underlie all forms of treatment and their application to all diseases are given in Lesson 24.

QUESTIONS—LESSON 25

1. What is Symptomatology?

2. Why is it necessary to study Symptomatology?

3. What is the difference between Symptomatology and Diagnosis?

4. Briefly outline the historical method of examination.

5. Briefly outline the analytical method of examination.

6. When can a direct diagnosis be made?

7. When is it necessary to make a differential diagnosis?

8. When should a provisional diagnosis be made?

9. Upon what does prognosis depend?

10. What must be known about the patient to enable you to apply the correct treatment?

EXTENSION COURSE
IN CHIROPRACTIC
AMERICAN UNIVERSITY
CHICAGO, Ill., U.S.A.

LESSON 26

SYMPTOMS OF ACUTE
CONSTITUTIONAL DISEASES

Fever is not a disease but a name applied to a group of symptoms that are present when there is an increase in the body temperature due to perverted metabolism, toxemia or some disturbance of the heat-regulating mechanism. In addition to the increase of the mouth temperature above 98 6/10, any or all of the following symptoms may be present: malaise, thirst, anorexia flushed face, hot and dry skin, scanty, dark urine, costiveness, delirium, and rapid pulse and respiration.

The fever may begin, especially in acute cases, with a Chill. The patient shivers and the skin is cold, but the internal temperature of the body is raised. Chills may also occur at intervals during the course of the fever.

The term Continued Fever means that the temperature throughout the illness remains well above normal and the daily changes in temperature are not greater than one degree. The fever is remittent when the fever remains persistently above normal but varies one or more degrees during the day. Fever is said to be. Intermittent when there are periods of fever separated by intervals in which the temperature is normal.

Septicemia (Blood Poisoning) is an acute constitutional disorder characterized by a localized superative inflammation. There is "Fever," usually ushered in by a chill, Leukocytosis, sweats and great prostration. Careful search will usually reveal the source of the toxins.

Pyemia is an acute constitutional disorder in which there is a formation of abscesses. There is a remittent fever, with recurring chills and sweats. Marked emaciation and prostration are present. The diagnosis is made by the finding of the abscesses.

Typhoid State is a term used to describe a group of symptoms that usually accompany Typhoid Fever, but may be present in any severe acute toxemia. There is fever and great prostration and the pulse becomes very rapid and soft. The tongue is dry and brown, the teeth and lips are coated. The patient has a low, muttering delirium and is in a semi-comatose condition. The eyes may be open, but he does not see (Coma vigil). He slips to the foot of the bed and picks at the bed clothes.

Influenza is an acute constitutional disorder characterized by inflammation in various organs of the body. The respiratory, gastrointestinal, and the nervous systems are usually most affected, producing symptoms characteristic of the acute disorders of these systems. There is a severe backache, the bones ache and the number of white cells in the blood are diminished, in addition to the symptoms of fever. The most important diagnostic symptom is the extreme weakness which is out of all proportion to the severity of the other symptoms.

Typhoid Fever is an acute constitutional disorder characterized by ulceration of the lymph glands of the small intestines, enlargement of the spleen, and granular degeneration in other organs. The onset is insidious with headache, anorexia, diarrhea, constipation and malaise. The fever usually rises each evening and falls each morning, the temperature each day being slightly higher than on the preceding day. As the disease progresses the abdomen becomes tender, there are frequent evacuations of fecal matter resembling pea-soup. Small red spots (Roseola) appear on the abdomen. At the end of the first week the spleen becomes enlarged and marked nervous symptoms develop. If the disease is improperly treated it progresses to the "Typhoid State" and all of the above symptoms are intensified. The ulcers may perforate the intestinal wall producing death from shock and hemorrhage.

Yellow Fever is an acute constitutional disease occurring principally in warm climates where the sanitation is neglected. The onset is sudden with all the symptoms of "Fever" and the patient is very much prostrated. The skin has a peculiar yellow color (Jaundice), the pulse is slow, and vomiting is usually present. There may be hemorrhages into the skin or mucous membrane. Albuminuria is present very early in the disease and is often severe.

Dengue is an acute constitutional disease of unknown pathology. The invasion is sudden with fever and pains in the muscles, bones and joints. The joints become red and swollen. A diffuse red skin eruption usually appears the first day. After two or three days the fever suddenly falls and the symptoms subside, except for some stiffness and soreness in the limbs. After an interval of two to four days the symptoms first present return, although they are usually less severe.'

Malaria is a chronic constitutional disorder characterized by recurring acute attacks of chills, fever and sweating. These attacks may occur every forty-eight, seventy-two or ninety-six hours. The onset is sudden with a rapid rise of temperature followed by shivering and violent shaking. The chill lasts from ten minutes to two hours while the thermometer in the mouth shows a temperature of 104 to 106. It is followed by a hot stage in which the face is flushed, the skin is red and hot, and there is great thirst, throbbing headache and a full bounding pulse. This stage lasts one-half to five hours. The sweating stage lasts two to four hours; the entire body is covered with profuse perspiration and the fever and other symptoms gradually subside. Between the acute attacks the patient feels nearly well but is anemic, debilitated, the skin is discolored and the spleen is enlarged.

Measles is an acute constitutional disease of childhood. There is no characteristic pathology. The onset is gradual with coryza, conjunctivitis, and fever. The eruption appears on the fourth day and consists of dark red, soft papules arranged in crescentic patches. After two or three days the fever gradually subsides, the rash disappears and the skin peels off in fine branny scales. Small, bluish spots on red base (Koplik's Spots) appear on the inside of the cheek opposite the molar teeth before the rash appears and when found will establish the diagnosis of Measles. Bronchopneumonia and Otitis media are the common complications.

German Measles is an acute constitutional disease of childhood with no characteristic pathology. The onset is gradual with malaise and mild fever. Scattered red papules appear the first day accompanied by pharyngitis and enlargement of the cervical glands. The eruption is brighter than that of "Measles" and less bright and larger than that of Scarletina.

Scarletina is an acute constitutional disease of childhood with no characteristic pathology. The onset is sudden with convulsions, lumbago and vomiting. The fever rapidly rises to 104 and the pulse is very rapid. The eruption appears the first day and rapidly spreads over the entire body. The skin is red and the rash appears like small red pieces of sand beneath the skin. There is pharyngitis, tonsilitis, usually severe, and a characteristic strawberry tongue. The fever subsides and the rash begins to disappear in three or four days. The skin peels off in large flakes. Albuminuria may be present. The common complications are Nephritis, Acute Uremia, Arthritis and Endocarditis.

Chicken Pox is an acute constitutional disease of childhood with no characteristic pathology. The onset is gradual with malaise and slight fever. Papules and vesicles Appear on the first day and reappear in crops. After two or three days the fever subsides and the eruption disappears.

Small Pox is an acute constitutional disease of childhood characterized by a skin eruption which is successively papular, vesicular, pustular and a crust and by a peculiar febrile course. The onset is sudden with headache, lumbago and vomiting. The fever is high until the rash appears when it and the other symptoms subside. Hard papules appear on the fourth day and change on the sixth day to vesicles with a depressed center. On the eighth day the vesicles become pustules and the fever returns and all of the first symptoms are aggravated. On the tenth day the pustules become crusts and inflammation of the skin and the temperature

Lesson 26: Symptoms of Acute Constitutional Diseases

gradually subsides. If the true skin has been destroyed, scars will be left when the crusts fall off. The common complications are Bronchopneumonia, Pleurisy, Laryngitis, Dysentery and Conjunctivitis.

Erysipelas is an acute constitutional disease characterized by rapidly spreading inflammation of the skin. The onset is sudden with fever. The eruption appears on the first day as dry, red, shiny, tense patches with sharply raised edges. The inflammatory areas heal in the center and spread on the circumference. The usual site is on the face.

Cerebro-Spinal Fever is an acute constitutional disease characterized by inflammation of the meninges of the brain and cord. The onset is sudden with chills, fever, vomiting and severe spinal pain. The muscles of the spine are spasmodically contracted, producing rigidity of the neck and back; the head is usually retracted. There is a noisy delirium which may be followed by coma. Symptoms of irritation of the spine and cranial nerves (Hyperesthesia, and Muscular Spasm) appear to be followed later by Anesthesia and Muscular paralysis in the parts supplied by the effected nerves. When the thigh is flexed at right angle to the body the leg cannot be extended on the thigh (Kernig's Sign). Blindness, deafness, mental feebleness, and paralysis may remain after recovery from the acute attack.

Acute Poliomyelitis is a constitutional disease of childhood characterized by inflammation followed by degeneration and sclerosis of the anterior horns of the spinal cord. The onset is sudden with fever and possibly convulsions. On the third to the fifth day paralysis of some small group of muscles appears. Less often a whole arm or leg is affected. The paralysis is lower neuronic in character (See diseases of the Nervous System) and is followed by atrophy. There is always some tendency to improvement after the acute attack, and under proper treatment, the muscles can in a great majority of cases be restored to their former usefulness.

Mumps is an acute constitutional disease of childhood characterized by inflammation of the parotid glands. The onset is gradual with mild fever and swelling in front of and below one or both ears. There is difficulty in mastication and swallowing. The common complications are Orchitis, Ovaritis and Mastitis.

Acute Tonsilitis is a constitutional disease characterized by inflammation of the tonsils. The throat is hot, dry and congested. The tonsils are swollen and reddened and are covered with small yellowish spots. Occasionally, there is suppuration in the tonsil or in the surrounding tissues (Quinsy). Mastication is difficult and there is dyspnea and dysphagia.

Diphtheria is an acute constitutional disease characterized by fibrinous inflammation of the tonsils, pharynx or larynx. The onset is gradual with mild fever and stiffness of the neck. The glands behind the angle of the jaw become tender and swollen and the pharynx, larynx, tonsils or soft palate become reddened and swollen. A whitish membrane appears upon the effected part as a small patch and rapidly grows until it covers a large area. The membrane is removed with difficulty, leaves a raw bleeding surface, and reappears after removal. Swallowing and mastication are painful and if the pharynx or larynx is involved there may be obstruction to respiration. Toxemia may be so severe as to produce marked prostration or coma. The common complications are Heart Failure, Bronchopneumonia, Nephritis and Paralysis.

Lesson 26: Symptoms of Acute Constitutional Diseases

Whooping Cough is an acute constitutional disease of children characterized by catarrhal inflammation of the respiratory mucous membranes. The disease is divided into two stages. In the first stage there is Coryza, Laryngitis and Pharyngitis and a loose cough. After one or two weeks the cough becomes paroxysmal and consists of a number of short rapid expiratory efforts followed by a deep, loud inspiration which gives the cough the characteristic whoop. During the cough the face becomes red, the eyes swollen and protruding and the child may vomit. The most common complication is Bronchopneumonia.

Acute General Tuberculosis is a constitutional disease characterized by the formation of tubercles in many parts of the body. The onset is gradual with Anorexia, Debility and Emaciation. Fever is irregular, but is usually higher in the afternoon than in the morning. The face is flushed when the fever rises and the patient may sweat profusely as the fever goes down. Toxemia is severe and the patient may die in from one to three weeks. A positive diagnosis can be made only by finding the tubercle bacillus in the secretions or discharges

Rheumatic Fever is an acute constitutional disease characterized by severe inflammation of the joints. The onset is usually sudden with pain in one or more joints and fever. The joints become red, hot, swollen, painful and tender. The inflammation may subside in one joint and reappear in another. The urine is scanty, highly acid, and contains an excess of urates. There is marked anemia and the patient sweats profusely. Endocarditis is the common complication.

Tetanus is an acute constitutional disease with no characteristic pathology. It usually follows a punctured or incised

353

wound. The onset is sudden with rigidity of the neck, jaw and face. The muscles become spasmodically contracted and the spasm extends to the muscles of the trunk and extremities. The pain is severe. The spasm of the muscles of mastication holds the teeth firmly together (Lockjaw). There is fever and rapid pulse and respiration. The mind remains clear until death, which may occur within a few days.

DIAGNOSIS OF ACUTE CONSTITUTIONAL DISEASES

These diseases are usually classified in medical books as "Infectious Diseases" because it is commonly believed that they are caused by bacterial infection. The exact relationship of the bacteria to the disease is still a matter of dispute. As the body as a whole is affected, these diseases may be 'called Constitutional Diseases.

An increase of the bodily temperature accompanies all of these diseases. When the temperature is raised several other symptoms are also present. These are included under the term "Fever" (see above). The presence or absence of fever, the type of fever, and the relationship of the fever to the other symptoms are of considerable importance in the diagnosis of these diseases.

Many of these diseases have a skin eruption; each disease has an eruption of a different type and is also accompanied by different symptoms so that the diagnosis is usually easy if care is taken to make a thorough examination.

In the United States, Typhoid Fever, Tuberculosis, Septicemia and Pyemia are the only diseases that have a fever running more than two weeks without a period of normal temperature. If the patient has had a fever for this length of time you may be reasonably sure that he has one of these disorders.

Septicemia can be diagnosed by the presence of the local suppurative inflammation; in Pyemia, abscesses may be more difficult to discover. The symptoms of Tuberculosis will be given in the lesson on Chronic Constitutional Diseases. Typhoid Fever is not difficult to diagnose when the disease runs the characteristic course. If you take a thorough history and make a careful examination, you should have no difficulty in differentiating these three conditions.

Yellow Fever, Dengue and Malaria are very rarely found except in those patients living or who have lived in the Southern States. The symptoms are so characteristic that no mistake should be made in their diagnosis.

When the rash peculiar to the disease is present and is accompanied by the other cardinal symptoms of that disease no difficulty should be experienced in diagnosing any of the exanthematous diseases. Many times, however, the rash is not characteristic and the disease does not run the typical course, making diagnosis difficult if not impossible.

So far as treatment is concerned, it is not absolutely necessary that a correct diagnosis be made, 'but an effort should be made to name the disorder whenever possible as the quarantine regulations regarding them are different. That these diseases are contagious has not been definitely proven, but it is best to be on the safe side and keep the sick person away from the well ones as much as possible. It should be remembered that these diseases are most contagious in their early stages and it is at this time that diagnosis is most difficult.

If the patient has a spotted, pimply rash with healthy areas of skin between the patches of eruption, fever and running from the nose it is usually safe to make a diagnosis of Measles. The rash of German Measles may resemble that of measles very much, but in this disorder there is sore throat and the glands of the neck are enlarged.

The eruptive spots of Scarlet Fever are much smaller than those of the above two diseases and the whole skin is reddened. The sudden onset with the rash appearing the first day will aid in distinguishing it from Measles. The differentiation between it and German Measles must be made by the character of the rash and the relative mildness of the latter disease.

A well-developed case of Small-Pox need not be mistaken for Chicken-Pox or any other disorder, but in some cases the eruption and the fever do not run the typical course. A valuable point of difference in the early stages is that in Chicken-Pox the papules and vesicles are present at the same time and recur in crops. In Small-Pox the eruption is either papular, vesicular or pustular, depending upon the stage of the disease; the three types of skin lesions do not occur all at the same time. The rash is usually the first symptom of Chicken-Pox, but it does not usually occur before the fourth day of Small-Pox; it is most abundant on the trunk in the former, and on the face in the latter disease.

In Erysipelas the whole surface of the affected part of the skin is inflamed and reddened. Although the face is usually affected, the inflammation may appear on any part of the body.

The skin lesions of Cerebro-Spinal Fever are not always present; they are due to small hemorrhages into the skin. The surface of the skin is not raised.

The roseola of Typhoid Fever is due to a temporary dilatation of the small arteries in the vessels of the skin. These spots can be made to disappear by stretching the skin or by pressure upon it.

If the patient has an acute constitutional disorder that cannot be called by any other name, a diagnosis of Influenza is usually made. The most important diagnostic symptom of this disorder is that the prostration is greater than the other symptoms seem to justify.

TREATMENT OF ACUTE CONSTITUTIONAL DISORDERS

The general principles of treatment given in Lesson 24 may be followed in treating these diseases in addition to whatever special treatment may be necessary in each disease.

In Septicemia, Pyemia and Tetanus the abscesses should be opened and the suppurating wounds should be cleaned and drained; hyperemia should be used as a local treatment. Special attention should be paid to the abdomen in Typhoid; the neck and chest in Measles; the neck and kidneys in Scarletina; the spine in Cerebro-Spinal Fever; the neck in Mumps, Tonsilitis, Diphtheria and Whooping Cough, and the affected joints in Rheumatic Fever.

PROGNOSIS

The prognosis of these disorders depends very largely upon how early the proper treatment is instituted and the vital resistance of the patient at the time of the attack.

If rational treatment is used from the beginning, the prognosis will be good in all of them except Septicemia, Pyemia, Tetanus, Yellow Fever, Malaria, Cerebro-Spinal Fever, and Diphtheria; the prognosis in these diseases is doubtful. In Acute General Tuberculosis and the Typhoid State the prognosis is bad.

QUESTIONS—LESSON 26

1. What is Fever?

2. Give the symptoms of Typhoid Fever.

3. Give symptoms of Measles.

4. Give symptoms of Cerebro-Spinal Fever.

5. Give symptoms of Whooping Cough.

6. How would you differentiate between Typhoid Fever and Influenza?

7. How would you differentiate between Scarletina and German Measles?

8. How would you differentiate between Small Pox and Chicken Pox?

9. Briefly outline the treatment of Acute Constitutional Diseases.

10. If the patient had the following symptoms what disease would you suspect:—Raised temperature, Chilliness, Hot and dry skin, Constipation, Rapid pulse and Respiration, Papular eruption, Sore throat and Headache?

EXTENSION COURSE
IN CHIROPRACTIC
AMERICAN UNIVERSITY
CHICAGO, Ill., U.S.A.

———

LESSON 27

CHRONIC CONSTITUTIONAL DISEASES

Diseases in which the pathology is not confined to any particular organ, system or structure are called Constitutional. When the disorder is accompanied by a perversion of the normal activities of the body cells, it is called "Metabolic." If it is caused by the absorption of poisons from without or that are generated within the «body, it is called an "Intoxication." When accompanied by micro-organisms in the blood, it is an "Infection."

The diseases given in this lesson should be carefully studied and their symptoms kept constantly in mind as many supposed local diseases are really local manifestations of constitutional disorders. Some diseases may affect many different organs and tissues and, while the local symptoms depend upon the particular structure affected, the general symptoms are always practically the same, irrespective of the seat of the disorder. The most important of these diseases are: Rheumatism, Gout, Alcoholism, Septicemia, Tuberculosis and Syphilis. Their constitutional symptoms are given in this lesson. When dealing with symptoms of these diseases of the individual organs in subsequent lessons, the symptoms given in this lesson will not be repeated in detail but will be included under the term of "General Symptoms of Tuberculosis," or "Syphilis" or whatever disease may be under discussion.

SYMPTOMS OF CHRONIC CONSTITUTIONAL DISEASES

Lithemia is a chronic disorder due to some disturbance of the metabolism or elimination of the end-products of protein digestion. These "purine bodies " (uric acid, etc.) are present in excessive quantities and produce muscular and articular pains, headache, neuralgia, skin eruptions, dyspepsia, bronchitis, high blood pressure and scanty, dark, highly acid urine which contains an excess of uric acid.

When some of the above symptoms are present with those of "Gouty Arthritis" the disorder is called Gout. If the symptoms of "articular" or "muscular" rheumatism accompany the above symptoms the condition is known as Rheumatism.

Diabetes Mellitus is a nutritional and metabolic disorder characterized by an excess of sugar in the blood. In addition to the excessive amount of urine containing sugar there is a voracious appetite, inordinate thirst and a progressive loss of weight and strength.

Diabetes Insipidus is a chronic disease characterized by a persistent passage of large quantities of urine of low specific gravity but otherwise normal. The thirst is excessive and the skin is dry, but there are no other symptoms of Diabetes Mellitus.

Acidosis is a condition which may complicate Diabetes Mellitus. It is due to some disturbance of the carbohydrate metabolism and is usually brought on by the use of too much fat or protein and too little carbohydrate in the diet.

The symptoms of its presence are Dyspnea, Headache, Delirium, Fever, Rapid Pulse, Sweetish Odor of the Breath, Drowsiness or Coma. Acetone will be found in the urine at the time of attack and for some days previous to it.

Uremia is a name applied to a group of symptoms that occur when the kidneys are unable to eliminate certain poisonous waste materials from the body. It usually accompanies Nephritis. Examination of the urine will show that there is a decreased amount of urea and that albumin is present. The patient is drowsy, has difficulty in breathing and the skin is cyanotic or may have a peculiar color. Headache, vertigo, diarrhea and vomiting are usually present and the breath has urinous odor. The attack may be acute, in which case all of the above symptoms will be aggravated and the patient sinks into a coma.

Obesity is a condition in which there is a persistent excessive accumulation of fat that cannot be reduced by a correct diet or proper exercise.

Scurvy is a chronic, nutritional disorder due to lack of inorganic salts or vitamins in the food. There is weakness and anemia, the gums are soft and spongy, and there is a tendency to hemorrhages in the mucous and serous membranes and into skin. The diagnosis can be made from the prompt relief that follows the use of fresh fruits and vegetables.

Lesson 27: Chronic Constitutional Diseases

Colon Toxemia is a condition in which there is retention of fecal matter in the colon and a consequent absorption of the toxins of proteid putrefaction. Practically any symptom may be produced; the following are the most common: headache, vertigo, lassitude, insomnia, dyspepsia, skin eruptions, stomatitis, pharyngitis, indicanuria and foul alkaline stools. The diagnosis is made by the relief of the symptoms when the constipation is overcome.

Carbohydrate Toxemia is a disorder caused by the use of an excessive amount of carbohydrate food. The symptoms are those of "Lithemia" (see above) except that there is an excess of large oxalate crystals in the urine instead of uric acid as in lithemia. The urine must be examined while fresh.

Acid Food Toxemia : The use of an excessive amount of acid-forming foods may decrease the alkalinity of the body fluids and tissues and produce a large variety of symptoms. The following symptoms are the most common: nervousness, lassitude, insomnia, headache, neuralgia, muscle and joint pains, dyspepsia, flatulency, constipation, skin eruptions, catarrhal discharges, increased acidity of the urine. The diagnosis is made by the change in the degree of acidity of the urine and relief of the symptoms when a decreased amount of acid-producing foods are used. A list of acid and alkaline foods will be given in Lesson 57.

Alcoholic Toxemia : Prolonged use of alcoholic drinks may produce sclerosis or fatty degeneration of the heart, liver, kidneys, stomach, brain or arteries. The nose and face are red, the eyes watery and bloodshot. There is a chronic gastritis characterized by morning vomiting. A tremor of the hands and tongue may be present and there is insomnia and mental restlessness.

363

Lead Toxemia is caused by the absorption of the metal through the mouth, lungs or skin. It produces degeneration of the kidneys, arteries, nerves and muscles. The principle symptoms are anemia, a blue line on the gums, constipation and intestinal colic with vomiting. When the nerves are affected it produces a peripheral neuritis, most often of the median nerve. The anemia is characterized by a granular degeneration of the red cells. The symptoms of "Arteriosclerosis," "Dyspepsia," or "Nephritis" may be present.

Morphine and Cocaine Poisoning is caused by the habitual use of either of these drugs. The most prominent symptoms are a sallow skin, tremors, restlessness, insomnia, mental deterioration and moral degeneration. There is an irresistible craving for the drug.

Septic Intoxication is a name applied to a group of symptoms that occur when there is an absorption into the blood of bacteria or their toxins. There are chills and irregular fever and the patient is usually prostrated. Examination of the blood shows a leukocytosis. Careful search usually reveals the presence of abscesses or infection of some organ or part of the body.

Tuberculosis is a chronic disease characterized by the formation of tubercles, or nodules. These tubercles break down and form abscesses which may become infiltrated with connective tissue or calcium salts. Practically any organ or tissue of the body may be affected; the constitutional symptoms are the same regardless of the location of the lesion. The special symptoms due to the involvement of the different organs will be considered when the disease of those organs are discussed.

Lesson 27: Chronic Constitutional Diseases

The general symptoms are fever (with morning remissions), night sweats, hectic flush, debility, anemia, progressive loss of flesh, dyspepsia, leukopenia and lymphocytosis. A positive diagnosis can be made only by finding the tubercle baccilli in the sputum, stool, urine or discharges.

Syphilis is a chronic disease having three stages, each accompanied by different pathological changes and symptoms. The primary stage is characterized by the formation of the chancre, which is a superficial ulcer having a hard indurated base. It usually occurs upon the external genitals but may be found upon any part that comes in contact with syphilitic discharges. It usually appears from fifteen to twenty-five days after exposure.

The Secondary stage is characterized by skin eruptions and shallow ulcers in the mucous membrane of the mouth and throat. There may be inflammation of the iris, the synovial membranes or the periosteum. These symptoms occur six to twelve weeks after the appearance of the chancre.

The Tertiary stage is characterized by infiltration of connective tissue or the formation of gumma (nodules) which may break down and form ulcers. Practically any tissue or organ of the body may be affected. A positive diagnosis can be made only by finding the syphilitic bacteria. The Wassermann test is by no means infallible. The symptoms present when the different organs are involved will be given when diseases of that organ are considered.

Malaria is a chronic constitutional disorder characterized by the presence of the malarial parasite in the blood. There is an enlargement of the spleen, anemia, debility and cachexia. During the active stage there are paroxysmal, periodic attacks of chills, fever and sweating. (See "Acute Constitutional Diseases.")

Rickets is a disease of children associated with malnutrition and is characterized by alterations in the bony tissues as well as various internal disorders. The characteristic pathological changes consist of the softening of the bones together with the formation of new bone which does not completely ossify. The articular ends of the long bones become enlarged and the bones become bent. The skull is enlarged and nearly square in shape. Bow-legs in children is usually due to Rickets. There are gastro-intestinal disturbances, anemia, loss of muscle tone and the bones of the legs are tender.

QUESTIONS—LESSON 27

1. What is Lithemia?

2. Give symptoms of Diabetes mellitus.

3. What is the cause of Acidosis during Diabetes mellitus?

4. What is Uremia?

5. Give symptoms of Morphine or Cocaine Poisoning.

6. Give general symptoms of Chronic Tuberculosis.

7. Give general symptoms of Chronic Syphilis.

8. What is Rickets?

9. Give symptoms of Malaria.

10. What is the cause of Scurvy?

EXTENSION COURSE IN CHIROPRACTIC AMERICAN UNIVERSITY CHICAGO, Ill., U.S.A.

LESSON 28

TREATMENT OF CHRONIC CONSTITUTIONAL DISEASES

The general principles of treatment given in Lesson 24 should be followed in the treatment of the chronic constitutional disorders. In addition to this, special measures may be used with the individual diseases. It is understood that in all cases, you should thoroughly examine the spine and correct whatever spinal lesions may be present.

The treatment of Diabetes Mellitus usually requires special attention to the diet. The patient should be fasted from three to seven days and then be given a diet that contains no carbohydrates for one week, the urine being examined every day to determine the percentage of glucose in the twenty-four hour specimen of urine. Then put him on a diet containing just enough carbohydrates to keep the glucosuria at, or below, the percentage it was when he was on a carbohydrate free diet. If correct treatment is used with the diet, it is usually possible to gradually increase the amount of carbohydrates the patient can take. In addition to the restricted

Lesson 28: Treatment of Chronic Constitutional Diseases

diet, you should stimulate elimination and metabolism, raise the vitality increase the activity of the pancreas and liver, overcome the constipation, and stimulate the seventh cervical vertebra.

When Acidosis makes its appearance, you should decrease the amount of fats and proteins in the diet and slightly increase the starches and sugars until the symptoms disappear. Special attention should tie paid to elimination.

Uremia is a serious condition and demands immediate and vigorous treatment. Prolonged hot baths or wet sheet packs should be used, together with repeated hot enemas. The patient should drink water freely. When the worst symptoms have been relieved, friction baths, massage and exercise may be used.

In Lithemia, meat, eggs and all foods containing purine bodies should be forbidden. Special attention should be paid to increasing the elimination and metabolism.

Scurvy, Rickets, Acid Food Toxemia, and Carbohydrate Toxemia are very largely due to improper diet and the treatment, of course, is to correct the diet. Fresh fruits and vegetables (especially green) are the most effective in Scurvy and Rickets.

In the Carbohydrate or Acid Food Toxemias the patient should be fasted and then should be put on a diet containing the minimum amount of the foods that have caused his trouble. Special attention should be paid to increasing the elimination and stimulating metabolism.

In Obesity the sugars, starches and fats should be reduced to the absolute minimum and the total amount of food should be no more than is absolutely required by the body. The proper amount and kind of exercise should be used and an effort should be made to stimulate metabolism and elimination.

The patient with Lead Toxemia should make every effort to protect himself from the absorption of the lead with which he comes in contact in his work. It is sometimes necessary to abandon the occupation that requires the handling of lead. Elimination should be stimulated, the blood should be purified, and the vital resistance should be raised. The treatment of Colon Toxemia will be considered under the head of "Constipation."

If the Toxemia is due to Morphine, Cocaine or Alcohol it should be gradually withdrawn while the elimination is increased and the vital resistance raised. A fast followed by the milk diet or vegetarian diet is of considerable value. Prolonged neutral baths or prolonged applications of moderate heat to the spine will tend to decrease the extreme nervousness and irritability.

The effective treatment of Septic Intoxication will depend altogether upon locating and removing the source of the infection. The toxins should be eliminated by the use of a fast, prolonged hot baths, hot enemas and water drinking. In addition to opening and draining the abscesses or suppurating wound, the blood supply to the affected part should be increased.

The general treatment of Tuberculosis is practically the same regardless of the organ or tissue affected. The patient should have abundance of fresh air and sunshine. He should rest in bed during the period of fever, but should exercise when there is no fever. Massage may be used as a substitute if the patient is unable to exercise. Every effort should be made to raise the vitality. The milk diet or the Salisbury meat diet are very good. The patient should not be stuffed with food, but should be cautioned against over-eating. Sun baths, air baths and ultra violet light are of considerable value. The entire spine should be thoroughly and carefully relaxed and any spinal lesions present should receive attention.

The treatment of Syphilis is very largely a question of purifying the blood, raising the vital resistance and increasing the elimination. The general principles of treatment as outlined in Lesson 24 may be followed.

The blood should be purified and the elimination increased in Malaria. The fever should be controlled with hydrotherapy, the spine should be relaxed and adjusted where necessary. Concussion of the second lumbar and the eleventh dorsal vertebra, will drive the parasites into the blood stream and increase the ability of the blood to destroy them.

PROGNOSIS OF CHRONIC CONSTITUTIONAL DISEASES

The prognosis as to life is good in all of these disorders with the possible exception of Uremia, Acidosis and Tuberculosis. The possibility of cure of the conditions depends altogether upon your ability to find and remove their causes before there has been too much destruction of vital tissue or the vitality of the patient is too low to react to treatment. They are all curable if correct treatment is instituted in time and they are all incurable if improper treatment is used or correct treatment is used too late in the disease.

Generally speaking, the prognosis in Scurvy, Rickets, Carbohydrate Toxemia, Acid Food Toxemia and Lithemia is good. The prognosis in Tuberculosis, Syphilis, Malaria and

371

Septic Toxemia is relatively bad. In the rest of these disorders the prognosis should be guarded.

QUESTIONS—LESSON 28

1. Why is it important that you thoroughly master the symptoms of the Chronic Constitutional Diseases?

2. How would you differentiate between Colon Toxemia and Acid Food Toxemia?

3. How would you differentiate between Alcoholic Toxemia and Lead Toxemia?

4. How would you differentiate between Uremia and Acidosis?

5. Briefly outline the treatment for Diabetes Mellitus.

6. Briefly outline the treatment for Uremia.

7. What is the most important thing to do in the Food Toxemias?

8. Briefly outline the general treatment of Tuberculosis.

9. Briefly outline the treatment for Alcoholic Toxemia.

10. What is the Prognosis in Chronic Tuberculosis?

CHIROPRACTIC

The Science of Spinal Adjustment

———

A SERIES OF LESSONS CORRELATING AND
SYSTEMATIZING THE KNOWLEDGE NECESSARY
TO PRACTICE CHIROPRACTIC

Nature's Greatest Ally

IN RESTORING DISEASED CONDITIONS OF THE
BODY TO PERFECT HEALTH, WITHOUT THE AID
OF DRUGS OR SURGERY

———

BOOK 8

DIGESTIVE DISORDERS

RESPIRATORY DISORDERS

BONE, JOINT, MUSCLE
and SKIN DISORDERS

Lessons 29, 30, 31, 32 and 33

———

ORIGINALLY PUBLISHED BY
AMERICAN UNIVERSITY
CHICAGO, ILLINOIS, U.S.A.

Organic MD Media
PO Box 50399
Palo Alto, CA 94303

First Published 1913, 1916
American University
Chicago, Ill, USA

Second Edition 2017
Published by OrganicMD Media
eBook Edition copyright © Organic MD Media 2017

Printed in the United States of America

Organic MD Media   2012 -

Chiropractic - The Science of Spinal Adjustment - Book 7

ISBN: 978-1-946036-07-0

Disclaimer

We are proud to republish this series of books on chiropractic medicine.

Originally published as a home-study course in 1913 by American University in Chicago, the 16 volumes give us an historical look at the theory and practice of chiropractic medicine in the early part of the 20th century.

This series is republished for historical interest only. The modern practice of chiropractic has advanced significantly in the century since these books were published. If you want to actually learn modern chiropractic techniques, please consult one of the many fine schools in this country.

The materials in these books are not intended to diagnose or treat disease. If you believe you are ill consult a licensed practitioner for care immediately. The publishers assume no liability for the use, misuse or nonuse of the materials in these books.

Thank you

EXTENSION COURSE IN CHIROPRACTIC AMERICAN UNIVERSITY CHICAGO, Ill., U.S.A.

LESSON 29

CONSTIPATION

Constipation is a condition characterized by prolonged retention of fecal material in the colon or rectum. The pathology of Constipation can be considered under three general heads: Atonic, Spastic, and Obstructive.

Diagnosis. Many people who are badly constipated will assure you that their bowels are perfectly normal. The patient's own word should never be taken seriously. With some persons it is normal to have a bowel movement every other day or even less frequently. It is a safe rule, however, to consider every patient who does not have at least one bowel movement a day as constipated.

If the fecal material is very hard or dry the patient is constipated, no matter how many movements he has a day. If the patient takes a tablespoonful of charcoal with a meal, its presence should be detected in the stool (black) not later than thirty-six hours after it is taken. If the daily bowel movement occurs in the morning, charcoal taken during the evening meal should appear in the stool of the second morning afterwards.

The patient is also constipated if the average amount evacuated every day does not correspond with the amount and bulk of the food taken. If it does not, there is an accumulation of fecal material somewhere in the intestinal tract. This can be diagnosed by the fact that the charcoal in the stool is present more than twelve hours after the time of its first appearance. Dry, hard lumps of the fecal material may accumulate in distended portions of the colon and remain there for long periods. These can be detected by restricting the patient's diet and using large, warm enemas for several days in succession.

Atonic Constipation is the most common type. The abdominal muscles are relaxed and flabby and oftimes the abdomen is distended with gas. Upon palpation, doughy masses can usually be felt along the course of the colon. Upon percussion, these fecal accumulations may be located by the dull sound they produce.

Spastic Constipation. In this type the patient complains of pain before and during the defecation. There is considerable straining at stool and the evacuation never seems to be satisfactory. It seems to the patient as if some fecal material was left in the rectum which cannot be expelled. Severe "Colitis" is invariably present in this disorder and is indicated by the passage of mucus with the stool together with the tenderness along the course of the colon (especially over the sigmoid on the left side).

The abdomen is not distended; when palpated the abdominal muscles are found to be hard and tense. The sphincter muscles of the anus are also spasmodically contracted. Upon deep palpation you can usually feel the contracted colon. It feels like a hard cord about one inch in diameter.

Obstructive Constipation cannot be always positively diagnosed, but is to be suspected when fecal matter can be palpated in the rectum or in the sigmoid flexure of the colon (just above the pubes). If a physical examination of the pelvis shows that the uterus is retroflexed, or that there is a pelvic tumor or an inflammatory exudate into the pelvic tissues, rectal obstruction is probably present. Rectal tumors or stenosis or a kink at the rectal-sigmoid junction or in the sigmoid (as seen through the sigmoidoscope) are evidences of obstruction.

An X-ray examination after the use of a bismuth meal or a bismuth enema is sometimes necessary in order to determine the presence, the location, or the nature of the obstruction.

CORRECTIVE TREATMENT
Practically all cases of all types of Constipation will be benefited by a week's Fast or Fruit Fast and by the Milk Diet. The fast gives the intestinal muscles a much needed rest and enables the patient to thoroughly clean his colon with enemas. The Milk Diet is a very effective means of strengthening the muscles of the bowels by increasing their nutrition. It is absolutely necessary that the patient have at least three bowel movements each day while taking the milk. This effect can usually be produced by some modification of the milk diet. Small quantities of milk taken with other foods will aggravate the Constipation.

The special treatment, of course, should be planned to produce an effect or a condition opposite to that present in the bowel. It is evident, then, that different types of constipation require different plans of treatment. Each type will be considered separately.

(a) Atonic

In addition to removing or correcting any condition in the body that may be interfering with the nerve or blood supply to the bowel muscles, much can be done to increase the tone and contractile power of the muscles. Generally speaking, any measure that Increases the Tone, Strength or Activity of the Deep Spinal Muscles of the Lumbar and Sacral regions or of the Muscles of the Abdominal Wall will, at the same time, have a similar effect upon the bowel muscles. The most effective measures are Exercise, Short Cold, or Prolonged Cool Applications, or the Slow Sinusoidal Current. Vibratory Stimulation, Massage and Osteopathic Stimulation of the Abdomen and the Lumbar Spine may also be used. Stimulation of the 2nd Lumbar Vertebrae by Electricity, Concussion, or Short Severe Pressures will cause the intestines to contract and thus directly affect the weakened muscles.

Cold enemas or very hot enemas (120 to 125 degrees) will also tone up the muscular coat of the Colon. The hot enema should not be retained longer than is absolutely necessary.

(b) Spastic

In this type, measures must be used that will Decrease the Activity or Produce Relaxation of the Bowel Muscles. Hot Sitz Baths (103 degrees, three to five minutes) or Prolonged Hot Applications to the Abdomen or to the Lumbar and Sacral Spine will produce relaxation and at the same time relieve pain.

The Therapeutic Lamp is very effective in these cases when applied to the Abdomen or to the Lumbar Spine. Abdominal massage may be used in some of these cases, but the movements must be very gentle. In many cases the condition is aggravated by massage. Prolonged Mild Traction of the Lumbar Region is also of value. Large (two quart) warm (105 degrees) enemas also tend to relax the spasms. They should not be continued over long periods as they tend to increase the Congestion of the Mucous Membrane of the Colon.

The High Frequency Effleurage is the most effective electrical application in these conditions. Stimulation of the 11th Dorsal Vertebrae will produce a relaxation of the Colon. Forcible Dilation of the spasmodically contracted Sphincter Muscle of the Anus produces immediate relief in many cases.

All Rough Manipulation of the Abdomen or Spine must be avoided. Do not use any measure that contracts muscles or stimulates nerves (except to the 11th Dorsal).

(c) Obstructive

If the obstruction to the peristaltic action of the Colon is due to an Accumulation of Fecal Material, this should be removed by the use of warm enemas. Abdominal massage while the water is in the colon assists in breaking up the fecal material. Prolapses of the Colon and other abdominal viscera must be overcome by strengthening the abdominal muscles and other appropriate measures. The Displaced Uterus and other organs that interfere with the movement of the bowels must be replaced.

Some of the cases of obstructive constipation will require surgical treatment. In a great many cases, however, operation can be avoided by treatment directed to the removal of all factors that tend to decrease the normal activity of the bowels, and the use of the palliative measures given below.

PALLIATIVE TREATMENT

In rare cases it is impossible to find or to remove the cause of the condition or it is impossible to directly affect the pathological condition of the colon. Under these circumstances, palliative treatment must be used.

Palliative treatment can also be used to prevent the toxic effects of the constipation while other treatment is being used. Palliative treatment should never be continued, however, any longer than is absolutely necessary.

Many practitioners have fallen into the vicious habit of using measures that give only temporary relief instead of planning and using some method of treatment that will make the patient independent of treatment.

Overcoming the lack of bowel activity by any of the palliative measures cannot be considered a cure of the condition. This should be constantly borne in mind.

Diet

Bulky or Stimulating Foods are perhaps the most effective of these palliative measures. Given below is a list of food classified according to their laxative power. By withholding all constipating food and feeding nothing but laxative food it is possible in most cases to produce bowel movement. Whole Cereals and Bran are the most used of these articles. . All vegetables (except potatoes and sweet potatoes) may be used. No radical changes should be made in the patient's diet immediately. It is best to forbid one or more of the constipating foods and substitute one or more of the laxative foods each day until the diet is composed very largely of the laxative foods.

A diet composed of Whole Cereals and Vegetables can be taken by the average individual and is usually effective. Some of the Sweet Fruits (figs, raisins, prunes, dried peaches, dried pears, etc.) are sometimes more effective than any other foods. The acid fruits are also very good, especially when taken at bed time or before breakfast.

Not all individuals are affected alike by the same food. A little experimentation on the part of the patient will soon teach him what foods produce the desired effect.

In extreme cases, Agar may be used. Agar (or Agar-agar) is a Japanese Seaweed which is practically indigestible. It absorbs water in the colon and forms bulky, moist, easily voided stool. It is perfectly harmless and half a pint a day can be taken usually without harm. It is best to take a tablespoonful or more at each meal rather than take it all at one time. It may be mixed with other cereals or taken by itself.

Sour Milk or Buttermilk are very good laxatives. Their use is especially desirable when Colitis is present, or where there are severe symptoms of Toxemia. Their prolonged use tends to destroy the Harmful Bacteria in the Colon and replace them with harmless bacteria which aid in the normal action of the Colon.

The patient must be warned about overeating. Overuse of any food, even laxative food, may produce indigestion and aggravate constipation. It is better to reduce the amount of non-laxative or constipating food than to increase the amount of the stimulating foods.

A glass or two of Hot Water before breakfast each morning will aid in re-establishing the regular movements with many individuals. Common Salt added to the water will increase its effectiveness. This measure should not be used over a long period as it will eventually produce some gastric disorder.

Exercise and Massage

All Active Exercises are good. Movements that Forcibly Bend or Twist the Lumbar Spine must be avoided in Spastic Constipation. Over-fatigue must be avoided in all cases. Outdoor Games or Sports are most desirable when the patient can partake of them. Rowing, Swimming, Tennis, Baseball and Basketball are especially good. Among the indoor games, Bowling, Hand Ball and Volley Ball are especially good. Slow Running, Walking or Horseback Riding can be used.

Special exercises that require the contraction of the Abdominal or Lumbar Muscles or cause pressure on the abdominal contents are especially good. All movements that involve Bending at the Waist or Twisting the Lumbar Spine are effective.

In Atonic Constipation the movements should be executed briskly and forcibly. In Spastic Constipation the movements must be made slowly and smoothly.

Massage is best just before breakfast. The exact technic is not of great importance. The abdomen must be Thoroughly and Deeply Kneaded, special attention being paid to the Colon. A very satisfactory abdominal massage may be had by the patient lying on his back and rolling a heavy croquet or iron ball around his abdomen. Deep Breathing exercises also produce a very good massage of the abdominal organs.

Hydrotherapy, Electrotherapy and Vibration

These measures can in many cases be used to overcome the primary pathology of Constipation. They can also be used as palliative measures. In this case, the object should be to Increase the Peristaltic Contraction of the Intestines.

Short Cold, Short Hot, or Alternate Hot and Cold Applications to the Abdomen or to the Lumbar Spine are very effective in promoting bowel activity. Any Stimulative Electric Current may be used. The Indifferent Electrode should be placed over the 2nd Lumbar Vertebrae while the Active Electrode should be moved about over the Anterior Surface of the Abdomen.

The Sinusoidal Currents (Slow, Surging, Superimposed, or Interrupted Rapid) are the Most Effective and Least Harmful. In extreme cases the Colon may be Filled with Water and then one Electrode used in the Rectum and the other one over the Colon.

Another way of applying the current is to use the Rectal Electrode in the Anus and a Tongue Depressor Electrode in the mouth. The Abdomen as a whole may be Vibrated by using an oscillator or by using a small hand Vibrator. Either Vibratory Stimulation or Vibratory Kneading may be used. The same treatment may be applied to the Lumbar Region of the Spine. It should be remembered that Over-Stimulation always results in Inhibition. The treatment should always be too short rather than too long.

Enemas

The injection of water into the colon is a very valuable measure in the treatment of constipation, if it is properly used. If improperly used, it is productive of a great deal of harm. The temperature, amount of water, and manner of administration should be governed by the effects desired.

The position of the patient when the enema is taken is not of a great deal of importance. Careful X-ray examination has shown that the water will reach the upper end of the colon (cecum) with the patient in any position if the douche can is held at least twelve inches above the highest part of the colon and sufficient water is used. The erect or sitting position is the least desirable as much more force is required to fill the colon. A long colon tube need not be used—a short rectal tip will answer all purposes.

If it is desired to simply wash out the accumulated fecal material from the colon, it can be done very effectively by using two quarts of warm water (105 degrees) passed slowly into the colon. The patient may lie on his back as this is usually the most comfortable position. The bottom of the douche can should be not more than twelve inches above the anus. If any desire is felt to expel the water before all of it has passed in, the flow should be stopped a few moments. For cleansing the colon the water should be retained for ten or fifteen minutes. These enemas can be used to advantage during the first week of treatment in any form of constipation.

If it is desired to stimulate the peristaltic contraction of the colon or rectum the water must be either cold or very hot. If the water is very hot (120 or 125 degrees) is must not be retained a moment longer than absolutely necessary. Any amount from one

386

to four pints may be used. Sometimes it may be best to use the regular bulb (Davidson's) syringe instead of the fountain syringe. The intermittent pressure produced by the bulb syringe is of value in promoting peristalsis. Cold enemas '(60 to 80 degrees) may be used where they do not produce pain. Sometimes a very small injection of cold water into the rectum is all that is necessary to initiate peristalsis.

Enemas given for the purpose of stimulating bowel activity should always be given at the time that the bowels should normally move. In most individuals this is early in the morning just before, or just after breakfast. An effort should always be made to move the bowels before the enema is given. If the bowels cannot be moved or if the evacuation is insufficient, the stimulating enema can then be used.

Psychotherapy

Suggestive treatment should be used with two objects. First of all you must overcome the patient's idea that artificial means are necessary to move the bowels. Many patients use artificial means simply because they think their bowels will not move without them.

You must also impress the patient with the idea that your treatment is going to overcome his constipation and that his bowels will move as soon as this is done. He should be instructed to visit the toilet every morning and attempt to move his bowels whether he has a desire to do so or not.

QUESTIONS—LESSON 29

1. What is Constipation?

2. Name the three types of Constipation and give Pathology of one.

3. Give diagnostic signs of c Constipation.

4. Give diagnostic signs of Spastic Constipation.

5. What should be the object of your therapeutic measures in the treatment of Atonic Constipation?

6. When should Palliative Treatment be used?

7. Name a few of the foods that may be used in the treatment of Constipation.

8. What kind of exercises should be used in Atonic Constipation?

9. What Hydrotherapeutic Measures should be used in the treatment of Spastic Constipation?

10. Give directions for using Enemas for washing out the Colon.

EXTENSION COURSE
IN CHIROPRACTIC
AMERICAN UNIVERSITY
CHICAGO, Ill., U.S.A.

LESSON 30

SYMPTOMS OF DISEASES OF THE STOMACH

Dyspepsia is not a disease, but is a name applied to a group of symptoms. These symptoms are of a general character and by themselves have no diagnostic value. They may occur in any of the diseases of the digestive organs. To avoid repetition the word "Dyspepsia" will be used in describing any disease that has some or all of the following symptoms: Abdominal pain or tenderness, Gastric or Intestinal distension, Heart burn, Acid eructations, Belching, Coated tongue, Foul breath, Sore mouth, Headache, Constipation, Diarrhea, Malaise.

Acute Gastritis is the acute inflammation of the mucous membrane of the stomach caused usually by some dietetic error. All of the symptoms of "Dyspepsia" may be present in addition to vomiting and marked pain and tenderness over the stomach.

Chronic Gastritis is characterized by increased secretion of mucus, changes in the gastric juice, weakening of the gastric muscle, and atrophy of the mucous membrane of the stomach.

389

The symptoms are those of "Dyspepsia" plus increased pain and tenderness in the middle line of the epigastric region, nausea, vomiting, diminished amount of hydrochloric acid, emaciation and spinal tenderness at the fifth, sixth and seventh dorsal vertebrae.

Gastric Ulcer is a condition in which there is a destruction of the localized area of the mucous membrane of the stomach. The ulcer may perforate the entire wall of the stomach. The pain (and tenderness) in Gastric Ulcer is severe and sharply localized. It is more intense just before and one or two hours after meals, and is usually relieved by eating or vomiting. The fifth, sixth and seventh dorsal vertebrae also show tenderness. The vomitus may be streaked with blood; blood may be found in the stool. The hydrochloric acid in the stomach contents is usually increased. The tender spot may be made to shift upward by concussion of the seventh cervical vertebrae.

Duodenal Ulcer is a condition similar to Gastric Ulcer except for the location of the lesion. The pain and tenderness are on the right of the middle line of the epigastrium. It is more intense two to four hours after meals. There may also be vomiting, increased hydrochloric acid and blood in the stools. The spinal tenderness is at the eighth and ninth dorsal. The pain in the abdomen may be relieved by concussion of the tenth dorsal vertebrae.

Gastric Cancer is a malignant growth that destroys the tissues of the stomach. It usually occurs after forty years of age in those individuals whose stomach is subject to constant irritation from Chronic Gastritis or improper diet. The pain is severe and continuous and is usually made worse by food. The vomitus resembles coffee grounds. Examination of the stomach contents may reveal decreased acidity and the presence of lactic acid and pieces of the tumor. There is anorexia, emaciation and cachexia. The tumor may be discovered by palpation or by taking an X-ray picture. When the tumor can be palpated, the case is usually too far advanced for any treatment to be of avail. The prognosis is unfavorable, unless treatment is instituted very early in the disease.

Gastrectasis or Gastric Dilatation is an abnormal permanent increase in the capacity of the stomach with loss of tone of its muscular walls. In addition to the symptoms of "Dyspepsia" there is vomiting of undigested food that has been eaten on a previous day. If the abdomen is shaken later than six hours after meals a splashing sound will be heard. Percussion will show that the lower border of the stomach is too low. Stimulation of the seventh cervical vertebrae may relieve the symptoms.

Gastric Neuroses. There may be motor, sensory and secretory disturbances of the stomach without anatomical lesions of that organ. These disorders are caused by some interference with the activity of the nerves that supply the stomach. For this reason they are called "Neuroses." They can be relieved by nerve stimulation or inhibition. A large percentage, of so-called stomach diseases are Neuroses, but a Neurosis should be diagnosed only when a very thorough examination and study of the case has proven that no anatomical lesions of the stomach are present.

DIAGNOSIS OF DISEASES OF THE STOMACH

All diseases of the stomach have many symptoms in common. Dyspepsia is not a disease but is a name given to a group of symptoms. When this term is used in describing some disease of the digestive or other organs (e.g. kidneys) it is understood that the patient has several or all of these symptoms. Abdominal pain and tenderness are common to all abdominal disorders so

391

have no diagnostic value unless there is some peculiarity as to time, intensity, location, relation to meals, etc. These factors are considered with each separate disease.

First study "Gastritis" and then compare the other diseases of the stomach with it, noting how each one differs from it. The pain and tenderness (in Gastritis) are located in the stomach region and are more intense than in dyspepsia. The loss of weight is due to the interference with nutrition. Diminished hydrochloric acid can be diagnosed only by examining the contents of the stomach. The pain of Gastric Ulcer is very characteristic; the patient usually points to the painful spot with one finger, and the area of tenderness is very small. In Duodenal Ulcer the pain occurs later and it and the tenderness are located over the duodenum instead of the stomach. It is well to remember that stimulation of the tenth dorsal vertebrae by concussion will relieve the pain of duodenal ulcer but not that of gastric ulcer.

Carcinoma of the stomach is to be suspected when the pain is severe and continuous and the patient is emaciated, anemic and has a peculiar discoloration of the skin (Cachexia). The vomitus is characteristic. The vomiting of the food of a previous meal and the presence of a splashing sound when the stomach is shaken (when it should be empty) are sufficient evidence upon which to base a provisional diagnosis of Dilatation.

A great many of the stomach disorders are not accompanied by any changes in the stomach itself but are due to some disturbance of the nervous impulses to the stomach. It should be remembered that the stomach is very easily influenced by disturbances elsewhere in the body (pelvic disorders, constipation, eyestrain, etc.) and that Constitutional Diseases (Anemia, Tuberculosis, Uremia, Diabetes

392

or Nervous Diseases) may interfere with digestion and cause symptoms referable to the stomach. In every case, however, the stomach should be carefully examined to be sure it is not diseased. Prolapse of the stomach and intestines accompanies many digestive disorders. The characteristic shape of the abdomen is easily noted on inspection.

SYMPTOMS OF INTESTINAL DISORDERS

Diarrhea is not a disease, but is a term used to describe a condition in which there is excessive frequency or fluidity of the stools. There is also thirst, the skin is dry, the urine is scanty, and if the diarrhea is long continued the patient becomes emaciated and debilitated and secondary anemia appears.

Intestinal Colic is a condition produced by the spasmodic contraction of the intestinal muscles due to irritation of the intestinal mucous membrane or of the nerves that supply the intestinal muscles. The onset is sudden with a severe pain of a tearing, twisting and bearing-down character most marked in the middle of the abdomen. The pain can usually be relieved by pressure. In severe attacks the skin is cold, the pulse is rapid, the features are pinched and there may be nausea, vomiting and tenesmus. The abdomen is usually distended with gas.

Intestinal Indigestion is a functional disorder due to some disturbance of the intestinal secretions or activity of the intestinal muscles, or both. In addition to the symptoms of "Dyspepsia" there is pain in the middle line of the umbilical region. The pain is usually two to six hours after meals. There may be constipation or diarrhea and undigested food is found in the feces. The condition may be acute or chronic. In the former the symptoms are more severe and of shorter duration.

Acute Enteritis is an acute catarrhal inflammation of the small intestines. The onset is sudden with severe intestinal pains moving from one part of the abdomen to the other. The pain is intermittent and followed at intervals by a sudden extreme desire to empty the bowels. There is diarrhea and the stools may contain mucus.

Chronic Enteritis is a chronic inflammation of the mucous membrane and intestines usually accompanied by atrophy of the muscular walls. There is diarrhea with indigested food in the stools and pain and tenderness over the small intestines. There is spinal tenderness at the 11th and 12th dorsal and the 1st lumbar vertebrae. The patient is usually, emaciated and anemic.

Tubercular Enteritis is a chronic constitutional disorder in which the primary pathology is in the intestinal tract. The symptoms are those of "Enteritis" plus those of "Tuberculosis."

Colitis is a chronic inflammation of the colon characterized by inflammation or atrophy of the mucous membrane and hyperplasia and loss of tone of the muscular layer. It is usually caused by chronic constipation. In addition to the symptoms of constipation, which is usually of the spastic type, there is painful defecation, tenderness over the colon, and the stools are mixed with, or covered with mucus.

Acute Appendicitis is an acute inflammation of the vermiform appendix. The inflammation may be catarrhal, ulcerative, suppurative or gangrenous in type. The onset is sudden with cramp-like pains in the middle of the abdomen which later become localized in the right inguinal region which becomes tender. There is nausea, vomiting and fever. Constipation is nearly always present. In severe cases the symptoms of peritonitis are present. If an abscess is formed the fever becomes irregular and is accompanied by chills and sweats, and all of the symptoms are aggravated. Examination of the blood will show a leukocytosis. If the contents of the appendix escape into the abdominal cavity the symptoms are those of collapse.

Chronic Appendicitis usually follows acute attacks or may be due to chronic constipation. There are recurring attacks of pain and tenderness in the right iliac fossa with fever, vomiting and constipation. Examination of the spine will show tenderness on the right side of the second lumbar vertebrae.

Dysentery is an acute inflammation of the mucous membrane of the large intestine which may be accompanied by ulceration. The onset is sudden with fever, abdominal pain, and diarrhea. There is a constant desire to defecate; the stools contain mucus and blood may be present. There is tenderness over the colon and from the 2nd to the 4th lumbar vertebrae. The patient rapidly becomes emaciated and debilitated.

Proctitis is a chronic catarrhal inflammation of the mucous membrane of the rectum, usually due to constipation or habitual use of enemas and purgatives. There is a burning pain in the rectum, tenesmus, and the passage of feces containing mucus, pus or blood. The anal sphincter is painfully contracted. The mucous membrane is reddened, thickened and ulcerated. The spinal tenderness is at the fifth lumbar, or second or fourth sacral vertebrae.

Hemorrhoids, or Piles, is a name applied to a permanent distention and engorgement of the rectal veins accompanied by weakening of their walls or some obstruction to the return flow of the blood. The common causes are constipation and diseases of the liver. There is a feeling of fullness in the rectum and defecation is painful and may be followed by bleeding. Rectal examination shows soft, spongy, red or bluish tumors outside or just inside the anal sphincter.

Acute Intestinal Obstruction may be due to hardened feces, foreign bodies, gall stones, or to the slipping of one part of the intestine into another. The symptoms are a sudden onset of abdominal pain which becomes continuous and severe, repeated vomiting, at first of the stomach contents and finally of fecal matter, and absolute constipation. The abdomen usually becomes distended with gas. Occasionally the obstruction can be palpated. The face is pinched, the skin cold, tongue dry, thirst marked, the urine scanty or suppressed, the pulse rapid and feeble and the temperature may be subnormal. Unless relieved death will occur in two or three days.

Chronic Intestinal Obstruction is usually due to a cancer of the intestines, but may be due to the same causes that produce acute obstruction. There is a gradual increasing constipation that cannot be relieved by the usual methods of treatment. The feces are ribbon-shaped or in small round masses. Abdominal pain and tenderness with distension are present. It is usually possible to palpate the mass producing the obstruction.

Intestinal Carcinoma is usually situated in the rectum. The mass gradually encircles the bowels and eventually blocks the passage. The symptoms are those of "Intestinal Obstruction" plus those of "Proctitis" in addition to the symptoms that may be caused by the pressure of the growing mass in the pelvis. The patient is anemic, debilitated and cachexic.

Intestinal Neuroses. Many disorders of the intestinal tract are not accompanied by the structural changes in the bowel but are due to some interference with the nerve impulses to the intestines. There may be motor, sensory, or secretory disturbances. Neuroses are usually diagnosed by exclusion, although a point in favor of this condition would be the relief obtained by nerve inhibition or stimulation. You should make sure that there is no pathological condition present before you call it a neuroses.

Gastro-Enteroptosis is a term applied to the prolapse of the abdominal contents due to a relaxation of the abdominal muscles or loss of tone of the supporting tissues of the viscera. There are symptoms of "Dyspepsia" which can be relieved by the use of an abdominal support. When the patient stands erect, there is protrusion of the lower abdomen with retraction of the upper abdomen. Physical examination of the abdomen will show that the stomach and intestines are displaced downward.

DIAGNOSIS OF DISEASES OF THE INTESTINES

"Diarrhea" and "Constipation" are names applied to groups of symptoms which may be present in intestinal or constitutional disorders, or diseases of other organs. These terms will be used in describing other diseases.

"Intestinal Indigestion" should be studied before the other intestinal diseases. The interval between taking food and the appearance of the pain, and the presence of undigested food in the feces are the most important symptoms. In "Enteritis" the pain

397

is more intense and the small intestines show tenderness upon pressure. If the disorder is severe enough to interfere with nutrition, the patient will be anemic and emaciated. "Tubercular Enteritis" is to be suspected if the general symptoms suggest Tuberculosis but can be positively diagnosed only by a microscopic examination of the feces. In "Dysentery" the diarrhea and constitutional symptoms are more severe and there is a constant desire to defecate (Tenesmus) and a gripping pain in the abdomen (Tormina). The tenderness is not general. Colitis can be differentiated from dysentery by the presence of constipation and mucus in the stools.

A constipation that persists and grows worse in spite of treatment suggests "Intestinal Obstruction." If the symptoms of obstruction are accompanied by symptoms of pressure upon other organs, blood vessels or nerves a "Tumor" should be suspected. You must make a careful examination to be sure that the supposed intestinal tumor is not some other abdominal organ or due to fecal matter. "Chronic Appendicitis" is much less common than is generally thought. Most supposed cases are really colitis and their symptoms can be relieved by washing out the colon. Study "Gastric Neuroses" above with "Intestinal Neuroses." The only sign of diagnostic value in "Tape Worm" is the finding of parts of the worm in the stools.

TREATMENT OF DISEASES OF THE STOMACH AND INTESTINES

The general principles of treatment as given in Lesson 24 should be followed whenever they may be applied. Constipation is quite frequently present in all these disorders and should be treated when present (see Lesson 29). The spinal lesions are almost invariably present and should be found and corrected.

Lesson 30: Digestive Disorders (Continued)

The diet is a very important factor in all diseases of the stomach and intestines and every patient should be instructed as to the proper amount and kind of food to be taken. In acute conditions and in stubborn chronic conditions the fast should be used followed by the diet that seems to be indicated in that case. The Milk Diet is very effective in most of the stomach and intestinal disorders. This plan of treatment can be used in Dyspepsia, Gastritis, Intestinal Indigestion and Enteritis.

Diarrhea should be treated with a fast and enemas and the bowels should be flushed by drinking large quantities of water. The lower dorsal and the lumbar spine should be thoroughly relaxed and any spinal lesions present should be corrected. Prolonged pressure applied to the muscles over the tenth dorsal to second lumbar vertebrae will inhibit the excessive bowel activity. In addition to these measures you may use rapid sinusoidal, high frequency, or faradic electricity, the lamp, prolonged hot or prolonged cool applications over the abdomen or the lumbar region or the spine. Rectal dilatation, abdominal massage and deep breathing are also effective.

Gastric and Duodenal Ulcer and Tubercular Enteritis are more intractable. The patient should be given absolute rest until the disorder is brought under control. A fast is usually essential; this may be followed by a Milk Diet. Stimulation of the tenth dorsal vertebrae will relieve the pain in duodenal ulcer and tend to overcome the irritation that produces it. A patient with tubercular enteritis should be given the general treatment for tuberculosis. (See Lesson 28.)

The diet should be restricted to the minimum quantity in the treatment of Gastrectasis and Gastro-enteroptosis. The stimulation of the first to the third lumbar, seventh cervical and fifth to eighth dorsal vertebrae will contract the stomach and intestines and increase the tone of their muscular walls. The slow sinusoidal current, abdominal exercises and deep breathing are also valuable. Some cases require the use of an abdominal support while treatment is being given. The abdominal support should be used no longer than is absolutely necessary, as it tends to weaken the abdominal muscles.

Gastric and Intestinal Carcinoma are not usually diagnosed until it is too late for any treatment to be of avail. When they have progressed so far that the tumor can be palpated, it is usually desirable to remove them surgically. This does not cure the patient but will usually prolong his life and relieve his suffering.

Colitis, Appendicitis and Proctitis can be treated according to the principles outlined above. Special attention should be paid to the constipation which is invariably present.

In Hemorrhoids you should find and remove the cause of the venous stasis. Lower abdominal breathing, special pelvic exercises and prolonged cool sitz baths may be used to decrease the amount of blood in the pelvis. The local treatment depends somewhat upon the type of hemorrhoid present. Rectal dilatation, vibration, sinusoidal or high frequency currents may be tried. The positive galvanic current with a copper rectal electrode is often effective when all other measures fail.

Acute Appendicitis, Acute Enteritis and Dysentery may be treated according to principles outlined under "Acute Constitutional Diseases" in addition to measures recommended for the chronic disorders of the same organs.

PROGNOSIS OF DISEASES OF THE STOMACH AND INTESTINES

Generally speaking the prognosis in these disorders is relatively good except in Gastric or Intestinal Cancer, Intestinal Obstruction, Tubercular Enteritis and Colitis. The prognosis in Cancer is bad; that in Tubercular Enteritis, Intestinal Obstruction and Colitis is doubtful.

It is understood, of course, that possibility of relief or cure depends altogether upon the use of correct treatment before there has been too much destruction of vital tissue, or the vitality of the patient is too low to react to treatment.

QUESTIONS—LESSON 30

1. What is Dyspepsia?

2. Give symptoms of Gastric Ulcer.

3. Give symptoms of Gastric Cancer.

4. How would you diagnose Gastritis from Duodenal Ulcer?

5. Give symptoms of Chronic Enteritis.

6. Give symptoms of Colitis.

7. How would you diagnose Dysentery from Intestinal Indigestion?

8. Give treatment for Gastric Ulcer.

9. Give treatment for Chronic Appendicitis.

10. Give treatment for Diarrhea.

EXTENSION COURSE
IN CHIROPRACTIC
AMERICAN UNIVERSITY
CHICAGO, Ill., U.S.A.

LESSON 31

SYMPTOMS OF DISEASES OF THE LIVER

Pancreatitis. Diseases of the pancreas are rare and it is almost impossible to diagnose them when they are present, as they have no really characteristic symptoms. In the acute type the onset is sudden with intense abdominal pain, tenderness and vomiting. The upper left quadrant of the abdomen is distended and tympanitic. The patient soon passes into a state of collapse and may die within three days. In the chronic variety there is paroxysmal pain, abdominal distention, "Dyspepsia" and "Diarrhea." The stools contain an excess of fat. Spinal tenderness at the eighth and ninth dorsal may aid in diagnosis.

Jaundice is not a disease but a name applied to a group of symptoms that are present when there is obstruction to the outflow of bile from the liver or gall bladder or a breaking down of the liver substance. In the Obstructive Type the skin and mucous membranes are yellow. There is "Dyspepsia," "Constipation" with pale, foul stools and bile in the urine. There is a tendency to hemorrhage, the skin itches, the pulse is slow, and the patient is

403

blue and despondent. In the Toxemia Type the skin and mucous membranes are yellow and hemorrhages may occur. There is vomiting, delirium and a rapid pulse. There may be convulsions.

Hepatic Congestion is due to an increased amount of blood from the portal vein or inferior vena cava. The former is called active congestion and is usually caused by dietary excesses (especially sugars, starches and alcohol). The symptoms of active congestion are dyspepsia, nausea, vomiting, constipation, headache, malaise. The liver is enlarged and tender and there may be "Jaundice." Passive congestion (venous obstruction) has symptoms similar to active congestion, but usually less severe. If due to a valvular lesion of the heart, pulsation may be felt over the liver.

Acute Yellow Atrophy is characterized by degeneration and atrophy of the liver cells and a decrease in size of the liver as a whole. In addition to the symptoms of "Dyspepsia," there is a severe jaundice (toxemic), hemorrhages from the mucous membrane, convulsions followed by coma. Death usually occurs within a week.

Atrophic Cirrhosis of the Liver is a chronic disease characterized by the increased amount of connective tissue in the liver with degeneration of the liver cells and decreased size of the liver. It occurs most often in alcoholics. The onset is gradual and no symptoms may be produced until there is considerable obstruction to the flow of the blood from the portal vein through the liver. This produces a progressive ascites and "Gastritis." There may be vomiting of blood or blood in the stools. "Hemorrhoids" are usually present. The patient becomes emaciated except the abdomen which becomes enlarged. "Jaundice" is slight or absent. The liver is diminished in size and its surface is roughened.

Hypertrophic Cirrhosis is a chronic disease of the liver characterized by an increased amount of connective tissue with enlargement of the liver. The onset is gradual with a progressive "Jaundice." The liver becomes enlarged and is the seat of periodic pain which is accompanied by fever. Physical examination shows that both the liver and spleen are enlarged and smooth. There are digestive disturbances and symptoms of toxemia but no ascites.

Amyloid Liver is characterized by an albuminous degeneration of the liver substance. It usually accompanies prolonged suppuration elsewhere in the body. There may be no symptoms except the smooth, painless enlargement of the liver and spleen. There is no Jaundice, ascites or pain. The symptoms of "Dyspepsia" may be present.

Fatty Liver is characterized by fatty degeneration or infiltration of the liver. It usually accompanies obesity, chronic wasting diseases, anemia, or toxemia. The symptoms may be absent and are never very severe. The diagnosis is made upon the presence of a smooth, soft, painless enlargement of the liver without enlargement of the spleen. There is no jaundice or ascites.

Liver Abscesses may follow inflammation and suppuration in other abdominal organs or be a primary disease. There may be one or several abscesses. The symptoms are those of "Septic Intoxication" with hepatic pain and tenderness. The liver is usually enlarged upward. The spinal tenderness is on the right side of the sixth, seventh and eighth dorsal vertebrae.

Carcinoma of the Liver is usually secondary to carcinoma in some other portion of the digestive tract. It rarely occurs before 40. There is a continuous pain with emaciation, debility, and cachexia. The symptoms of dyspepsia are present and there is a progressive, irregular, nodular enlargement of the liver. If untreated the disease terminates with death in six to eighteen months.

Syphilis of the Liver occurs in the third stage of "Syphilis." There is a hard nodular enlargement of the liver with a history of or constitutional symptoms of syphilis.

Acute Cholecystitis is an inflammation of the mucous membrane lining the gall bladder and the bile duct. The symptoms are those of "Dyspepsia" plus those of "Obstructive Jaundice." There is tenderness over the gall bladder and at the ninth and tenth dorsal vertebrae.

Chronic Cholecystitis is characterized by inflammation and thickening of the walls of the gall bladder and bile duct. The symptoms are pain, tenderness and rigidity at the tip of the ninth rib with fever, vomiting and obstructive jaundice. If the gall bladder becomes sufficiently enlarged, it may be palpated as a soft, elastic, movable tumor.

Cholelithiasis. Stones may be formed in the gall bladder or the bile duct. This condition usually follows or accompanies "Cholecystitis" and cannot be diagnosed from it unless one of the stones is small enough to pass through the duct in which case it will probably produce "Hepatic Colic." It is possible for a patient to have gall stones for many years with no symptoms.

Hepatic Colic is a name applied to a group of symptoms that occur when the stone attempts to pass through the bile ducts. There are sudden intense pains in the right upper quadrant of the abdomen which may radiate to the right shoulder, vomiting and prostration. There is fever with chills and profuse sweating. The vomiting is severe. The pain is usually intermittent but may become continuous. Jaundice is usually present and the gall bladder is enlarged and tender. The urine contains bile and the stools are pale and may contain gall stones. The spinal tenderness is at the ninth and tenth dorsal vertebrae.

DIAGNOSIS OF DISEASES OF THE LIVER

Most diseases of the liver are accompanied by enlargement. The differentiation of these diseases will depend upon the size, shape, consistency, etc., of the liver as well as the associated symptoms (jaundice, pain, enlargement of spleen, etc.). Hypertrophic cirrhosis presents the most symptoms in common with other diseases of the liver so it should be studied first. The liver is always enlarged downward except in Abscess.

Atrophic Cirrhosis differs from the other hepatic diseases in that the liver decreases in size. In the beginning it may resemble cancer of the liver, but it can be differentiated by its slower progress, slight pain and absence of jaundice until very late in its course. Later, the diminished size of the liver will make the diagnosis clear. Gall Stones cannot be distinguished from inflammation of the Gall Bladder except when the patient has attacks of "Biliary Colic."

TREATMENT OF DISEASES OF THE LIVER

The general plan of treatment given for diseases of the stomach and intestines can be followed in the treatment of many of the diseases of the liver.

In Obstructive Jaundice, whatever is interfering with the outflow of the bile must be removed. There is usually an accompanying Cholecystitis and Cholelithiasis which should receive the proper treatment. In Toxemic Jaundice, your efforts should be directed towards elimination of the toxic material and purification of the blood. The liver should be treated if necessary.

If the Hepatic Congestion is due to dilatation of the splanchnic vessels, the diet should be restricted, (especially carbo-hydrates) abdominal exercises and massage and prolonged cool sitz baths should be used. Concussion of the fifth to the eighth dorsal vertebrae will constrict the splanchnic vessels. If the accumulation of the blood in the liver is due to a cardiac condition, the heart should receive appropriate treatment. Stimulation of the first to third lumbar vertebrae is also of value.

Acute Yellow Atrophy should be treated according to the plan given under "Acute Constitutional Diseases." Atrophic Cirrhosis and Hypertrophic Cirrhosis require restricted diet, (limited fats and carbo-hydrates) fruit diet, fast followed by "Milk Diet", abdominal massage, abdominal breathing, waist exercises and slow sinusoidal current to abdomen in addition to whatever general treatment may be necessary. The middle dorsal vertebrae and lower ribs should receive attention. Applications of prolonged heat from the fifth to the twelfth dorsal vertebrae will increase the amount of blood in the liver and will increase the activity of the liver cells as well as tend to promote absorption of the abnormal tissue.

In Amyloid and Fatty Liver, the causes should be found and treated in addition to the treatment suggested for Cirrhosis.

Syphilis of the Liver and Liver Abscesses should receive the appropriate general treatment in addition to that for Cirrhosis. The Therapeutic Lamp may be used. Not much can be done for Carcinoma of the Liver as it is usually discovered too late for any treatment to be effective. You should increase the elimination and raise the vitality and may use the therapeutic lamp. The ultra violet light is more effective in this condition than the ordinary incandescent lamp.

Cholecystitis and Cholelithiasis should be treated with the fast, enemas and prolonged cool applications over the fifth to tenth dorsal vertebrae. Prolonged application of heat may be used over the gall bladder. Stimulation of the sixth dorsal vertebrae will contract the gall bladder, and may force the stones out. If the stones are large and are causing considerable trouble an operation may be required but the case should not be operated until after other measures have been given a thorough trial. In Hepatic Colic a hot sitz bath or prolonged applications of moderate heat and prolonged moderate pressure at the ninth and tenth dorsal vertebrae will dilate the bile ducts and relieve the pain.

PROGNOSIS OF DISEASES OF THE LIVER
The possibility of cure in Jaundice and Hepatic Congestion is good if the cause can be found and removed. In Cirrhosis, Amyloid or Fatty Liver, Hepatic Syphilis or Abscesses, Cholecystitis

and Cholelithiasis the prognosis is doubtful. Carcinoma of the Liver is usually hopeless.

QUESTIONS—LESSON 31

1. What is Jaundice?

2. Give symptoms of Atrophic Cirrhosis of the Liver.

3. Give symptoms of Carcinoma of the Liver.

4. Give symptoms of Cholelithiasis.

5. What is Hepatic Colic?

6. How would you diagnose Hypertrophic Cirrhosis from Liver Abscess?

7. Briefly outline the treatment of Jaundice.

8. Give treatment for Gall Stones.

9. What is the treatment for Atrophic Cirrhosis?

10. What is the prognosis of Carcinoma of the Liver?

EXTENSION COURSE
IN CHIROPRACTIC
AMERICAN UNIVERSITY
CHICAGO, Ill., U.S.A.

LESSON 32

SYMPTOMS OF RESPIRATORY DISORDERS

Acute Bronchitis is an acute catarrhal inflammation of the larger and medium sized bronchi. It may be caused by the breathing of dust or irritating vapors, or it may be secondary to disorders in other parts of the respiratory tract, or to circulatory disorders. The symptoms are coryza, pain behind the upper portion of the sternum, cough with muco-purulent sputum and fever. Auscultation over the larger tubes will reveal dry and moist rales and increased breath sounds.

Chronic Bronchitis is a chronic inflammation of the medium and larger bronchial tubes. The symptoms are similar to those of acute bronchitis but less severe.

Bronchiectasis is a chronic condition characterized by weakening of the bronchial walls and dilatation of the tubes. It is usually secondary to other lung diseases. There is a cough which raises a large amount of thin, very foul sputum. Percussion of the chest will show an area of dullness over the affected tubes. After

412

the sputum has been raised this dullness will be changed to hyper-resonance.

Bronchial Asthma is a chronic disorder characterized by a spasmodic contraction of the bronchial tubes or swelling of the mucous membrane lining them. Emphysema and Chronic Bronchitis are usually present in long standing cases. The principle symptom is a sudden attack of a severe inspiratory dyspnea during which there is cyanosis, sweating, cold extremities and a small rapid pulse. The patient cannot lie down during the attack. The attack usually occurs in the early morning hours and lasts from a few minutes to several hours. During the attack there is a dry cough which gradually becomes moist with the raising of a thin sputum containing small round masses. Between the attacks there is a wheezing cough and dry rales over the whole chest. "Emphysema" and "Bronchitis" are usually present with the characteristic symptoms of these two disorders.

Broncho-Pneumonia is an acute inflammation of the small bronchial tubes and the air cells of the lungs. It is usually secondary to some acute constitutional disorder. In addition to the symptoms of fever there is dyspnea, chest pains, cyanosis and a cough with muco-purulent sputum. Physical examination shows rapid respiration which may be accompanied by a grunt during expiration, increased vocal fremitus, broncho-vesicular breathing, and fine rales over the body of the lungs. Percussion may reveal small areas of dullness scattered over the lungs.

Lobar Pneumonia is an acute, exudative inflammation of one or more lobes of the lungs with a general toxemia. The onset is sudden with a chill, high fever, chest pain, rapid and difficult breathing. There is a cough which raises a rusty or blood-streaked sputum. The face is flushed and the patient lies on the affected side. The pulse rate is increased and the respiration is proportionately very rapid. The physical signs during the first stage are decreased chest movement on the affected side, decreased resonance and increased breath sounds with fine rales. During the second stage there is increased dullness, fremitus and bronchial breathing. The area of dullness corresponds to the location of one or more lobes of the lungs. The disease usually terminates suddenly on the fifth, seventh and ninth day.

Acute Pulmonary Tuberculosis may have the symptoms of either "Lobar" or "Bronchial Pneumonia" plus a hectic fever, severe prostration, night sweats and rapid emaciation. It is usually accompanied by "Pleurisy." It can be diagnosed from Pneumonia only by the presence of T. B. bacilli in the sputum.

Chronic Pulmonary Tuberculosis is a chronic constitutional disorder characterized by the formation of tubercles in the lungs. The symptoms vary with the stage of the disease. **Incipient Tuberculosis** has cough with a muco-purulent sputum, chest pain, impaired resonance, increased breath sounds and fine, moist rales. In the **Moderately Advanced Stage** the sputum becomes more profuse and contains small coin-like masses; there may be hemoptysis. The areas of impaired resonance become dull, breathing becomes bronchial and there are coarse, bubbling rales. In the **Advanced Stage** cavities are formed and the areas formerly dull become hyper-resonant. Vocal fremitus is increased and there is amphoric breathing. All stages are accompanied by the constitutional symptoms of tuberculosis and the T. B. bacillus may be found in the sputum.

414

Pulmonary Fibrosis is a chronic inflammation of the supporting tissue of the lungs resulting in an increased production and subsequent contraction of the connective tissue and obliteration of the air spaces. The symptoms are cough, dyspnea, unsymmetrical and diminished chest movement with flattening of the chest wall, dullness and increased breath sounds. The contraction of the lungs usually displaces the heart.

Pulmonary Syphilis is a chronic constitutional disorder in which the lungs are principally affected. The physical signs are the same as those of Pulmonary Tuberculosis and there is a history and constitutional symptoms of "Syphilis."

Pulmonary Abscess is usually secondary to other diseases of the lungs. The physical signs are those of "Pulmonary Tumor" followed by those of the advanced stage of "Tuberculosis." The sputum is profuse, very foul and contains fibrous tissue and pus. The symptoms of "Septicemia" are present.

Pulmonary Gangrene is usually secondary to other lung disorders. The symptoms are those of the preceding disorder plus a horribly offensive breath and sputum containing stinking lung tissue. The physical signs are those of the third stage of "Pulmonary Tuberculosis."

Pulmonary Tumor is usually secondary to malignant tumors of other parts. In addition to pressure symptoms (see above) there is an area of dullness and increased vocal fremitus. A positive diagnosis can be made only by an X-ray examination or microscopic examination of pieces of the tumor.

Emphysema is a chronic condition characterized by a permanent dilatation of the air vesicles with atrophy of their walls. The chest is large and barrel-shaped. Percussion reveals an increased resonance and an extension of the lung borders behind their normal limits. There is dyspnea with a prolonged expiration. The second pulmonic heart sound is accentuated. "Bronchitis" is usually present.

Pulmonary Edema or **Congestion** is usually secondary to some interference with the circulation or to heart failure. There is dyspnea, cough with a bloody, frothy expectoration (may be hemoptysis) and fine, moist rales. Heart Disease or weakness is usually present.

Acute Pleurisy is an acute inflammation of the serous membrane lining the thorax and covering the lungs. The inflammation is fibrinous at first, usually changing later to an effusion which may become purulent. The onset is sudden with sharp pain usually in the lower portion of the chest. There are chills, followed by a rapid rise of temperature. Breathing is difficult and restrained due to the pain it produces. There is a dry cough, During the first stage there is diminished movement of the affected region of the chest and a friction rub may be heard. During the second stage the interspaces bulge, the heart is displaced, percussion shows flatness which changes its location with the position of the patient. The vocal fremitus and breath sounds are absent. If effusion becomes purulent (Empyema) the symptoms of "Septicemia" will be present.

Chronic Pleurisy may follow acute pleurisy or diseases of the lung tissue. The symptoms are diminished chest movement, friction rub, bulging inner spaces or flattening of chest wall, diminished vocal resonance and absence of breath sounds. There may be chest pain.

Chronic Empyema has the symptoms of "Chronic Pleurisy" plus those of Septic Intoxication. Positive diagnosis can be made only by tapping the pleural cavity and examining the fluid obtained.

Mediastinal Tumors may be mistaken for diseases of the lungs. The principle symptoms are those due to pressure (see above "Pressure Symptoms"). Physical examination of the chest will show abnormal dullness behind the sternum and an X-ray examination will reveal the tumor.

DIAGNOSIS OF DISEASES OF THE RESPIRATORY ORGANS

Physical diagnosis is absolutely necessary in differentiating the various respiratory diseases from each other as well as from other diseases. You should review Lesson 23 before taking up the study of these diseases and should refer to it whenever necessary to a thorough understanding of the symptoms given in this lesson.

Cough is sudden explosive expiration caused by some irritation of the sensory nerve endings usually in the mucous membranes of the respiratory tract. It should be borne in mind, however, that this irritation may be located elsewhere (for example, ear, stomach). Pressure of tumors, etc., upon the respiratory organs or the nerves that supply them may also produce cough. When the cough is accompanied by the raising of sputum it is called a moist cough; when no fluid is raised, it is a dry cough.

Sputum may vary in its several characteristics according to the abnormal conditions present. The special types of sputum accompanying each disorder will be mentioned' when that disorder is discussed.

Hemoptysis must be differentiated from Hematemesis. When the blood is from the lungs, it appears suddenly and frequently follows coughing. It is preceded by a salty taste in the mouth. The blood is bright red in color and may be intimately mixed with mucus. It is alkaline in reaction. Hemoptysis may be caused by injury or disease of the lung or pleura, rupture of an aneurism or it may be due to vicarious menstruation.

Dyspnea is a common symptom in lung disorders. This symptom is discussed in Lesson 23 A's section on the "Physical Signs" of the lungs.

Some disorders of the lungs as well as those of the other thoracic organs may produce symptoms from the effect of pressure upon certain structures. When the term "Pressure Symptoms" is used in describing diseases of the chest it will be understood that any or all of the following symptoms may be present: cough, dyspnea, dysphagia, aphonia, displaced apex beat, diminished breath sounds, diminished vocal fremitus.

When the patient complains of any of the following symptoms you should suspect some disease of the respiratory organs and a thorough examination of them should be made: cough, expectoration, hemoptysis, dyspnea, chest pain, cyanosis, loss of weight and strength, night sweats and fever. It should be remembered that many of the changes in the breath sounds and percussion sounds are purely functional and may be made to disappear by concussion of the third and fourth dorsal or the seventh cervical vertebrae, or by rubbing the chest with a towel.

As "Chronic Pulmonary Tuberculosis" in its various stages presents most of the symptoms that are present in other diseases of the lungs you should first study this disorder until you thoroughly understand it and then compare the other lung diseases with tuberculosis and note the difference between them. It should be noted that the symptoms of tuberculosis vary with the stage of the disease. The symptoms of the advanced stage are seldom found as the patient usually dies before they appear. A positive diagnosis of tuberculosis of the lungs should never be made unless the constitutional symptoms are present or the tubercular bacillus is found on the sputum.

Passive Pulmonary Congestion resembles tuberculosis in the first stage, but does not have the constitutional symptoms and it is always accompanied by symptoms of heart weakness. Pulmonary Abscess has the chest symptoms of the second stage of tuberculosis plus the foul sputum and the general symptoms of infection. Gangrene in the beginning may also resemble moderately advanced tuberculosis. The diagnosis of Pulmonary Syphilis will depend upon the presence of the general symptoms of Syphilis. Pulmonary Fibrosis can be differentiated from tuberculosis by the greater retraction of the chest walls, the relative mildness of the chest symptoms and the absence of the constitutional symptoms of tuberculosis.

Tumors of the lungs are almost always malignant, and are accompanied by the constitutional symptoms of malignancy. Unless tumors produce pressure upon the vessels, nerves or other structures in the chest the local symptoms will resemble those

419

of the second stage of tuberculosis except that the sputum is different. Bronchiectasis can be differentiated from tuberculosis by the sputum and the fact that the affected area shows dullness on percussion before the spasm of coughing and hyper-resonance after it.

Emphysema can be diagnosed from other lung diseases by the characteristic shape and movement of the chest. When emphysema is accompanied by periodical attacks of severe, expiratory dyspnea the condition is called Bronchial Asthma. In this condition the patient inhales freely, but has great difficulty in exhaling—all other forms of Asthma have both inspiratory and expiratory dyspnea. Chronic Pleurisy can be differentiated from Tuberculosis by the greater dullness (flatness) over the affected area and the absence of breath sounds and of tactile fremitus. Empyema has more intense constitutional symptoms than pleurisy.

TREATMENT OF DISEASES OF RESPIRATORY ORGANS

The Acute Diseases of the Respiratory Organs can be treated according to the principles given in Lesson 24 ("Acute Constitutional Disorders"), plus prolonged hot applications over the chest or prolonged cool applications over the upper dorsal spine to decrease the pulmonary congestion.

The Chronic Diseases of the Lungs, Bronchi and Pleurae may be treated according to the general principles given in Lesson 24, together with whatever special treatment may be necessary. Breathing exercises, movements to increase the size and flexibility of the chest and mobility of the dorsal vertebrae may be used effectively in these diseases.

Lesson 32: Respiratory Disorders

In Bronchitis, Bronchiectasis, Pneumonia, Pulmonary Edema or Congestion, the object of treatment should be to decrease the amount of blood in the lungs and to overcome the interference with the circulation through them. Prolonged cold applications to the upper dorsal spine, use of the lamp or prolonged moderate heat to the front and sides of the chest (avoid spine) and concussion of the seventh cervical vertebrae are all effective for this purpose.

If the patient has Hemoptysis he should be put at absolute rest in bed and allowed no food. In addition to the prolonged cold applications to the upper dorsal spine you may use prolonged moderate heat to the lumbar spine and deep, prolonged pressure over the eighth to the twelfth dorsal vertebrae, prolonged hot sitz bath and any measure that will lower the blood pressure.

Success in the treatment of Bronchial Asthma depends altogether upon finding and removing the cause of the attacks. You should thoroughly relax the neck and upper dorsal region of the spine and chest. Any neck, spinal, or rib lesions should receive attention. The diet should be restricted and constipation should be overcome. The patient should have plenty of fresh air and sunshine and should be given breathing exercises. Stimulation of the third and fourth dorsal and the fourth and fifth cervical vertebrae will aid in preventing attacks.

Pulmonary Fibrosis, Syphilis and Gangrene can be treated in the same way as Bronchitis (see above). Pulmonary and Mediastinal Tumors are usually malignant and little can be done for them except to relieve the symptoms. In Pulmonary Abscess and Empyema, the "Septic Intoxication" should be treated. An operation may be necessary, but should not be used until other measures have been given a thorough trial.

Chronic Pulmonary Tuberculosis is really a constitutional disease and should be treated as such (see section on "Chronic Constitutional Diseases"). In addition to the general plan of treatment an attempt should be made to increase the size and flexibility of the thorax. Spinal and rib lesions are usually present and they should be adjusted. Considerable success has been obtained in the treatment of this disorder by the use of hyperemia. Concussion of the tenth dorsal vertebrae and prolonged hot applications to the upper dorsal spine will increase the amount of blood in the lungs. The ultra violet light on the chest and back and the inhalation of ozone are of considerable value.

PROGNOSIS OF RESPIRATORY DISORDERS
As with diseases of other systems, the prognosis depends very largely upon your ability to find and remove the cause of the trouble or to correct the primary pathology before there has been too much destruction of the lung tissue.

The prognosis is good in acute disorders (except Tuberculosis) and in Chronic Bronchitis, Bronchial Asthma and Chronic Pleurisy. The prognosis is bad in Acute Pulmonary Tuberculosis, Pulmonary Gangrene, Pulmonary Tumor and Advanced Tuberculosis. In the remaining respiratory disorders the prognosis should be guarded.

QUESTIONS—LESSON 32

1. Give symptoms of Chronic Bronchitis.

2. What is Bronchial Asthma?

3. Give symptoms of Lobar Pneumonia.

4. Give symptoms of Chronic Pleurisy.

5. Give symptoms of the advanced stage of Chronic Pulmonary Tuberculosis.

6. How would you diagnose Bronchiectasis from Pulmonary Tumor?

7. How would you diagnose Pulmonary Fibrosis from Chronic Pleurisy?

8. Give treatment of Chronic Pulmonary Tuberculosis.

9. Give treatment of Chronic Bronchitis

10. Give treatment of Bronchial Asthma.

EXTENSION COURSE
IN CHIROPRACTIC
AMERICAN UNIVERSITY
CHICAGO, Ill., U.S.A.

LESSON 33

DISEASES OF THE BONES, JOINTS, MUSCLES AND SKIN

Fracture is a sudden breaking of a bone due to direct or indirect violence. There will be a history of an accident and inspection will show some deformity of the part. Usually one end of the bone may be moved independently of the other end, allowing an unusual amount of mobility of the free end. The function of the injured part will be interfered with; there is usually pain and symptoms of inflammation. If the two ends of the bone are in contact, movement may produce a grating sound. Many times an X-ray picture is necessary for a positive diagnosis.

Acute Osteomyelitis is an acute suppurative inflammation of the bone marrow. The onset is sudden, a chill, high temperature and severe pain in the affected part. The part becomes swollen, infiltrated and congested. The pulse is rapid and small and delirium soon comes on. When pus forms, the skin over the abscess pits on pressure (edema). If proper treatment is not begun immediately the disease is usually rapidly fatal.

424

Osteo-Periostitis is an inflammation of the bone and the periosteum. There is a deep-seated, aching pain (and tenderness) which is worse in bed. The bone is enlarged and the surface may be roughened. An X-ray picture shows an increase in the amount of bone tissue.

Tubercular Osteo-Periostitis is characterized by the formation of tubercles which break down and destroy the bone tissue. In addition to the constitutional symptoms of Tuberculosis, there is a dull pain, worse at night, and muscular contraction and atrophy. Palpation of the bone will reveal a soft, fluctuating swelling. The abscess may break through the skin and form a sinus. An X-ray picture will show a destruction of, or thinning of, the bone tissue.

Rickets is a constitutional disease accompanied by changes in the bones (see Lesson 27).

Bone Sarcoma produces a circumscribed, painful enlargement with the constitutional symptoms of malignancy. An X-ray picture will show the nature of the growth.

Dislocation is the displacement of the articular ends of bones to such an extent that the articular surfaces are not in contact. The condition is usually produced by violence, but may be congenital or produced by extreme relaxation of the ligaments. The joint is deformed and there is limitation of its movement. Palpation will show that the articular head is absent from its normal position and in an abnormal position. An X-ray picture may be necessary for a positive diagnosis.

Laceration of Ligaments (Sprain) is a condition in which the ligaments have been injured by sudden force or prolonged strain. There is a history of accident and the symptoms of inflammation are present. The movement of the joint is decreased and painful.

Arthritis is inflammation of the synovial membrane and surrounding structures of a joint. In addition to the common symptoms of inflammation, the joint movement is limited and painful. Palpation may reveal the presence of fluid or an increase in the amount of connective or bone tissue. When the Arthritis is accompanied by the constitutional symptoms of "Lithemia" it is called "Articular Rheumatism." In Tubercular Arthritis the symptoms resemble those of tubercular Osteo-Periostitis except for the location of the symptoms.

Ankylosis is a condition in which there is a growth of bone tissue between the articular ends of two bones forming the joint. It is to be suspected when there is absolutely no movement in the joint, but a positive diagnosis can be made only from an X-ray picture. False Ankylosis is due to a shortening of the ligaments or an increased amount of connective tissue around and within the joint.

Myositis is an inflammation of a muscle, due usually to an accumulation of toxic material. In addition to the usual signs of inflammation, there is severe pain which is aggravated by contraction or stretching of the muscle. When Myositis is accompanied by symptoms of "Lithemia" it is called "Muscular Rheumatism."

Muscular Laceration is a condition in which the substance of the muscle has been injured by sudden violent contraction or by overstretching of the muscle. There is a history of trauma and the symptoms of "Myositis."

Paralysis is a condition in which the muscle has wholly or partially lost its contractile power. It is usually a symptom of a nervous disorder. The muscle may be lengthened, relaxed, soft, flabby and atrophied (Lower Neuronic, or Flaccid Paralysis), or it may be contracted, hardened and show little atrophy, (Upper Neuronic, or Spastic Paralysis).

Skin Diseases may be divided according to their etiology into three classes:

Irritative Skin Diseases are due to the action of some irritating gas, liquid, or other substance upon the skin, or to temperature extremes, pressure, friction, dry air, etc. These irritants may produce practically all of the lesions that effect the skin. The diagnosis is made by the finding of the source of irritation and the relief of the disorder when the irritant is removed.

Infective Skin Diseases are due to the presence of animal or vegetable parasites in the skin. These disorders are named, according to the parasite present: Scabies, Pediculosis, Sycosis, Ringworm, Impetigo, Boils, etc.

Symptomatic Skin Diseases are merely manifestations of an internal derangement. The great majority of the skin diseases fall in this class. The most common forms are known by the names of Eczema, Urticaria, Pemphigus, Acne, Psoriasis, Carbunculus, Forunculosis, Purpura, Herpes, etc.

427

TREATMENT OF DISEASES OF THE BONES, JOINTS, MUSCLES AND SKIN

The treatment of Fractures and Dislocations requires special training and an extended experience, so it is best for the drugless practitioner to turn these cases over to a competent surgeon when the diagnosis has been made. Unsatisfactory results sometimes follow even the best treatment. Dislocations and Fractures are the cause of more malpractice suits than all other disorders combined. The emergency treatment of these conditions will be given in the lesson on "First Aid."

In the remaining diseases of these structures the general principles of treatment outlined in previous lessons may be followed. The acute disorders of these structures will require rest, removal of the irritation, or the interference with the blood or nerve supply to the part, in addition to the use of prolonged moderate heat, gentle massage and Swedish Movements. In the chronic Bone, Joint and Muscular Diseases, you must find and remove whatever may be causing or aggravating the condition. The affected part may be treated by the use of prolonged moderate heat (Therapeutic Lamp, hot packs, dry hot air, etc.) massage and Swedish Movements, exercise, vibration and high frequency current may be used. The object of your treatment should be to stimulate the circulation through the part, to promote absorption of the abnormal tissue present and to restore as far as possible the function of the part.

In Laceration further injury to the joint may be prevented by the use of a bandage or other support until the acute symptoms have subsided. The bandage must be removed once or twice a day while the joint is treated with heat, kneading and passive

428

movements. As the condition improves, the bandage should be loosened so that it gives less support to the joint. If the joint is tightly bandaged and the bandage remains continuously on it for a week or more, there will probably be considerable limitation of movement of the joint.

Tubercular diseases of the bones or joints may be treated the same as the chronic inflammations of the same structure in addition to the constitutional treatment for Tuberculosis. The ultra-violet light is especially good in these conditions. Sometimes an operation is necessary to remove the dead bone that acts as an irritant and prevents healing.

Sarcoma is usually too far advanced when discovered for any treatment except operative removal to be of avail. The patient must have constitutional treatment. The ultra-violet light may be used.

Acute Osteo-Myelitis is a serious disease and requires immediate and active treatment. The general treatment outlined for acute constitutional diseases may be followed in addition to prolonged applications of heat to the affected part. If the symptoms continue to grow worse under the treatment, a surgeon should be called to open and drain the abscess.

The treatment of Paralysis must find and correct the cause of the loss of control over the muscle. In Upper Neuronic Paralysis the muscle may be stretched, kneaded or be treated with prolonged vibration, prolonged moderate heat, slow sinusoidal or high frequency current. In Lower Neuronic Paralysis the measures should be used to increase the tone of the muscle. Massage may be of some value in increasing the nutrition of the muscle, but vibratory stimulation, rapid or slow sinusoidal current, interrupted galvanic current, faradic current, short cold, or alternating hot and cold applications will be more effective.

In the Irritative Skin Diseases the irritant must be found and removed or the skin must be protected from its action. Bran baths or prolonged neutral baths, high frequency effleurage, and the therapeutic lamp are of some value in relieving the symptoms. If the skin disorder is due to the presence of a Parasite, efforts should be made to destroy the parasite. Sometimes chemical poisons are necessary, but the ultra-violet light, the high frequency sparking, sunlight, X-ray or the positive galvanic current with a copper electrode will usually kill them. No treatment of the Symptomatic Skin Diseases will be permanently effective unless directed to the constitutional condition that is producing the skin symptoms. Every effort should be made to increase the elimination, purify the blood and raise the patient's vitality in addition to the treatment advised for the irritative skin diseases. The therapeutic lamp, ultra-violet light and high frequency current may be used.

The Prognosis of the above disorders depends almost entirely upon your ability to find and remove their cause and to use the proper treatment before the disease has progressed beyond the possibility of cure. The prognosis of Tubercular Bone and Joint Diseases and Acute Osteo-Myelitis should be guarded; that of Sarcoma is bad.

QUESTIONS—LESSON 33

1. Give diagnostic signs of Fracture.

2. Give diagnostic symptoms of Acute Osteo-Myelitis.

3. Give diagnostic signs of Dislocation.

4. Give symptoms of Articular Rheumatism.

5. How would you diagnose an Irritative Skin Disease?

6. Give treatment of Laceration of Ligaments.

7. Give treatment of Tubercular Osteo-Periostitis.

8. Give treatment of Symptomatic Skin Diseases.

9. How would you treat Muscular Paralysis?

10. What is the prognosis of Bone Sarcoma?

CHIROPRACTIC

The Science of Spinal Adjustment

———

A SERIES OF LESSONS CORRELATING AND
SYSTEMATIZING THE KNOWLEDGE NECESSARY
TO PRACTICE CHIROPRACTIC

Nature's Greatest Ally

IN RESTORING DISEASED CONDITIONS OF THE
BODY TO PERFECT HEALTH, WITHOUT THE AID
OF DRUGS OR SURGERY

———

BOOK 9

HEART DISEASES

URINARY DISEASES

FEMALE PELVIC DISEASES

NERVOUS DISEASES

MISCELLANEOUS DISEASES

Lessons 34, 35, 36, 37 and 38

———

ORIGINALLY PUBLISHED BY
AMERICAN UNIVERSITY
CHICAGO, ILLINOIS, U.S.A.

Organic MD Media
PO Box 50399
Palo Alto, CA 94303

First Published 1913, 1916
American University
Chicago, Ill, USA

Second Edition 2017
Published by OrganicMD Media
eBook Edition copyright © Organic MD Media 2017

Printed in the United States of America

Organic MD Media   2012 -

Chiropractic - The Science of Spinal Adjustment - Book 9

ISBN: 978-1-946036-08-7

Disclaimer

EXTENSION COURSE
IN CHIROPRACTIC
AMERICAN UNIVERSITY
CHICAGO, Ill., U.S.A.

——————

LESSON 34

——————

SYMPTOMS OF HEART DISEASES

Acute Pericarditis is an acute inflammation of the serous membrane surrounding the heart. In the fibrinous or dry type the symptoms are slight and may be absent. There is usually a slight pain over the heart and auscultation will reveal a to-and-fro friction sound caused by the rubbing together of the two layers of the pericardium. When effusion takes place there is dyspnea, precordial distress, and rapid pulse. Percussion shows that the cardiac dullness is increased; the area of dullness is triangular with the base below. The heart sounds are weak and muffled. Fever is present.

Chronic Pericarditis may be fibrinous with adhesion of the two layers of the pericardium or the pericardial sac may be filled with fluid. The symptoms are similar to those of acute pericarditis.

Acute Myocarditis is characterized by degeneration of the muscular tissue of the heart. It occurs usually in the acute

435

constitutional diseases. There is heart pain, dyspnea, fever, and marked prostration. The heart action is irregular and feeble, the heart sounds are weak, and there may be a shortened silent period or a "Gallop Rhythm."

Chronic Myocarditis is characterized by an infiltration of connective tissue or fatty degeneration of the muscular substance of the heart. It is caused usually by prolonged toxemia. There is palpitation, dyspnea, heart pain and a rapid, weak, irregular pulse. The heart sounds are weak and irregular and the symptoms of Dilatation or Venous Stasis may be present.

Angina Pectoris is a chronic condition characterized by acute attacks brought about by a spasmodic contraction of the heart muscle. The attack is sudden with intense pain over the heart. The pain radiates down the left arm. The patient remains absolutely motionless. The chest is constricted and there is a feeling of suffocation and impending death. The attack may last a few seconds or minutes and end in syncope. Sudden death may occur during or following an attack.

Acute Endocarditis is an acute inflammation of the endothelial lining of the heart. It usually accompanies or follows one of the acute constitutional diseases. The symptoms may be slight or absent, but usually consist of precordial distress, dyspnea, rapid, weak, irregular pulse, and valvular murmurs. Acute dilatation may occur.

Chronic Endocarditis may follow Acute Endocarditis or prolonged toxemia. The endocardium covering the valves is principally affected resulting in a distortion or destruction of the valves. The heart hypertrophies and there are cardiac murmurs and changes in the intensity of the heart sounds. "Dilatation" or "Venous Stasis" may be present. When some one or more of the heart valves are primarily affected, the condition is named according to the valve affected and the nature of the lesion.

Cardiac Dilatation is a condition in which the heart is enlarged through a weakening and relaxation of its muscular walls. Physical examination will show an enlarged cardiac dullness with displaced apex beat. The impulse at the apex is weak, irregular and diffuse. The heart sounds (and pulse) are weak and irregular in time and force. The symptoms of "Broken Compensation" and "Venous Stasis" are always present.

Cardiac Neuroses. In many of the so-called heart diseases there is no organic change in the heart itself. The disturbances of the rate, force, time or regularity of the heart beat are due to some interference with the nerve impulses to or from the heart. The cardiac neuroses can be positively diagnosed only by the absence of physical changes in the heart itself and by the fact that the symptoms can be relieved by spinal stimulation or inhibition.

Venous Stasis occurs when there is a backing up of the venous blood because of a decrease in the pressure in the arteries or to some interference with the flow of the blood to or through the heart. The symptoms vary according to the region of the body most affected. Any or all of the following symptoms may be present: Vertigo, Syncope, Insomnia, Pulsating jugular veins, Cough, Dyspnea, Hemoptysis, Rales, Cyanosis, Large, pulsating, tender liver, Dyspepsia, Edema, Albuminuria.

DIAGNOSIS OF DISEASES OF THE HEART

The differential diagnosis of the various diseases of the heart depends very much upon the physical signs present in these disorders (See Lesson 23A). From the standpoint of treatment and prognosis it is far more important to determine the functional capacity of the heart than the site and nature of the physical changes that may be present in the heart (see "Condition of Heart" in Lesson 23 A). Attention is called again to the importance of the location, nature and regularity of the apex beat in diagnosis of cardiac diseases. If the apex beat is in its normal position and regular in time and force, the heart may, for all practical purposes, be considered normal.

If you desire for your own satisfaction to know just what structural changes have taken place in the heart or which valve is affected, you may auscultate the sounds produced by the valves. The heart murmurs are not difficult to detect when they are present, but it is extremely difficult to determine absolutely whether the murmur is functional or organic and which valve is producing the murmur. So far as prognosis and treatment are concerned the information obtained from auscultation of the murmurs is of little practical value. The most valuable information can be obtained by determining the functional condition of the heart ("Condition of the Heart," Lesson 23 A).

"Endocarditis," with the accompanying valvular lesions, is the most common heart disorder and, as it produces symptoms that are also present in the other heart diseases, it should be studied and understood first. Afterward you may study the other heart diseases comparing them with endocarditis and noting the difference between them.

Lesson 34: Heart Diseases

Valvular lesions can be positively diagnosed only by auscultation of the heart sounds. The different lesions of each valve are distinguished from each other and from lesions of the other valves by the time of the murmur (systolic or diastolic) and by its location. The direction of the enlargement and the changes in the intensity of the sounds also vary with the character and location of the valves affected.

The pulse is characteristic in the aortic lesions. Valvular lesions very rarely produce symptoms of other parts unless the heart is incapable of maintaining circulation up to the requirements of the body. When the circulation begins to fail the signs of venous stasis appear. These are given above. Lesson 23A should be carefully studied with this lesson. It should be borne in mind that the presence of heart murmurs alone does not prove that the valves are diseased as the great majority of murmurs are purely functional. A lesion of any valve of the heart will produce changes in the sound of some other valve as well as in the valve affected and is always accompanied by "Hypertrophy" of the heart.

When the strength of the heart muscle does not increase proportionately with the work the heart has to do "Dilatation" and "Broken Compensation" will be present. It should be noted that venous stasis is always present in broken compensation and broken compensation is always present in dilatation. If the heart is capable of doing the work required of it there will be no symptoms of Venous Stasis, Broken Compensation or Dilatation.

Angina Pectoris can be distinguished from other diseases with precordial pain by the general appearance, attitude and sensations of the patient during an attack. The function of the heart is very often disturbed through influences acting upon the cardiac nerves or their centers in the brain and cord producing the "Cardiac Neuroses." These can be positively diagnosed only by the absence of the organic changes in the heart itself and by the relief from the symptoms that follows stimulation or inhibition of the centers that control the heart

TREATMENT OF HEART DISEASES

Acute Pericarditis, Acute Myocarditis and Acute Endocarditis can be treated according to the general principles of treatment for Acute Constitutional Disorders (Lessons 24 and 26). The patient should be at absolute rest in bed until all danger of cardiac failure has passed. After the most marked symptoms have subsided, it will be-well to use massage and Swedish Movements (cautiously) for some time before the patient is allowed to get out of bed. Prolonged hot applications over the heart will relieve the pain and reduce the congestion of the heart, but may tend to increase the rate and decrease the strength of the heartbeat. If the bad effect on the heart action cannot be overcome by concussion of the seventh cervical vertebrae, prolonged moderate pressure or prolonged moderately cold applications over the second to fourth dorsal vertebrae, the hot applications must not be used. Prolonged cool packs (not below 60) will relieve the cardiac congestion as well as slow and strengthen the heartbeat. They may relieve the pain as well as the hot applications. It should be remembered that cold is a vital depressant and it should not be used except when necessary. Hot sponge baths (sponging one part of the body at a time) may be used if other forms of hot baths have a bad effect upon the heart action.

Spinal lesions are invariably present and they should be corrected, but you should be very careful about giving a thrust or using any rough manipulation around the upper dorsal vertebrae when there is danger of sudden heart failure. You should thoroughly but carefully relax the neck and upper dorsal spine and use light thrusts until you learn just what effect your treatment has upon the heart.

Chronic Pericarditis, Chronic Myocarditis and Chronic Endocarditis can be treated alike. The neck, spine and ribs should be thoroughly examined and any lesions present should be corrected. An effort should be made to decrease the demands upon the heart— severe cases will require rest in bed. If the blood pressure is high it should be lowered. The diet must be restricted to the minimum amount needed by the body; constipation must be overcome. The habits should be regulated; no alcohol or tobacco should be used. Short cold sponge baths followed by friction should be used daily. Prolonged hot baths usually tend to weaken the heart action and should be avoided.

Properly graduated exercises are the most effective of all methods of treatment and should be used in every case as soon as the patient's condition will permit. He should first be given mild exercises for small muscle groups. As the heart gains in strength larger muscles may be exercised and more strenuous movements may be attempted. It is usually best for the patient to exercise for short periods several times a day. In every case he must stop his exercise just as soon as the heart begins to beat irregularly, cyanosis appears, breathing becomes difficult or there is a feeling of faintness. He should avoid any exercises or work that puts a sudden strain upon the heart. During the exercises the breathing must be full, deep and unrestricted. The breath should never be held under any circumstances. In addition to the specific treatment outlined above, every effort should be made to increase the patient's vitality and to eliminate the toxic material that is producing the cardiac disorder.

Cardiac Dilation, Broken Compensation and Venous Stasis should be treated by putting the patient at rest in bed until compensation is established. An effort should be made to normalize the activity of the nerves supplying the heart and to decrease the amount of work it has to do by lessening the resistance to the flow of the blood through the peripheral vessels. If there is congestion in any part of the body it should be overcome. Prolonged neutral or prolonged cool baths and deep breathing may be used.

When compensation is established you may use Massage, followed by Swedish Movements, and then graduated exercises. The massage should be very carefully given to avoid exciting the heart and increasing its work. Only the extremities should be treated during the first treatment. If no bad effect is produced on the heart, the abdomen may be included in the second treatment. Each succeeding treatment may include more of the body. You should be very careful in massaging the spine, especially the upper dorsal region. As the patient improves you may add Swedish Movements to the massage treatment. Within a short time the patient should be able to sit up for a short period each day. This period should be increased daily and eventually he may be allowed to stand and to walk about. As the heart muscle increases in strength he may be allowed to walk greater distances each day and the graduated exercises may be taken.

The treatment of Valvular Lesions will depend upon whether compensation is good or broken. If the compensation is broken, the treatment outlined above for broken compensation should be used. If the compensation is good, you may follow the plan of treatment suggested for Myocarditis, paying special attention to measures that will increase the vital resistance of the patient and the strength of the heart muscle. The diet should be restricted and the patient should avoid dissipations and sudden severe strains.

In Angina Pectoris the cause of the nerve irritation should be found and removed. Stimulation of the third and fourth dorsal will usually stop an attack and daily use of this measure may prevent attacks. Prolonged hot applications to upper dorsal spine are also of value. The patient should avoid excitement, fatigue and emotional disturbances. The treatment of Cardiac Neuroses is to find and remove the cause of the abnormal nerve activity. Spinal treatment and Hydrotherapy may be used to control the activity of the heart. Deep breathing is also very good.

PROGNOSIS OF HEART DISEASES

The prognosis of the acute cardiac disorders is good if proper treatment is instituted in time. In Angina Pectoris the prognosis is bad, although the patient's life may be prolonged for many years. In the remaining cardiac diseases the prognosis is doubtful as to complete cure, but they need not necessarily shorten the patient's life if he is willing to co-operate with you and to do the things necessary to keep the heart muscles in good shape and avoid doing those things that will injure the heart.

If the heart is compensated and is able to do all the work demanded of it by the patient's occupation, you may assure him that it will not necessarily shorten his life if proper treatment is used and he takes the proper amount and kind of exercise.

QUESTIONS—LESSON 34

1. Give symptoms of Acute Pericarditis.

2. Give symptoms of Chronic Myocarditis.

3. What are the diagnostic signs of Chronic Endocarditis?

4. Give the symptoms of Venous Stasis.

5. What is Cardiac Neurosis?

6. Give treatment of Acute Myocarditis.

7. Give treatment for Angina Pectoris.

8. Why should exercise be used cautiously in Heart Disease?

9. What is the Prognosis of Chronic Endocarditis?

EXTENSION COURSE
IN CHIROPRACTIC
AMERICAN UNIVERSITY
CHICAGO, Ill., U.S.A.

LESSON 35

SYMPTOMS OF URINARY DISORDERS

Acute Parenchymatous Nephritis is an acute inflammation of the epithelium of the tubules of the kidneys. It usually arises as a complication of some acute constitutional disorder, but may be due to cold and exposure or the persistent use of irritating substances. In addition to fever, there is nausea, vomiting and dull pain over the kidneys. There is a frequent passage of scanty, dark colored, albuminous urine containing casts and blood. Dropsy soon appears, beginning first in the face. Anemia and weakness are pronounced.

Chronic Parenchymatous Nephritis is a chronic inflammation of the tubules of the kidneys, due usually to a prolonged toxemia. The urine is scanty, turbid and of high specific gravity. Much albumin and many casts are present. The patient has dyspepsia, diarrhea and difficulty in breathing. He is anemic and debilitated. Dropsy, especially of the lower eyelids and face, is present. When the disease progresses so far that the kidneys are unable to eliminate the toxins they should, "Uremia" appears.

445

Chronic Interstitial Nephritis is characterized by an increase in the amount of connective tissue in the kidneys with a decrease in the size of the kidney. It may be due to chronic heart disease, high blood pressure or toxemia. The urine is increased in amount and is clear and of low specific gravity. Albumin or casts may or may not be present. The patient may complain of dyspepsia, vertigo, dyspnea and headache. The skin is dry. High blood pressure and cardiac hypertrophy are usually present.

Suppurative Nephritis is characterized by inflammation and destruction of the kidney substance with the formation of pus. The kidney is enlarged and tender. There is pain in the lumbar region and frequent passage of acid urine containing blood and pus. The symptoms of septic intoxication are present.

Uremia may accompany any of the above kidney diseases when the function of the kidneys is seriously impaired. It may be of gradual onset and is then called Chronic Uremia. (See Lesson 27.) Acute Uremia begins suddenly, usually with convulsions, followed by coma. There may be nausea, vertigo, vomiting and fever. The urine is scanty with low specific gravity and diminished amount of urea. The respirations and pulse are rapid. The breath has a urinous odor.

Nephrolithiasis is a condition in which stones are formed in the kidneys. The stones may be present for a long time without producing any symptoms, but usually there is lumbar pain, made worse by exercise, blood and pus in the urine and the kidney is tender. An X-ray picture will show the stones. If the stone is small it may pass down the ureter and cause "Renal Colic."

Renal Colic is due to a spasmodic contraction of the ureter caused by the irritation of a small stone attempting to pass through it. The attack is sudden with an agonizing pain in the back which radiates along the ureter to the pubic region. Micturition is frequent and painful. The face is pale, the skin is cloudy and clammy. There is nausea, vomiting and faintness. The attack may terminate suddenly when the stone escapes into the bladder. If the stone does not pass through the ureter, the attack may recur.

Renal Cancer produces a continuous lumbar pain, renal tenderness, recurrent hematuria, anemia, emaciation and cachexia. Palpation will reveal an enlarged malformed kidney. An X-ray picture may be necessary to confirm the diagnosis.

Acute Cystitis is an acute inflammation of the mucus membrane of the bladder. The onset is abrupt with chills and fever. Micturition is frequent but the urine is voided drop by drop and its passage is followed by vesical tenesmus. There is dull pain over the bladder and a burning sensation along the urethra. The urine is cloudy, alkaline reaction and is filled with epithelial cells, pus and blood.

Chronic Cystitis is a chronic inflammation, ulceration, and hypertrophy of the mucus membrane of the bladder. The muscular wall may be hypertrophied or degenerated. The symptoms are vesical pain, frequent passage of foul, turbid, alkaline urine containing mucus, blood and pus.

DIAGNOSIS OF URINARY DISORDERS

The differential diagnosis of these conditions usually depends very largely upon the changes produced in the urine which should be examined whenever kidney or bladder diseases are suspected. The urinary changes and the method of examination are given in Lesson 23 B.

It should be remembered that changes in the urine do not always indicate kidney or bladder diseases, as diseases of other organs or constitutional diseases may produce pathological urine or the abnormal elements in the urine may be due to the patient's diet. Neither are all kidney diseases always accompanied by abnormal urine (for example, Chronic Interstitial Nephritis may show no urinary changes at certain time). The other local and general symptoms must always be considered with the urinary findings.

Chronic Parenchymatous Nephritis should be studied first and then the other kidney diseases compared with it. As dyspepsia is a common symptom in any form of Nephritis, the urine should be examined in all cases of chronic indigestion. It will be seen when comparing the interstitial form of nephritis with the parenchymatous form, that in the latter the principal symptoms relate to the kidney (abnormal urine and dropsy), and in the former, the symptoms are manifested principally in the circulatory organs (heart and blood pressure).

Suppurative Nephritis includes the conditions usually called Pyelitis, Pyelonephritis and Pyronephrosis. The urinary findings are those of parenchymatous nephritis plus the presence of pus in the urine. Nephrolithiasis has the symptoms of Suppurative Nephritis plus the X-ray findings, the aggravation of the lumbar pain by exercise, and the renal colic.

TREATMENT OF DISEASES OF THE URINARY ORGANS

Acute Parenchymatous Nephritis can be treated according to the same plan that is used for the acute constitutional disorders. An effort should be made to increase the activity of the skin so that some of the toxic material, normally eliminated through the kidneys, may be eliminated through the skin. Hot sponge baths, hot sheet packs, or a hot blanket pack may be used. If the patient can stand it, he may be put in a bath tub. The patient should eat no food, with the possible exception of fruit juices, until the condition is under control. He should be encouraged to drink an abundance of water. During convalescence they may take the "Milk Diet." The lower dorsal region of the spine should be thoroughly but carefully relaxed and any subluxation present should be adjusted. You should avoid any procedures that tend to dilate the vessels of this region of the spine, as it will increase the amount of blood in the kidneys and aggravate the condition.

Acute Cystitis may be treated practically the same as Acute Nephritis. Hot applications may be used over the bladder to relieve the pain and the spasmodic contraction of the sphincter. The treatment of Chronic Uremia has been given in Lesson 27. Acute Uremia will require more vigorous treatment. The patient should be immediately placed in a hot bath or a hot blanket pack, large hot enemas should be given, and prolonged application of heat over the lower dorsal region of the spine should be used to increase the activity of the kidneys.

Chronic Parenchymatous Nephritis, Chronic Interstitial Nephritis, Suppurative Nephritis and Renal Tuberculosis may all be treated according to the same plan. They are usually caused,

449

or at least aggravated, by the prolonged presence of toxic material in the blood (Toxemia). Your efforts should be directed towards eliminating this toxic material, preventing the intake or formation of more toxins and lessening the work required of the kidneys. The diet is very important. No irritating or stimulating food or drinks should be allowed, and it is usually best to reduce the amount of protein in the diet to the minimum. An excess of salt should be avoided. The waste products of meat are especially bad and the patient should avoid broths, beef tea and similar preparations.

Special attention should be paid to the lower dorsal region of the spine. In addition to the correction of any lesions that may be present, prolonged hot applications or concussion of the 10th dorsal vertebrae may be used in the interstitial form. In the Parenchymatous or Suppurative form the amount of blood in the kidneys should be decreased by concussion of the 12th dorsal, prolonged cool applications over the lower dorsal region and similar measures.

Nephrolithiasis may require a surgical operation if the stone is large and is producing much trouble. Correction of the diet may prevent an increase in size or the formation of new stones. Analysis of the urine may give a clue as to the composition of the stone. If this can be determined the patient should avoid the foods that contain an excess of those minerals. Every effort should be made to restore and maintain the normal blood and nerve supply to the kidneys.

In Renal Colic the patient should be put in a hot sitz bath or a hot pack used over the abdomen, lower dorsal and lumber regions of the spine. Adjustment of any subluxations present in the lower dorsal region and prolonged pressure over the contracted spinal muscles will relieve the pain and the spasmodic contraction of the ureter.

Renal Cancer will require constitutional treatment to overcome the toxemia and to restore the normal composition of the blood. When discovered, the disease has usually progressed too far for treatment to be of avail. The pain may be relieved by spinal treatment or by the use of the lamp or hot applications.

Chronic Cystitis may be treated practically the same as Chronic Parenchymatous Nephritis. If there is retention of urine in the bladder, a catheter must be used. Every precaution should be taken to prevent infection of the bladder by an unclean catheter. If there is some obstruction to the outflow of the urine it must be overcome. The lamp or hot applications may be used over the pubic and perineal regions, but should not be used over the lumbar region. Hot sitz baths (105 degrees) may be used, but they should not be prolonged beyond five minutes.

PROGNOSIS OF DISEASES OF THE URINARY ORGANS

The prognosis of these disorders depends, of course, very much upon whether or not their causes can be found and removed. If this can be done early enough in the disease, the prognosis will be good in all of the urinary disorders with the possible exception of Nephrolithiasis, Cancer and Movable Kidney.

The prognosis in Suppurative Nephritis, Renal Tuberculosis and Chronic Cystitis should be guarded. They are relatively more difficult to relieve than the other disorders of the same organs. If hypertrophy of the muscular wall of the bladder has occurred in Chronic Cystitis, the prognosis is bad as to complete cure. If there

451

is a stone of any size in the kidney, it is not probable that you will be able to get rid of it although the patient's symptoms may be-relieved.

The prognosis is bad in Cancer as the disease is usually beyond help when it is discovered. Acute Uremia is a dangerous condition and the patient may die in spite of all that can be done.

QUESTIONS—LESSON 35

1. Give symptoms of Acute Parenchymatous Nephritis.

2. Give symptoms of Chronic Interstitial Nephritis.

3. What symptoms would make you suspect Uremia?

4. What is Renal Colic?

5. Give symptoms of Chronic Cystitis.

6. How would you diagnose Cystitis from Nephritis?

7. Give treatment of Chronic Parenchymatous Nephritis.

8. Give treatment of Uremia.

9. What is the Prognosis of Renal Cancer

EXTENSION COURSE
IN CHIROPRACTIC
AMERICAN UNIVERSITY
CHICAGO, Ill., U.S.A.

LESSON 36

DISEASES OF THE FEMALE GENERATIVE ORGANS

Although a knowledge of the exact-pathology present in the pelvis will be of considerable aid in the treatment of these disorders, drugless treatment may be very successfully applied without knowing exactly which of the reproductive organs is affected or the exact condition of the affected organs. The same general principles underlie the treatment of practically all of the female pelvic diseases.

The symptoms of the more common diseases of these parts will be given as well as whatever special treatment may be needed for each one. If you are unable to diagnose the exact condition, you may apply the general plan of treatment given below with assurance that favorable results will be secured in a large percentage of the cases.

While any of the etiological factors given in Lesson 22 may produce diseases of the pelvic tissues, some of them are more prone to do so than others. The normal circulation through the pelvis is maintained by the respiratory movement of the lower abdominal wall. Anything that interferes with this respiratory movement may produce pelvic stasis or congestion which may be accompanied by any or all of the pelvic diseases.

Lesions of the lumbar spine, sacrum, innominates or coccyx are almost invariably present and they may interfere very much with the nerve or blood supply to the pelvis. Eyestrain, nervous irritability, general toxemia, general debility, malnutrition or anemia may produce pelvic symptoms. A great many of the so-called pelvic diseases are due entirely to constipation-and a loaded colon and cannot be relieved until the constipation has been overcome.

Dysmenorrhea. Normal menstruation may produce malaise and mild symptoms in the pelvis. When the pelvic symptoms are severe enough to amount to actual discomfort the condition is called Dysmenorrhea.

Dysmenorrhea is divided into four types, depending upon the principal pathology present. It is not always possible to distinguish between these four types, but an effort should be made to do so, as it will assist you in treatment.

Neuralgic Dysmenorrhea is produced by nerve irritation. There is an intermittent sharp pain in the lumbar region, groin and thighs most severe before and at the commencement of the menstrual flow. The breasts are painful.

Congestive Dysmenorrhea is caused by the tension produced in the uterus, by the accumulation of blood in that organ. There is a continuous dull pain in the sacral region and pelvis before and throughout the period. Some relief is experienced when the flow is free.

Obstructive Dysmenorrhea is caused by anything that interferes with the discharge of blood from the uterus (Malposition, Malformations, Tumors, etc.). There are intermittent, cramp-like pains just above the pubic symphysis. They are present before and during the flow.

Membranous Dysmenorrhea is caused by the discharge of the greater portion of the lining of the uterus at one time. There is a severe, cramp-like pelvic pain beginning before and ceasing with the expulsion of the membrane.

Pelvic Congestion. Practically all pelvic diseases are caused, aggravated or accompanied by an increased amount of blood in the pelvis, or some interference with its circulation through the pelvic vessels. This circulatory disturbance may produce any of the diseases of the individual pelvic organs, or any of the' symptoms that are usually ascribed to the diseases of these organs. You are usually safe in assuming that some congestion is present whenever the patient complains of symptoms referable to the pelvis.

Uterine Displacements. The uterus has no constant position in the pelvis. Its location depends upon whether the bladder or the rectum, or both, are full or empty, and upon the position of the patient at the time of examination. The uterus may be displaced beyond its normal range of movement, but generally speaking, this displacement will produce no trouble unless the displacement is marked, the uterus is fixed in its abnormal position by pelvic adhesions, or remains for long periods in the same position because of the patient's posture (prolonged standing, etc.).

While the uterine ligaments and the muscles of the pelvic floor aid in supporting the uterus, the respiratory movement of the lower abdomen is the most important factor in maintaining the normal position of the pelvic organs. Any interference with the normal respiratory movement of the lower abdomen will interfere with the circulation of blood through the pelvis and allow the weight of the abdominal contents to fall upon the uterus and its appendages. If this persists over a prolonged period there will be weakening and relaxation of the ligaments allowing the uterus to become displaced enough to produce other pelvic disorders.

Uterine displacements are classified according to the direction of the displacement into retro-version, retro-flexion, lateral-flexion, prolapse, etc. It may sometimes aid in treatment to know the exact position of the uterus, but the treatment outlined below may be successfully applied without knowledge of the exact position of the uterus.

Vulvo-vaginitis is a term applied to inflammation of the mucous membranes lining the vulva and vagina. It is usually due to irritation, infection or uncleanliness. The symptoms are pain, swelling, itching, leucorrhea and dyspareunia. The mucosa is red, granular and hardened.

Endometritis is an inflammation of the membrane lining the uterus. It is due usually to an extension of inflammation from the vagina. The symptoms are leucorrhea and pelvic pain and the symptoms of "Congestive Dysmenorrhea." The cervix is eroded and there is a cervical discharge. The uterus is enlarged.

Metritis is an inflammation of the uterus accompanied by an increase in the amount of muscular or connective tissue. It may be the result of an extension of the inflammation from the vagina, pelvic stasis, child birth, or abortion. The symptoms are dull pelvic pain, menorrhagia, metorrhagia, leucorrhea and the symptoms of "Congestive Dysmenorrhea." The uterus is large and tender and may be hard or boggy. Micturition and defecation are usually painful.

Salpingitis is an inflammation of the mucous lining of the Fallopian tube. There is pain in the region of the tube especially after exercise, menorrhagia, leucorrhea and symptoms of "Congestive Dysmenorrhea." Palpation may reveal an enlarged, hardened tube.

Pyosalpinx is suppurative inflammation of the tube due usually to extension of inflammation from below. It is not, as commonly thought, always due to gonorrhea. There is a constant tubal pain, leucorrhea (pus), symptoms of "Septic Intoxication" and a history of pelvic infection. An enlarged, smooth, tender, fluctuating mass may be found extending laterally from the uterine fundus.

Ovaritis (Inflammation of the Ovary) is quite frequently diagnosed, but is a very rare disorder. The symptoms are constant pain in the groin, aggravated by standing, "Congestive" or "Neuralgic Dysmenorrhea" and reflex nervous disturbances. Palpation will show the ovaries enlarged and tender.

Ovarian Abscess has the symptoms of "Ovaritis," but more severe, in addition to those of "Septic Intoxication." There may be a history of pelvic infection.

Lesson 36: Diseases of the Female Generative Organs

Pelvic Cellulitis is characterized by a simple or a suppurative inflammation of the connective tissue of the pelvis producing abscess, formation or adhesions of the pelvic structures. There is a constant severe pelvic pain aggravated by micturition, defecation and movement. The uterus and appendages are fixed in their positions which may be normal or abnormal. There is an inflammatory mass behind or at either side of the uterus.

Pelvic Peritonitis is a simple, or suppurative inflammation of that portion of the peritoneum that covers the pelvic organs. The symptoms are those of severe "Cellulitis" plus abdominal distension, rigidity, thighs flexed on abdomen, anxious expression and a rapid, weak, small irregular pulse.

Uterine Fibroma or Myoma. Tumors of fibrous or muscle tissue may be formed in or upon the uterine wall. It is possible for them to be present for a long time without producing symptoms of any kind. The most common symptoms are pelvic pain, uterine hemorrhage, serous, purulent or bloody discharge and symptoms due to pressure upon other pelvic structures. The uterus has an irregular enlargement with a hard rounded mass in or upon the body. An X-ray picture will show the tumor.

Uterine Carcinoma or Sarcoma. These malignant tumors usually appear after forty. The presence of a persistent uterine hemorrhage should make you very suspicious of their presence. Eventually they produce severe, constant pain that is not usually relieved by the usual measures. There is a very foul discharge, symptoms due to pressure and the constitutional symptoms of "Cachexia." It usually affects the cervix of the uterus, appearing as a rapidly growing, nodular, friable mass which bleeds easily. An X-ray picture will show the tumor. A microscopic examination of a portion of the tumor is usually necessary to establish a diagnosis of Malignancy, but this procedure is not entirely free from danger.

Ovarian Cyst may produce no symptoms until it becomes very large. The symptoms are those due to pressure upon the other pelvic structures. It may reach an enormous size, producing a marked distension of the abdomen. Palpation will reveal a tense, smooth, fluctuating tumor free from the uterus.

Pregnancy may be confused with any of the pelvic diseases. The symptoms are amenorrhea, enlargement of the breasts, morning nausea, bladder irritability and abdominal enlargement. Pelvic examination will show the uterus to be enlarged and soft, the cervix softened and a bluish discoloration of the vagina. A positive diagnosis can be made only after the six months when there will be fetal movement, fetal heart sounds, quickening, uterine contraction and ballottement. An X-ray examination will show the fetal skeleton.

Extra Uterine Pregnancy has the early symptoms of normal "Pregnancy," but with a return of menstruation and cramp-like pains. There is a hard, tender mass beside or behind the uterus. It always terminates by rupture with severe pain, shock and collapse.

Puerperal Sepsis is a suppurative inflammation of the uterus and other pelvic structures following childbirth. It is usually due to lack of cleanliness on the part of the attendant, or retention of some of the fetal membranes. The local symptoms vary with the extent of the infection. There is usually severe pelvic pain and a foul discharge, in addition to the symptoms that accompany the diseases of the individual organs. The constitutional symptoms are chill, fever, rapid pulse, delirium and prostration. Constipation is usually present and defecation is difficult and painful.

Urethritis is an inflammation of the urethra. There is frequent, painful micturition and urethral discharge. The urethra is tender 'and the external meatus is reddened.

Gonorrhea is a suppurative inflammation of any part or all of the genito-urinary tract. The symptoms will vary with the organ or tissue affected. A positive diagnosis can be made only by finding the gonococcus in the urine or in the urethral, vaginal or cervical discharge.

Syphilis. The primary sore or chancre usually appears on some portion of the external genitalia. It is a painless, shallow ulcer with a hard base. It may appear first as a small pimple or as a slight erosion of the skin. The inguinal glands are enlarged and hard.

Chanchroid is a painful, deep, punched-out, ragged-edged ulcer with an abundant discharge. There is usually more than one. The inguinal glands are enlarged, painful and usually break down and ulcerate.

TREATMENT OF PELVIC DISORDERS

These diseases are practically always accompanied by spinal lesions, which should be found and corrected. In addition to this, you must locate and remove any etiological factor that may be operating outside or within the body (see above and also Lesson 22).

One of the most important of the etiological factors is the restriction of the lower abdominal respiratory movement (see

461

above). This can be corrected by teaching the patient the normal movement of the abdomen during respiration. Movements of the thighs and of the chest with the patient lying on her back on a slanting board (head low) also aid in lifting the pelvic organs and in accelerating pelvic circulation. The patient should be instructed to avoid prolonged standing and positions that flex the lumbar spine or interfere with respiration. Rest in bed may be necessary in extreme cases.

Pelvic Congestion will require lower abdominal breathing, special pelvic exercises (see above), prolonged hot sitz baths, prolonged cold sitz baths, alternate hot and cold sitz baths, prolonged applications of cold to the lumbar and sacral spine, cold vaginal douches or the use of slow sinusoidal current. Spinal lesions, eyestrain, constipation and bad sexual habits should be corrected.

Uterine Displacements will require treatment similar to that outlined for congestion, with the exception of the hot sitz bath and hot applications, which should not be used for any length of time. Stimulation of the 1st to the 3rd lumbar vertebrae or use of the slow sinusoidal current with a uterine-elevator electrode are of considerable value. If the pelvic floor is torn, it may be necessary to repair it. The knee-chest position for five to ten minutes several times a day will aid materially in replacement. Not much results from treatment can be expected if constipation is present and the fecal material is allowed to accumulate in the pelvic colon.

Neuralgic Dysmenorrhea will require treatment of whatever is producing the nerve irritation. Spinal lesions are the most common causes, and, of course, should be found and removed. For the relief of the pain you may use cold sitz baths, the therapeutic lamp, rapid sinusoidal or high frequency current, prolonged vibration or prolonged hot applications to the lumbar and sacral spine.

Obstructive Dysmenorrhea will require the removal of any malformation, malposition, new growth, or adhesions that may be obstructing the menstrual flow. Hot sitz baths or alternating hot and cold sitz baths, cold vaginal douches, or alternate hot and cold vaginal douches may be used.

Endometritis, Congestive Metritis, Salpingitis, Ovaritis, and Subinvolution may be treated similarly to "Pelvic Congestion." Pyosalpinx, Ovarian Abscess, Pelvic Cellulitis, Pelvic Peritonitis and Puerperal Sepsis may be treated in the same manner as "Pelvic Congestion," in addition to the treatment necessary for the "Septic Intoxication" (See Lesson 28.)

Uterine Fibroma and Carcinoma and Ovarian Cyst will require the treatment for "Pelvic Congestion," general elimination, purification of the blood and raising the vitality. The positive galvanic current is of some value in Fibroma. The ultra violet light may destroy the carcinoma if used in time. All three of these conditions may require an operation if neglected too long. When Extra-Uterine Pregnancy is diagnosed, the patient should be sent to a surgeon immediately.

The treatment of Gonorrhea is that of the inflammations of the affected organ plus general eliminative procedures. When the condition is acute, the patient should be at rest in bed. Ultra-violet light is of considerable value in these cases.

Chanchroid and Chancre usually require no treatment except cleanliness. The therapeutic lamp may be used. The general treatment for Syphilis (see Lesson 28) should be used when a chancre is present. Successful treatment of Amenorrhea will depend altogether upon your ability to find and correct the cause. The menstrual flow may be temporarily established by the use of very hot sitz baths (fifteen minutes), prolonged hot applications to the lumbar and sacral spine, manipulation of the lumbar region, hot vaginal douches and the therapeutic lamp.

PROGNOSIS OF FEMALE PELVIC DISORDERS

Prognosis, of course, depends very largely upon the correct treatment being instituted early enough in the disease. Cases that have been operated upon will be harder to cure or relieve than those that have not been so mutilated. It may not be possible, in all cases, to restore the pelvic structures to their normal condition, but you will be able in a very large percentage of cases to bring about sufficient change to make the patient free from symptoms.

The prognosis of Carcinoma is bad, but by no means hopeless. It will be best for the beginner to turn these over to a more experienced practitioner. Fibroma and Ovarian Cyst do not respond so readily to treatment as the other disorders. The prognosis in Pyosolpinx, Pelvic Cellulitis, Pelvic Peritonitis and Ovarian Abscess should be guarded. When Malposition or Prolapses of the Uterus is accompanied by laceration of the perineum, the prognosis as to cure is doubtful unless the pelvic floor is repaired.

QUESTIONS—LESSON 36.

1. Explain how tight corsets may produce Pelvic Diseases.

2. Give symptoms of Neuralgic Dysmenorrhea.

3. Give symptoms of Endometritis.

4. Give symptoms of Pelvic Cellulitis.

5. What would make you suspect Uterine Carcinoma?

6. Give symptoms of Urethritis.

7. Describe the appearance of Chancroid.

8. Briefly outline the treatment for Pelvic Congestion.

9. How would you treat Neuralgic Dysmenorrhea?

10. What is the Prognosis in Uterine Fibroma?

EXTENSION COURSE
IN CHIROPRACTIC
AMERICAN UNIVERSITY
CHICAGO, Ill., U.S.A.

LESSON 37

DISEASES OF THE NERVOUS SYSTEM

Many of the so-called diseases of the nervous system are the result of irritation of the peripheral nerves or interference with the circulation through the brain and cord or abnormal blood supply to the nerves or their ganglia. Practically all of the symptoms that may accompany diseases of the brain or cord may be produced by subluxations of vertebrae and other spinal lesions.

The spines of all patients having nervous symptoms should be carefully and thoroughly examined and all lesions present should be corrected. Even in those cases where there is a functional or a structural disease of the brain or cord much may be done through spinal treatment, which will restore the normal circulation through the brain and cord and remove the peripheral irritation.

While any of the etiological factors given in Lesson 22 may produce nervous disorders, spinal lesions, peripheral irritations, toxemia and excessive waste of nerve energy are the most important causes of these diseases. The nervous systems of some individuals are less stable than that of others, making it possible for slight causes to bring on serious disturbances when they would have no effect upon the more normal individual. Persons with an irritable nervous system are said to be of the "Neurotic Temperament."

SYMPTOMS OF NERVOUS DISORDERS

Hysteria is a functional disease of the nervous system characterized by alterations of character and disposition without failure of intellect and by motor or sensory disturbances without organic diseases of the brain or cord. It is due to an oversensitive nervous system plus some local or general irritation. Practically any mental, sensory, motor, secretory or special sense symptoms may be present. The patient may have exaggerated convulsions followed by an incomplete coma. When the symptoms are not justified by the physical or laboratory findings, a provisional diagnosis of Hysteria may be made. A positive diagnosis of Hysteria should be made only when a very complete history and a thorough examination of the patient reveals nothing that may be responsible for the symptoms.

Neurasthenia is a functional disorder of the nervous system caused by a deficient supply or an excessive expenditure of nerve energy. Any or all of the symptoms of any functional or organic diseases of any organ or part may be present. There is insomnia, melancholia, hypochondriasis and a marked tendency on the part of the patient to exaggerate the severity of his symptoms. The mental and physical exhaustion and irritability are the most important diagnostic symptoms. A diagnosis of Neurasthenia should be made only after a complete history and a thorough examination has failed to disclose anything that may be producing the symptoms.

Chorea (St. Vitus' Dance) is a functional disorder of the nervous system occurring most often in children. It is due to a neurotic temperament plus a local or general irritation of the nervous system. It is characterized by involuntary, irregular, spasmodic movement of the muscles and limbs. There is also incoordination, irritability and constipation.

Epilepsy is a functional disorder of the nervous system characterized by a sudden loss of consciousness usually preceded by general convulsions. It is caused by a reflex irritation or general toxemia in a person with a hyper-sensitive nervous system. The convulsions are preceded by some peculiar sensation which is called an Aura. The patient drops down suddenly after uttering a piercing shriek. All of the muscles are contracted, the body rigid and the eyes fixed. The hands are clenched and the chest is immobile. The pupils are dilated. After about thirty seconds the muscles of the face and body begin to alternately relax and contract, the extremities are tossed wildly about and the tongue may be severely bitten. There may be involuntary evacuations of the urine or feces. After two or three minutes the patient lapses into unconsciousness, which may last for several hours.

Paralysis Agitans is a functional disorder of the nervous system due to a premature aging of the nervous system, superinduced by a waste of nerve energy. It occurs usually after fifty years of age. The patient has a characteristic posture. The body is flexed at the hips, the face is immobile, the fingers have a peculiar, coarse, irregular tremor. The patient moves along by shuffling one foot after the other. He seems to be constantly falling

468

forward. The muscles show weakness and rigidity. As the disease progresses, the tremor may extend to the arms, shoulders, head or even to the entire body.

Tetany is a condition characterized by muscular spasms usually of the hands or feet with increased excitability of the muscles and nerves. The localized spasms occur at irregular intervals and may last from a few seconds to several hours. Passive movement of the affected part is painful.

Apoplexy is a hemorrhage into the brain substance accompanied by pressure degeneration of the brain cells. Most often it affects the motor area of the cortex, producing "Hemiplegia." It is caused by a prolonged toxemia, which produces a degeneration of the vessel walls. The onset is sudden with a profound coma, snoring respiration, slow and full pulse and turning of the eyes to one side. Examination will show that an arm and leg or one side of the face is paralyzed. The unconsciousness may last for many hours and end in death. If the patient regains consciousness the leg, arm or face, or all three, remain paralyzed. After a few weeks, the paralyzed muscles become hard and rigid.

Cerebral-Thrombosis is the formation of a clot of blood in one of the vessels of the brain. There is headache, vertigo and convulsions followed by Hemiplegia of gradual onset. The paralysis is of the upper neuronic or spastic type.

Cerebral-Embolism is a sudden plugging of a vessel by a particle floating in the blood stream. There is a sudden Hemiplegia accompanied by a slight or short coma and a weak pulse. Later the mind becomes impaired.

Cerebral-Meningitis is an inflammation of the membranes covering the brain. It may be due to injury, infection, toxemia, or extension of inflammation from other parts. There is fever, headache, vomiting, optic neuritis, strabismus, irritability, pain over the cranial nerves, followed by anesthesia, spasms or paralysis of the muscles supplied by the cranial nerves. The disease may be acute or chronic. In the former the symptoms are more severe but of shorter duration.

Brain Tumor is a new growth in the brain substance. It produces severe headache not relieved by the usual measures, vertigo, vomiting without nausea, optic neuritis and a slow, full pulse. The pressure of the tumor produces mental, motor, sensory or special sense disturbances, depending upon its location in the brain.

Brain Abscess is a localized suppurative inflammation of the brain substance. Its symptoms are those of "Septic Intoxication" plus the symptoms of brain tumor.

Hydrocephalus is a condition produced by an excessive accumulation of the cerebro-spinal fluid. It is usually congenital. The skull is enlarged, there is mental deterioration and the development of the child is slow.

Jacksonian Epilepsy is a name applied to localized muscular convulsions without loss of consciousness. It is due to irritation of the nerve cells in the cortex of the brain.

Cerebral Atrophy (General Paralysis) is a chronic disorder characterized by degeneration of the cerebral cortex and atrophy of the substance of the cerebrum. The symptoms are dementia, hallucinations of grandeur and delusions of persecution. There are also tremors of the lips and tongue and a slow slurring speech. In the late stages there is complete paralysis of all the voluntary muscles and loss of control of defecation and micturition.

Insanity is a mental disorder characterized by changes in character and habits, melancholia, mania, illusions, delusions, hallucinations and dementia.

Bulbar Sclerosis (Bulbar Paralysis) is a chronic sclerosis and degeneration of the motor nuclei in the medulla and degeneration of some of the motor nerves. It produces a lowered neuronic (flaccid) paralysis of the lips, tongue, pharynx or larynx. There is atrophy of the tongue, speech disturbances, dysphagia, dyspnea and cardiac irregularity.

Dorsal Sclerosis (Locomotor Ataxia) is a chronic disorder characterized by inflammation of the posterior nerve roots followed by degeneration of the posterior sensory columns of the cord. The symptoms are divided into three stages. In the First Stage there are lightning pains along the course of the spinal nerves. The knee reflexes are lost, there is loss of control of micturition and the Argyll-Robertson pupil is present. In the Second Stage there is ataxia of the lower extremities, neuralgic pains in the different organs and the gait is characteristic. The feet are separated and the patient raises the foot very high, throws it outward and forward and allows it to fall suddenly to the ground in an awkward manner. In the Last Stage the patient is bed-ridden, completely paralyzed, the mind is vacant and there is involuntary evacuations-of urine and feces.

Transverse Sclerosis (Myelitis) is a chronic degeneration and sclerosis of several or all of the motor tracts, sensory columns or gray matter of the cord. It is due to toxemia or infection. Practically any of the symptoms of any disease of the cord may be produced. There are usually hypoesthesias and muscular spasms, followed by anesthesia and paralysis of the part supplied from the affected region of the cord. The micturition and defecation reflexes are disturbed. Diagnosis is made by exclusion, that is, if it is not some other disorder of the nervous system, it is called Myelitis. The condition may be acute or chronic. In the former the symptoms are more severe and of shorter duration.

Acute Anterior Polio-Myelitis is an inflammation followed by degeneration of the anterior portion of the gray matter of the cord. There is sudden paralysis of a small group of muscles during an acute febrile attack. The paralysis is lower neuronic (flaccid) in type, and is accompanied by atrophy.

Chronic Anterior Polio-Myelitis (Progressive Muscular Atrophy) is a sclerosis and degeneration of the anterior horns of the cord. Muscular strain or fatigue may be an exciting cause. The onset is gradual with weakness and wasting of the muscles of the hands and later of the arms and shoulders. There is pain, muscular twitching and sensory disturbances. The legs may be similarly affected late in the disease.

Lateral Sclerosis (Spastic Paraplegia) is a chronic sclerosis and degeneration of the lateral motor tracts of the cord. The onset is gradual, with a feeling of heaviness and weakness in the limbs, progressing to complete paralysis of both legs. There is also jerking and twitching with cramps and stiffness of the muscles of the limbs. The gait is typically spastic. The legs drag behind and are

472

thrown stiffly forward, the toes dragging against the ground and the patient having a tendency to fall forward. The contraction of the muscles may become so great that no movement is possible. Sensation is unaffected.

Posterior and Lateral Sclerosis (Ataxic Paraplegia) is a chronic sclerosis and degeneration of the posterior sensory columns and of the lateral motor tracts of the cord. The onset is gradual, with weakness and incoordination of the limbs. The patient reels or sways if the eyes are closed (Ataxia). The knee jerk is increased and there is muscular rigidity and spasms. Eventually both limbs become paralyzed.

Disseminated Sclerosis (Multiple Sclerosis) is a chronic disorder characterized by a formation of isolated patches of connective tissue in the brain or cord producing degeneration of the nerve cells and fibers. There may be headache, vertigo, convulsive attacks, ataxia, spastic gait and paralysis of any group of muscles. The diagnostic symptoms are a tremor made worse by voluntary movement, involuntary movement of the eyeballs, and a peculiar jerky speech.

Spinal Cavities (Syringomyelia) is a chronic affection characterized by dilatation of the central canal of the cord or formation of the cavities in the cord substances. The symptoms are very irregular and include motor and sensory disturbances and atrophy of the affected muscles. The diagnostic symptoms are loss of the pain and temperature sense with retention of the sense of touch.

Spinal Meningitis is an inflammation of the membranes covering the cord and usually extending to the spinal nerve roots.

473

It is due to toxemia, infection or an extension of inflammation from adjacent structures. The symptoms are fever, spinal pain and rigidity, shooting pains over the spinal nerves, followed by anesthesia and muscular spasms, followed by paralysis of the muscles supplied by the spinal nerves from the affected region of the cord. When the thigh is flexed at right angles to the trunk the leg cannot be extended on the thigh (Kerlig's Sign). The disease may be acute or chronic. In the former, the symptoms are more severe and of shorter duration.

Compression of the Cord may be the result of Trauma, or of new growth within the spinal canal. There is hyperthesia, and muscular spasms followed by anesthesia and paralysis of all parts supplied by the spinal nerves leaving the cord below the affected region.

Neuralgia is a functional disorder of a nerve characterized by a paroxysmal pain that radiates over the course of the nerve to its area of distribution. It is caused by irritation of the brain or cord centers or of any division of the spinal nerve. There is numbness, tingling, shooting pains and muscular spasms. The pain is usually relieved by pressure.

Neuritis is an inflammation of a nerve or its sheaf caused by irritation, poisoning or disturbed circulation of the nerve or of its centers in the brain or cord. There is continued pain, increased by pressure. In the later stages, there are motor sensory and trophic changes in the parts supplied by the nerves.

Nerve Degeneration may follow "Neuritis" or inflammation or degeneration of the brain or cord centers of the nerve. There is anesthesia, trophic disturbances and a flaccid paralysis and atrophy of the muscles.

Spinal Nerve Irritation is a functional disturbance of the spinal nerve, produced usually by subluxated vertebrae or similar spinal lesions. The nerve irritation may produce practically any motor, sensory, secretory, visceral or special sense disturbance. The diagnosis of this condition is made from the fact that the symptoms disappear in a short time when the lesions of the spinal column are removed or when nerve inhibition is used.

DIAGNOSIS OF DISEASES OF THE NERVOUS SYSTEM

In this group of disorders it is much more important to know the location, nature and extent of the lesion than to know the name of the disease. This can be learned only by careful study of the symptoms present.

Muscular spasms, hyperesthesia or paresthesia indicate irritative lesions of the spinal or cranial nerves, their cord centers or the motor tracts or sensory columns above the cord centers. Flaccid Paralysis, Atrophy or Anesthesia indicate destructive lesions of the spinal or cranial nerves or their cord centers. Spastic Paralysis indicates a destructive lesion of the motor tract above the cord center of the affected muscle.

Increased skin, tendon or visceral reflexes indicate irritative lesions of the spinal or cranial nerves, of their cord centers, or irritative or destructive lesions of the motor tracts above the cord centers. Decreased reflexes indicate destructive lesions of the spinal or cranial nerves or their cord centers.

The table given in Figure 7 of Lesson 13 shows the segments of the spine that control each muscle, skin area or reflex. The location of the motor, sensory or reflex symptoms will show you which segments of the cord are affected. If muscles are affected you will know that the lesion affects the motor fibers; if sensation is affected, the sensory fibers are affected. If the reflexes are abnormal, it may be because either the motor or sensory fibers are affected (see above).

If the symptoms are those of irritation of the nerve tissue (see above) it indicates congestion or inflammation; if the symptoms of destruction of the nerve tissue are present (see above) it indicates sclerosis of, or pressure upon, the nerve tissue.

TREATMENT OF DISEASES OF THE NERVOUS SYSTEM

A great many symptoms that are supposedly due to diseases of the Nervous System are in reality produced by lesions of the spinal muscles, ligaments and bones and will disappear when these lesions are corrected. In every one of these cases you should thoroughly examine the spine and correct any lesions present.

The acute disorders of the nervous system may be treated according to the plan laid down for the treatment of Acute Constitutional Disorders in addition to prolonged hot baths to decrease the congestion of the cerebral and spinal tissues.

In Hysteria, Neurasthenia, Chorea, Epilepsy, Paralysis, Agitans and Tetany you must search for and remove the causes of the extreme irritability of the nervous system, the lesions that are interfering with normal nerve activity or circulation of the spinal cord and brain, and prevent excessive waste of nervous energy.

Lesson 37: Diseases of the Nervous System

You should also use measures to purify the blood, to increase elimination, to raise the vital resistance and to decrease the activity of the nervous system. Thorough relaxation of the spine and adjustment of any lesions present should be used in every case. Prolonged applications of moderate heat or moderate cold to the spine, prolonged warm or neutral baths, deep breathing exercises and rectal dilatation may be used.

In the Chronic Diseases of the Cord you must determine the region of the cord that is affected (by the location of the motor, sensory and reflex symptoms). This region of the spine should be thoroughly relaxed and any lesions present corrected.

When the symptoms show irritation of the nerve cells or fibers, the amount of blood in the spinal cord must be decreased by five to ten-minute applications of moderate heat over the whole length of the spine, prolonged mild traction or prolonged mild kneading of the spinal muscles or by the use of prolonged hot baths.

When the symptoms indicate destruction of the nerve tissue you should use measures to increase the amount of blood in the affected region of the cord. Hot applications (water, lamp, etc.) over the affected region of the spine will increase the amount of blood to the spinal cord and tend to promote absorption of the fibrous tissue, and regeneration of the nerve tissue. Not more than one-fourth of the spine should be treated at one time and the treatment must be continued fifteen to thirty minutes. The appropriate constitutional treatment must also be used.

The treatment of Neuralgia, Nerve Degeneration and Spinal Nerve Irritation is that of the underlying causes. In addition to the removal of the spinal lesions, you may use prolonged moderate pressure, prolonged concussion, prolonged moderate heat, prolonged cold, the lamp, vibration or any prolonged mild electrical current along the course of the nerve or over its posterior primary division (between the laminae of the vertebrae). In extreme cases you may freeze the nerve. In Neuritis you may use practically the same measures as used for Neuralgia except pressure, vibration and faradic current, which usually aggravate the condition. The high frequency effleurage is of value in many cases.

Not much can be done in the brain disorders except to remove any interference with the circulation through the brain and to apply appropriate constitutional treatment. Measures for the relief of the motor and sensory symptoms may be used.

PROGNOSIS OF DISEASES OF THE NERVOUS SYSTEM

As with other diseases, the possibility of cure and the time required depends very largely upon your ability to find the cause of the patient's symptoms and to use the proper treatment before there has been too much destruction of nerve tissue.

Generally speaking, the prognosis depends upon the nature and the extent of the pathological condition present. Brain diseases are less affected by treatment than those of the cord and peripheral nerves. When there has been destruction of nerve tissue much longer treatment will be required than when the pathological changes are merely causing irritation of the nerve cells or fibers. Functional disorders respond much more rapidly to treatment than when there has been anatomical changes in the nerve tissue. The number of tracts or columns in the cord affected and the length of the region of the cord affected also influences prognosis.

These diseases are quite commonly thought to be incurable, but appropriate drugless treatment will cure a very large percentage of them.

QUESTIONS—LESSON 37

1. Why should the Spinal Column be thoroughly examined in all cases of Diseases of the Nervous System?

2. What is Hysteria?

3. What are the symptoms of Chorea?

4. Give symptoms of Brain Tumor.

5. Give the symptoms of Dorsal Sclerosis.

6. Give symptoms of Acute Anterior Poliomyelitis.

7. Give symptoms of Lateral Sclerosis.

8. Give treatment of Neurasthenia.

9. Give treatment for Sclerosis of the Lower Dorsal Region.

EXTENSION COURSE
IN CHIROPRACTIC
AMERICAN UNIVERSITY
CHICAGO, Ill., U.S.A.

LESSON 38

DISEASES OF THE EYE, EAR, NOSE AND THROAT

Conjunctivitis is an inflammation of the mucous membrane covering the eye and lining the eyelids. There is pain, or smarting, photophobia, epiphoria, congestion and a catarrhal or purulent discharge. There may be pink or gray elevations or ulcers upon the mucous membrane.

Keratitis is an inflammation of the cornea. There is pain, photophobia and the cornea is cloudy and opaque. The vision is usually much impaired. Ulcers may form.

Iritis is an inflammation of the iris usually due to toxemia or an extension of inflammation from adjacent structures. There are shooting pains, worse at night, and the vision is much reduced. The iris is muddy and discolored, the pupil is contracted, irregular and immobile. The aqueous humor is cloudy. The vessels surrounding the cornea are dilated.

481

Choroiditis, Retinitis and Optic Neuritis can be diagnosed only by the use of the ophthalmoscope, which requires special training. They all produce marked impairment of vision.

Glaucoma is a condition characterized by hardening of the eyeball due to an increased amount of fluid within the eye. There is pain, loss of vision, diminished power of accommodation and the patient sees halos around the lights he views. The cornea has a steamy appearance and the eyeball feels hard.

Amblyopia is a condition in which there is a failing of vision without apparent disease of any of the eye structures. It is due to toxemia or interference with the circulation of the eye.

Ammetropia is a condition in which there is a congenital malformation of the eyeball or some interference with the accommodation so that rays of light are not properly focused upon the retina. The symptoms are headache, nervousness, asthenopia, lacrimation and "Conjunctivitis." A positive diagnosis can be made only by examining the eye with test lenses.

Heterophoria is a condition in which there is an increased or decreased tone and contractile power of one or more of the eye muscles. If the difference between the tone of the muscle is very great, Strabismus is produced. Lesser degrees of muscular imbalance can be detected only by examination of the eyes with prisms and test lenses.

Otitis Media is a simple or purulent inflammation of the structures of the middle ear. There is pain, tinnitus aurium, vertigo and deafness. There may be a discharge through the auditory canal.

Mastoiditis is a condition in which the inflammation from the middle ear has extended to the cells in the mastoid process of the temporal bone. There is a deep-seated pain and tenderness behind the ear in addition to fever and the general symptoms of "Septic Intoxication."

Nerve Deafness is a condition in which the impaired hearing is due to some disorder of the inner ear or of the auditory nerve. It is distinguished from conductive deafness by the fact that a watch is heard better when placed against the skull behind the ear than it is heard when held lightly against the external ear.

Conductive Deafness is a condition in which the impaired hearing is due to some interference with the transmission of the sound waves to or through the middle ear. In this form, the watch is heard more plainly when placed on the skull than when held over the external ear.

Rhinitis (Nasal Catarrh) is an inflammation of the mucous membrane lining the nasal cavities. There is a discharge from the nose, obstructed respiration and headache. The different forms of Rhinitis can usually be distinguished only by an examination of the nasal cavities.

Nasal Malformations include tumors, deformed septum, enlarged turbinates, etc. The symptoms are similar to those of a severe Rhinitis. The diagnosis can be made only by an internal examination.

Hay Fever is a Rhinitis occurring at certain periods of the year, usually in the fall. It is due to a hyper-sensitive nervous system and an irritable nasal mucous membrane plus the presence of some irritating substance in the air. The symptoms are those of Rhinitis and Conjunctivitis.

Stomatitis is an inflammation of the mucous membrane of the mouth due to gastro-intestinal disorders or the ingestion of irritating substances. The mouth is sore and mastication and swallowing are difficult. The mucous membrane is inflamed and may be covered with ulcers, blisters or white elevated spots. In severe forms the gums are spongy and the teeth become loose.

Tonsilitis is a condition in which there is congestion, inflammation or hypertrophy of the tonsils. The tonsils are enlarged, painful and congested. Swallowing is difficult. Inspection will show the tonsils projecting beyond the pillars and they may be reddened or pale, depending upon the type of Tonsilitis.

Adenoids is a term applied to the hypertrophy of the lymph tissue in the posterior nasal pharynx. The interference with respiration causes mouth breathing and a nasal voice. A soft, spongy mass may be palpated in the nasal pharynx.

Pharyngitis is an inflammation of the mucous membrane lining the pharynx. There is cough, hoarseness and expectoration. The mucous membranes may be thickened and red or pale, dry and glossy or covered with ulcers.

Laryngitis is an inflammation of the mucous membrane lining the larynx. The symptoms are practically the same as those of Pharyngitis, except that examination of the throat with a laryngoscope will show that the larynx is affected instead of the pharynx.

TREATMENT OF DISORDERS OF THE EYE, EAR, NOSE, MOUTH AND THROAT

A large proportion of these disorders are caused, or at least aggravated, by muscular and bony lesions of the cervical spine which interfere with the blood and nerve supply to the affected parts. In all disorders of the head, the neck should be thoroughly and carefully relaxed and any lesions present should be corrected.

In all of the Eye Disorders, the eyes should be carefully examined for refractive errors or muscular imbalance and proper glasses fitted if necessary. Excessive use of the eyes must be avoided. Frequent washing of the eye with a solution of common salt (one teaspoonful to a quart) is of considerable value. The high frequency current may be used (cautiously) in the treatment of the Chronic Eye Disorders. Concussion of the seventh cervical vertebrae may help to relieve the symptoms. It should be remembered that many so-called diseases of the eye are merely symptoms of a constitutional condition.

The neck treatment outlined above may be used in the Ear Diseases. Prolonged hot applications, the therapeutic lamp, and the high frequency current may be used in Otitis media. In Nervous Deafness you may use any of the stimulating electric currents or vibratory stimulation to the ear or to the second and fourth or seventh cervical vertebrae. In Conductive Deafness you may use the therapeutic lamp, suction hyperemia, high frequency effleurage or vibration over or behind the external ear. Pulling the soft pallet forward and massage of the nasal pharynx is very effective, but should be very carefully done.

Many cases of Rhinitis are due to the effort of the body to eliminate toxins that should have been eliminated in other ways.

485

You, should increase the elimination, purify the blood and restrict the diet (especially limit cooked starches and sugars). In addition to the neck treatment, the nose may be washed with a warm salt solution (see above).

Diseases of the Mouth and Throat are many times secondary to diseases in other parts of the respiratory or digestive tract which should receive treatment. Through relaxation of the anterior neck muscles and prolonged moderate pressure with the finger at either side of the base of the tongue (finger inside) aids very much to relieve these conditions. Massage of the tonsil may' be used in the treatment of Congestive Tonsilitis. The high frequency or the negative galvanic current is of some value in Fibroid Tonsilitis.

MISCELLANEOUS DISEASES

Arterio-Sclerosis is a chronic condition characterized by infiltration of the walls of the arteries with connective tissue and calcium salts. The principal symptoms are headache, vertigo, high blood pressure and hardening of some of the peripheral arteries. The heart is hypertrophied, the second aortic sound is accentuated and Interstitial Nephritis is usually present. The presence of high blood pressure does not always indicate Artero-Sclerosis, as is quite commonly believed. A positive diagnosis can be made only by the finding of the hardened arteries.

Aneurysm is a permanent dilatation of an artery with degeneration of its walls. When the condition appears in the peripheral arteries it forms an enlargement along the course of the artery which has an expansile pulsation with heart beat. The principal symptoms of thoracic and abdominal Aneurism are those due to the pressure they cause upon the surrounding structures.

486

There will also be an area of dullness over the enlargement and an expansile pulsation may be felt on palpation. An X-ray picture is usually necessary for a positive diagnosis.

Varicose Veins are due to a permanent enlargement of the veins with degeneration of their walls. They are most common in the lower extremities. The veins are visible as large, tortuous cords, which may be hard. Ulcers may occur along the course of the vein.

Phlebitis is an inflammation of the walls of the veins. There is fever with pain, redness and edema along the course of the vein. Signs of venous stasis appear in the part drained by the vein. Palpation will show the vein to be hard and tender.

Lymphadenitis is an inflammation of the lymph glands due usually to an excessive amount of toxic material passing through them. The glands are enlarged and tender, but freely movable. Tubercular Adenitis is due to the formation of tubercles in the lymphatic glands, usually of the neck. The glands are swollen and adherent to the adjacent tissues. They may break down into discharging ulcers with thin undermined edges.

Adrenal Disease is usually tubercular. It produces drowsiness, extreme loss of strength, dyspepsia and heart weakness. The skin has a peculiar bronze color.

Myxedema is due to atrophy or removal of the thyroid gland. The skin is swollen and inelastic and does not pit on pressure. The temperature is subnormal. The patient has a stupid expression and mental deterioration.

Goiter is an enlargement of the thyroid gland, which may be due to congestion, increase in the bland tissue or an increased amount of fibrous tissue. Cysts or tumors may also be present in the gland. The gland is enlarged and may produce symptoms due to pressure upon the surrounding structures.

Exophthalmic Goiter is a constitutional disease in which the thyroid gland usually enlarges. There is protrusion of the eyeballs, tachycardia and a fine tremor of the hands.

Symptomatic Anemia is a decrease in the volume or coloring matter of the blood secondary to hemorrhage, toxemia, malnutrition or excessive loss of albumin. The skin and mucous membranes are pale, the patient is weak and complains of dyspnea, dyspepsia and palpitation of the heart. Examination of the blood will show that the red cells and hemoglobin are moderately reduced.

Chlorosis is a form of anemia occurring most frequently in young girls. It may be caused by improper diet, poor hygiene or anything that lowers the vitality or disturbs the activity of the blood-forming organs. Constipation is invariably present. In addition to the symptoms of "Symptomatic Anemia," there is a greenish-yellow skin and a perverted appetite. Examination of the blood will show that the hemoglobin is greatly, but the red cells are only slightly reduced.

Pernicious Anemia is a severe form of Anemia due to malnutrition, toxemia or defective elimination. In addition to the general symptoms of a severe "Symptomatic Anemia," there is a lemon-yellow skin and a tendency to hemorrhages. Examination shows the red cells greatly and the hemoglobin moderately reduced.

Leukemia is a form of Anemia in which the white blood cells are greatly increased. The symptoms are similar to those of symptomatic anemia except that the blood examination shows an enormous number of white blood cells.

Prostatitis is a condition in which there is congestion, inflammation or hypertrophy of the prostate gland. There is perineal pain and frequent painful micturition and the urine may be cloudy and contain shreds of mucus. Rectal examination will show the prostate to be enlarged and tender. If enlargement is very great, it will interfere very much with micturition. The patient usually has mental, nervous and sexual symptoms.

Orchitis is a simple or suppurative inflammation of the testicle usually secondary to inflammation in another part of the genital tract. There is scrotal pain, tenderness and swelling.

Varicocele is an enlargement of the scrotum due to dilatation of the veins. The swelling disappears when the patient lies down. The scrotum feels like a bag of worms.

Gonorrhea in the Male is a suppurative inflammation of the urethra which may extend to other genital structures. There is a urethral discharge, appearing three to five days after exposure. Micturition is frequent and painful and the urine is cloudy. The external urethral meatus is reddened. Chordae is usually present. When the condition becomes chronic the symptoms are less severe.

Chancroid and Chancre have been described under "Diseases of the Female Generative Organs."

Acute Peritonitis is an acute inflammation of the serous membrane lining the abdomen and covering the abdominal organs. It is usually secondary to inflammation of the abdominal viscera. The onset is sudden with a chill, fever, and a rapid small pulse which may be irregular. There is intense abdominal pain and tenderness. The patient lies motionless on his back with the thighs flexed on the abdomen. The abdomen is distended and the abdominal muscles are spasmodically contracted. Breathing is shallow and the diaphragm is immovable.

Chronic Peritonitis is accompanied by abdominal pain and tenderness, ascites and the abdominal muscles are contracted. There may be areas of impaired resonance and a friction rub may be heard. There are usually adhesions between the various abdominal organs or between them and the abdominal walls.

TREATMENT OF MISCELLANEOUS DISEASES

The treatment of Anemia is that of the underlying causes. In addition to this, the patient should have sufficient sleep, plenty of outdoor exercise in the sunlight and a diet that supplies the elements the blood needs. Every effort should be made to raise the vitality. Ultra-violet light, ozone, and concussion of the 11th dorsal and 2nd lumbar vertebrae will increase the number of red blood cells and the amount of hemoglobin in the blood.

In Goiter the neck should be thoroughly and carefully relaxed and any lesions present should be corrected. Concussion of the 7th cervical and measures to decrease the blood supply in the gland may be used except in Fibrous or Cystic Goiter. Vibration, high frequency and negative galvanic currents, hyperemia and massage may be used in the Fibrous Type. Cysts and tumors usually require an operation. Exophthalmic Goiter should receive the constitutional treatment advised for chronic constitutional diseases in addition to the neck treatment suggested above.

Thoracic and Abdominal Aneurism may be treated by concussion of the 7th cervical vertebrae. The patient should be cautioned about any severe or prolonged physical exertion. In Varicose Veins you must find and remove the cause of the obstruction to the circulation or the weakening of the vessel walls. An elastic bandage or stocking is sometimes necessary. Arterio-Sclerosis will require removal of the source of the toxic material and elimination of the toxins. The diet must be restricted.

The diseases of the Male Generative Organs may be treated in the same way as- similar disorders in other organs. Stimulation of the 12th dorsal vertebrae and the slow sinusoidal current applied to the rectum and urethra are of considerable value. The therapeutic lamp, hot sitz baths, and the general treatment advised for female pelvic disorders may be used.

A correctly fitted truss should be worn in Hernia. The shape and the composition of the pad is important. The small, hard, round pads tend to increase the size of the opening in the abdominal wall. A pad that is soft and elastic and extends well behind the hernial opening is much less harmful. Every effort should be made to strengthen the tissues of the abdominal wall and to relieve it of any undue pressure from within. The slow sinusoidal current and prolonged cool application are of value but dependence must be placed very largely upon proper exercises and breathing (special exercises will be given in the lesson on Medical Gymnastics). Some cases of hernia will require operation, but this should be delayed until other measures have been given a fair trial.

The above treatment should also be used after operation or the hernia may recur.

EMBRYOLOGY

This subject deals with the development of the individual from the human ovum until the termination of Pregnancy. The mature human ovum is a single, spherical cell about one-twenty-five- hundredth of an inch in diameter composed of a yolk and nucleus and two enveloping membranes. The ovum is produced in the ovary and is carried by the fallopian tubes to the cavity of the uterus. Impregnation, or the joining of the male spermatoza with the female ovum, may take place in the fallopian tube or in the uterus.

When conception, or impregnation, takes place the ovum becomes attached to the mucous membrane of the uterus and begins to go through the process of segmentation. The cell divides into two, these two into four, and so on until thousands of cells are formed. These cells are arranged in three layers from which, in the course of development, all of the tissues and parts of the body are formed.

The ovum receives its nourishment at first from the uterine mucosa, but soon develops a placenta, in which the fetal blood absorbs nutrition and oxygen from, and throws off waste materials into, the mother's blood.

The placenta is firmly adherent to the uterus and is connected to the child by the umbilical cord, which contains the blood vessels.

The fetal circulation differs from that of the adult in that only a very small portion of the blood passes through the lungs. There is an opening between the right and left auricle of the heart through which passes the blood that in the adult passes through the lungs. The blood from the placenta is carried by the umbilical vein to the liver and the inferior vena cava and returns to the placenta through the abdominal aorta and the umbilical artery.

OBSTETRICS

The management of cases of child birth requires special study and training and the Chiropractor should not attempt to handle these cases until he has had considerable experience under the direction of a competent teacher.

Pregnancy is the period between conception and labor and normally extends over a period of forty weeks, or nine calendar months. The symptoms of normal Pregnancy have been given under "Diseases of the Female Pelvic Organs."

The first symptoms to appear are suppression of menstruation, enlargement of the breast, bladder irritability and morning nausea. The positive signs do not appear until after the sixth month. They are fetal heart sounds heard on auscultation, fetal movements felt by the examining hand and the movement of a solid body in a fluid when sudden pressure is applied on the lower extremity of the fetus through the vagina (Ballottement).

Nephritis, eclampsia, constipation, hemorrhoids, uncontrollable vomiting and "Extra uterine Pregnancy" are the most common complications of Pregnancy.

Labor begins with the first labor pain and ends with expulsion of the fetus and fetal membranes. Under normal conditions it extends over a period of from two to sixteen hours and is not accompanied by any serious symptoms.

If the pelvis is deformed or too small, the child is too large, malformed or in an abnormal position or if there is some interference with the contraction of the uterus, labor may be delayed and may result in the death of the child or mother.

If the labor is uncomplicated, any good nurse can take care of the mother and child, but when complications are present, the services of an experienced and very capable physician are needed.

QUESTIONS—LESSON 38

1. Give symptoms of Iritis.

2. Give symptoms of Glaucoma.

3. Give symptoms of Mastoiditis.

4. Give treatment for Otitis Media.

5. Give symptoms of Exophthalmic Goiter.

6. Give symptoms of Pernicious Anemia.

7. Give symptoms of Acute Peritonitis.

8. Give briefly the treatment of Hernia.

9. Give the symptoms of Pregnancy.

www.ingramcontent.com/pod-product-compliance
Lightning Source LLC
Chambersburg PA
CBHW062149270326
41930CB00009B/1480